CANCER OF THE UTERINE ENDOMETRIUM – ADVANCES AND CONTROVERSIES

Edited by **J. Salvador Saldivar**

Cancer of the Uterine Endometrium – Advances and Controversies
Edited by J. Salvador Saldivar

Published by InTech

Janeza Trdine 9, 51000 Rijeka, Croatia

Publishing Process Manager Iva Simcic

Technical Editor Teodora Smiljanic

Cover Designer InTech Design Team

Additional hard copies can be obtained from orders@intechopen.com

Cancer of the Uterine Endometrium – Advances and Controversies,
Edited by J. Salvador Saldivar
p. cm.
ISBN 978-953-51-0142-0

For EU product safety concerns:
IN TECH d.o.o., Prolaz Marije Krucifikse Kozulić 3, 51000 Rijeka, Croatia,
info@intechopen.com or visit our website at intechopen.com.

Meet the editor

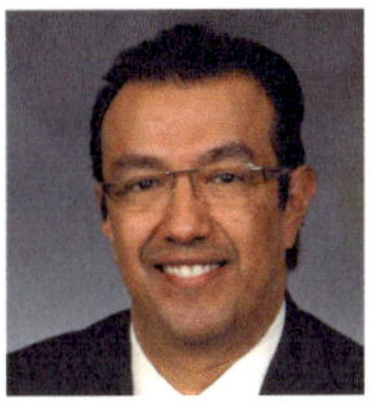

Dr J. Salvador Saldivar, MD, MPH, is an Assistant Professor in the Department of Obstetrics and Gynecology at Texas Tech University Health Sciences Center-Paul L. Foster School of Medicine in El Paso, Texas, USA. Dr Saldivar is Board Certified in Obstetrics and Gynecology. He received his medical degree from the University of Illinois at Chicago College of Medicine and completed his residency training in OB/GYN at Texas Tech University Health Sciences Center in El Paso. He received a Masters of Public Health from the University of Texas School of Public Health and training in gynecologic oncology at the MD Anderson Cancer Center in Houston, Texas. He finished his Clinical Fellowship in Gynecologic Oncology at the University of British Columbia and the British Columbia Cancer Agency in Vancouver, British Columbia, Canada. His areas of interests include genetic risk assessment in high risk gynecologic cancer families, minimally invasive robotic surgery, management of complicated gynecologic cancers and fertility-sparing surgery.

Contents

Preface

Cancer of the uterine endometrium is the most common gynecological cancer in developed countries, and the most common gynecologic cancer in the USA. Obesity, diabetes and a hyper-estrogen state are common risk factors associated with the majority of uterine cancer cases. Although most women with endometrial cancer are diagnosed at an early stage, it is still a significant cause of gynecologic cancer-related morbidity and mortality. The primary treatment of endometrial cancer is surgical, however, there still remains controversy regarding the survival benefit following complete lymphadenectomy. Further, the roles of combination chemotherapeutic agents, radiotherapy techniques and hormonal treatment are continually evolving.

This first edition of *Cancer of the Uterine Endometrium - Advances and Controversies* brings together an international collaboration of authors to attempt to address these issues. Effective treatment of any gynecologic cancer is best approached via a multidisciplinary model that includes physicians, scientists and oncologic personnel, among others, to improve the outcome for women. The book is divided into four sections in an attempt to emulate this multi-faceted model of collaboration: 1) Biology and Genetics, including hereditary endometrial cancer; 2) Modern Imaging and Radiotherapy; 3) Surgery and Staging; and 4) Therapeutic Strategies. Each section brings forth the most relevant and evidence-based information for the diagnosis and treatment of endometrial cancer. In addition, controversies regarding therapeutic strategies are addressed in the context of the latest clinical studies.

This book is not intended to cover the basics of endometrial cancer. For this, one should refer to a number of excellent gynecologic oncology textbooks. Rather, the vision of this book is an international expert collaboration of the most updated advances in the biology, genetics, diagnosis, imaging, and treatment strategies for cancer of the uterine endometrium. Ultimately, it is hoped that this opens a platform for which other authors may add their work in future editions of this book. It is meant for all learners who care for women with this gynecologic cancer. It is dedicated to our women patients, our best teachers.

Asst. Prof. Dr. J. S. Saldivar MD, MPH
Division of Gynecology Oncology,
TTUHSC-El Paso, Texas
USA

Part 1

Biology and Genetics

1

Molecular Biology of Endometrial Carcinoma

Ivana Markova and Martin Prochazka
Department of Medical Genetics and Fetal Medicine,
Palacky University Medical School and University Hospital Olomouc
Department of Obstetrics and Gynecology,
Palacky University Medical School and University Hospital
Czech Republic

1. Introduction

The term tumour is understood as a general denomination for newly formed tissue formation or cell populations in an organism that do not develop as a physiological response to external or internal stimuli, show abnormality signs and more or less escape the regulatory influence of the surrounding cells and organism. Currently, a general opinion has been accepted that tumours result from congenital or acquired genetic damage. Thus, the spectrum of formerly suggested theories of carcinogenesis has narrowed down to a single genetic theory. It is therefore necessary to emphasize that regardless of malignant growth being sporadic for the individual or recurrent for many family members as a hereditary trait, it is clearly a genetic disease.

2. Molecular principles of tumour genesis

The process of tumour development consists of several stages and is determined by the imbalance between the cell proliferation and cell death. The cells proliferate if they undergo a cell cycle and mitosis, whereas the destruction, due to a programmed cell death, removes cells from tissues through a standard DNA fragmentation process and cell suicide called apoptosis. These processes of cell division and cell death are regulated by a number of genes. According to the extensive research of several recent decades it is the mutation in genes controlling the cell proliferation and death that is responsible for cancer.

In most malignant tumours mutations appear in a single somatic cell in which, during subsequent division, genetic errors are cumulated, i.e. multistep carcinogenesis. More rarely, if the malignity occurs under the hereditary syndrome with tendency towards malignant tumours, the initial mutations causing cancer are inherited in the germinal line and are therefore present in every cell in a body. Different types of genes participate in the initiation of the tumorous process, e.g. genes coding proteins of signal pathways for cell proliferation, cell cycle regulators or proteins responsible for detecting and correcting mutations. As soon as the malignant growth is triggered by any mechanism, it develops as accumulation of other genetic changes through mutations of genes coding the cell apparatus that repairs damaged DNA and maintains cytogenetic stability. The damage to these genes results in further impairment in cascaded mutations of the increased number of genes controlling cell proliferation and repairing damaged DNA. The original clone of neoplastic cells may, in this way, develop into many sublines with a different degree of malignity. Thus, the cell clone able to survive is selected, i.e. clonal selection. Such tumorous cells generally acquire the ability of invasive growth and metastases.

Each malignant tumour is a mixture of cells with various characteristics as, during the excessive and mostly chaotic and imprecise division, other changes are cumulated and new characteristics acquired. Therefore, the metastatic cells do not reveal different genetic changes than the cells of the original tumour. However, all these cells emerged through the division of a single originally maligned cell and thus the tumour is termed as monoclonal.

The above indicates that the complex tumorous process involves a great number of genes. The main events starting from the carcinogenesis initiation stage to propagation and metastases include activation of proto-oncogenes, inactivation of tumour suppressor genes, microsatellite instability, aneuploidy and loss of heterozygosity (Kolář et al., 2003, Nussbaum et al., 2004).

3. Molecular biology of endometrial carcinoma prognostic factors

As already mentioned above, the tumour development is a multistage process. It embraces genetic changes, i.e. direct changes in DNA nucleotide sequence, epigenetic changes not altering the genetic code but affecting its expression (methylation of certain DNA bases or histone acetylation) and functional changes at the cell metabolism regulation or at the level of gene expression control and cell division. Considering genetic changes there are two most significant types of genes: proto-oncogenes and tumour suppressors.

3.1 Oncogenes

The foundations of the theory on existence of genes that may cause tumours (oncogenes) were laid in 1911 when Rous described a transmissible sarcoma in chickens. It was discovered that the transmissible etiologic agent of this tumour was a virus, denominated as Rous sarcoma virus (RSV). In broad terms, the oncogenes are all active genes able to cause or boost up tumorous transformation. There are two forms of oncogenes: viral-oncogene that forms a part of the retrovirus genomes causing tumours and cellular oncogene that develops by activation of the proto-oncogene. Proto-oncogenes are genes of standard eucaryotic cells coding proteins that are important for growth or differentiation of cells. They become potential oncogenes if, due to quantitative changes or qualitative changes in the structure of the actual gene or its protein product with a subsequent defect of a functional interaction with other genes, they are subject to an incorrect expression. The mechanisms of this incorrect expression vary:

a. point mutation when one or few nucleotides are deleted (deletion) or are, on the contrary, inserted (insertion, duplication) or substituted without a change in the number of nucleotides (substitution),
b. gene amplification,
c. gene deletion (loss of large sections of genes),
d. translocation of chromosomes when an entire chromosome is broken at a specific place and then it is connected to a different chromosome (typical for haematological malignities),
e. insertional mutagenesis when proto-oncogenes are activated through the insertion of retroviral promoters and enhancers (sequences determining the quantity of the respective gene to be generated, i.e. the quantity of protein produced).

As a consequence, the changes described above may result in an unregulated function or increased expression of the oncogene product and eventually to the stimulation of tumour growth. Under standard conditions, the oncogene products function as growth factors (int-1), hormones and receptors for growth factors and hormones (c-erbB-2), as well as proteins functioning as signal transducers (K-ras) and proteins binding DNA sequences to gene expression regulators, i.e. transcription regulatory factors (c-myc). A specific group includes oncogenes that inactivate tumour suppressor genes (E6 a E7) or inhibit the physiological process of cell renewal – apoptosis (bcl-2).

At the cell level, oncogenes play a dominant role, which means that under activation or increased expression one mutated copy (allele) is able to alter the cell phenotype from normal to malignant (Kolář et al., 2003, Nussbaum et al., 2004 , Ruddon, 2007).

Despite a large number of oncogenes known to be related to various malignancies, only certain ones are significant in endometrial carcinogenesis, e.g. bcl-2, c-erbB-2, K-ras, etc.

3.1.1 c-erbB-2

The c-erbB-2 oncogene (human cellular oncogene) is identical to HER2/neu (rat cellular oncogene). It codes a transmembrane glycoprotein receptor for a growth factor similar to EGRF (epidermal growth factor receptor). The difference is that the coding gene is located on chromosome 17q21-22 (EGRF on chromosome 7) and that the mRNA size of this gene is only 4.6 kb (for EGRF 5.8 - 10 kb). Under normal circumstances c-erbB-2 protein forms a part of signal transduction pathways and therefore regulates the cell growth, survival, adhesion, migration and differentiation, i.e. functions that are either intensified or, on the contrary, weakened in tumour cells.

In a number of tumours the increased expression of this oncogene is associated with poor prognosis. Its relationship is probably best understood in association with breast carcinoma when its amplification and increased expression occurs approximately in 15 to 20% of cases. The increased expression of this receptor in breast cancer is definitely related to the increased risk of recurrence and poorer prognosis (Kakar et al., 2000). From the clinical perspective, c-erbB-2 protein has been recently found important thanks to its ability to bind monoclonal antibody trastuzumab (Herceptin). Trastuzumab binds solely to the defective protein, i.e. only if the expression of the c-erbB-2 gene receptor has increased. Bound to the tumour cell it also functions as a "lighthouse" identifying the cell. Identified tumour cells are then attacked and killed by their own immunity cells. This prevents further uncontrolled growth of breast carcinoma tumour cells and thus increases the chances of survival (Adam et al., 2008). Recent studies have shown a better effect of trastuzumab in late-stage breast carcinoma. The effect in early stages remains controversial. Other problems lie in the usual development of the resistance of tumour cells to this antibody and last, but not least, its high price (Hudis, 2007). Trastuzumab has also been tested on other tumours with a demonstrated increased expression of c-erbB-2 gene, for instance, on serous papillary endometrial carcinoma (Santin et al., 2008). This preparation has been approved in a number of countries as a first-line therapy for primarily metastatic breast carcinoma - in the Czech Republic since 1 July 2001.

An increased expression of c-erbB-2 also occurs in different tumours, such as ovarian cancer, stomach cancer and endometrial carcinoma. In endometrial carcinomas an increased expression occurs in 10 to 40% of cases and is associated with negative prognostic factors, such as advanced stage of disease and lower degree of histological differentiation (Mariani et al., 2003). It is highly probable that the increased expression of this oncogene might be among the late events in the endometrial carcinoma carcinogenesis, whereas in serous carcinoma it concerns an early event developed de novo (Matias-Guiu et al., 2001). A negative prognostic impact of a c-erbB-2 expression has been documented in some, but not in all, trials and thus the clinical application of changes in expression of this factor remain ambiguous (Ferrandina et al., 2005, Morrison et al., 2006). The dissimilar outcomes of the respective studies may, to a great degree, be the result of so far non-uniform diagnostic procedures applying either the immunohistochemical methodology or FISH methodology or alternatively CISH methodology.

3.1.2 bcl-2

Proteins of the bcl-2 family belong among the significant regulators of apoptosis (for more see Chapter p53). The bcl-2 protein was discovered while studying the chromosomal translocations t(14,18) frequent in some lymphomas resulting in an increased expression of the bcl-2 gene and resistance to apoptosis. The bcl-2 protein family consists of both inhibitors and promoters of programmed cell death. At least 25 members of this family have been identified in mammals, whereas bcl-2 is the typical and best described representative of antiapoptotic proteins and in proapoptotic it is Bax. Many theories based on the experimental results have tried to explain the manner in which the proteins in this family regulate cell death. Originally, it was assumed that bcl-2 functions as an antioxidant transporting proteins through nucleous membrane. It has been recently discovered that it also regulates the activation of caspase-related proteases that are responsible for the final effector stage of apoptosis. Its other functions include the protection of cells against various cytotoxic effects, including various types of radiation and chemotherapy. The bcl-2 family proteins also belong among the important agents affecting chemosensitivity or chemoresistence. Thanks to their ability to block cell death induced by the anti-tumorous drugs bcl-2 may be considered as an important protein active in the development of multi-drug resistance (Wang, 2001).

The antiapoptotic factor bcl-2 derives its name from B-cell lymphoma 2; the respective gene lies on chromosome 18q21.3. This oncogene is not associated with cell proliferation but with cell death. By regulating the cell death, inhibiting apoptosis, it prolongs cell survival and thus contributes to the spread of tumorous process. Numerous studies have demonstrated its role in the oncogenous process of, for instance, melanoma, breast, prostate and lung carcinomas, and it also plays an important role in autoimmunity disorders and schizophrenia (Glantz et al., 2006, Li et al., 2006).

While studying the function of this gene in endometrial tissue, it was demonstrated that the immunohistochemical expression of bcl-2 typically changes during the menstrual cycle. During the proliferation stage of the cycle the expression is high and then during the secretion stage and menstruation it dramatically drops which proves that a bcl-2 expression is controlled by the regulatory mechanisms of sex hormones. It was further demonstrated that the bcl-2 expression grows in endometrial dysplasia, whereas it decreases in endometrial carcinoma. It is therefore probable that the increased expression of this oncogene may be one of the frequent events in endometrial carcinogenesis (Chen et al., 1999). Frequent studies demonstrate the loss of the bcl-2 expression correlates with poor prognosis, deeper invasion, advanced clinical stage and aggressive histological types (Erdem et al., 2003, Ohkouchi et al., 2002). The inversion relationship between the loss of expression and biological aggressiveness of the tumour seems to be an obvious paradox. The mechanisms of this down-regulation have not been exactly described yet. It seems that based on some experimental studies the bcl-2 expression is at least partially regulated by oestrogens and the tumour suppressor gene p53. For example, Popescu et al. discovered that in colorectal carcinomas the relationship of inverted correlation between bcl-2 and p53 is probably derived from the active bcl-2 down-regulation depending on other genes taking over the antiapoptotic function (Popescu et al., 1998). The antiapoptotic function of bcl-2 seems reduced depending on the alterations of other genes, including p53, which are normally involved in the regulatory mechanism of programmed cell death. Less differentiated and clinically more advanced endometrial carcinomas are often associated with the loss of oestrogen receptors and, on the contrary, an increased expression of the p53 gene, which may, to a certain point, explain the loss of the bcl-2 expression in these tumours. The bcl-2 expression, depending on steroid receptors, could facilitate the identification of high-risk tumours (Markova et al., 2010, Ohkouchi et al., 2002).

3.1.3 K-ras

The ras oncogene family embraces more than 100 members with various degree of homology of their effector region. There are 3 main groups of ras genes – K-ras, H-ras and N-ras and they belong among the group of oncogenes coding signal transducers. The K-ras oncogene is located on chromosome 12p12 and codes protein of molecular weight equal to 21 kD, forming a part of a signal transduction pathway modulating the cell proliferation and differentiation. Mutations of this oncogene result in the constitutional activation of this signal pathway with subsequent unregulated proliferation and reduced differentiating ability. Point mutations in codons 12 and 13 are found in about 10 to 40% of endometrial carcinomas and in approximately 16% of endometrial dysplasia cases (Cristofano & Ellenson, 2007). It may be concluded that a similar percentage of mutations of this oncogene in endometrial precancerous and malignant lesions mean that the activation of the K-ras gene is one of the early events in endometrial carcinogenesis. It seems that the K-ras gene mutations are more frequent in well differentiated carcinomas than in papillary serous and clear-cell carcinomas. However, in the majority of cases the mutations of the ras gene do not correlate with staging, grading and depth of myometrial invasion and therefore the significance of this marker in prognosis is so far controversial (Lagarda et. al, 2001).

3.1.4 C-myc

It belongs among nuclear proto-oncogenes and is the precursor for protein associated with nuclear chromatin. The C-myc gene is located on chromosome 8 and its product functions as a transcription factor. If stimulated by growth factors its expression increases ten to twenty times and it may be an important regulator of cell growth and oestrogen-induced differentiation. The c-myc levels are significantly higher in endometrium than in any other tissue compartments of the uterus. Recent studies have demonstrated an increased c-myc expression in 3 to 19% of endometrial carcinomas (type I) and the immunohistochemical staining for c-myc represented an independent prognostic factor (Geisler et.al., 2004).

3.2 Tumour suppressor genes

Genes contributing to malignancy in a completely different manner than oncogenes, i.e. through a loss of function in both alleles of a certain gene, are identified as tumour suppressor genes. They regulate cell division or are involved in contact inhibition of cell growth - they function as "safety fuses" which turn off the cell cycle if exposed to abnormal proliferation or damage to genetic information. Their protein products check the correctness and preciseness of division and are able to either correct the errors, "care takers", or prevent the cell from going to the next division stage, "gatekeepers". Other products are able to induce even cell death, apoptosis (e.g. p53). Any damage to these genes results in malignant growth as the cell escapes the control mechanisms, which allows for accumulation of secondary mutations of either proto-oncogenes or other tumour suppressor genes leading to a superiority of factors supporting growth, invasiveness and development of a tumour.

The types of tumour suppressor gene disorders are similar to those typical for oncogenes, such as point mutation, amplification, deletion, etc. A full gene or a larger section of a chromosome may get lost in tumour suppressor genes. This loss is manifested as so called loss of heterozygosity (LOH), see below.

While in oncogenes the tumour process may be initiated by damage to just one copy, the genes coding for the tumour suppressors are recessive, which means that the tumour suppressor gene is inactivated only if both its alleles are affected. Inactivation of just one allele is usually insufficient. This Knudson's two-hit hypothesis was applied for the first time to explain how tumours such as retinoblastoma occur in both hereditary as well as sporadic form (Knudson, 1971). In hereditary tumours the cells heterozygous for mutation include another functional copy of a tumour suppressor gene that is sufficient to maintain the normal cell phenotype. However, a cell that accidentally losses the function of the second, remaining, allele losses its ability to suppress the development of a tumour. This "second hit" most frequently concerns a somatic mutation and thus tumours in hereditary syndromes frequently develop repeatedly in the same tissue. On the other hand, in sporadic forms of malignancies resulting from a loss of the tumour suppressor gene only a single cell is probably affected by such a rare event, which means two hits in one cell. These tumours are usually monoclonal and the original tumour occurs in one place which may, however, subsequently widely metastasize. At present, the two-hit model is widely recognized as a basis for hereditary as well as sporadic malignant tumours caused by mutations making the cell lose the function of both copies of a tumour suppressor gene (Kolář et al., 2003, Nussbaum et al., 2004, Ruddon, 2007).

In endometrial carcinogenesis, mutations of various tumour suppressor genes have been shown, such as p53, PTEN, p16, p21, MLH1, MSH2, MSH6.

3.2.1 p53

The defects of this gene located on chromosome 17p13.1 belong among the most frequent in human tumours. It mostly concerns mutations of both alleles of somatic cells but hereditary mutations of one allele have been described as well, which significantly increases the risk of the second allele mutation and subsequent development of a tumour. Members of families suffering from one allele mutations of the p53 gene are faced, based on epidemiological studies, with a 25 times higher occurrence of malignant tumours than other population (i.e. Li-Fraumeni syndrome).

The p53 gene codes for nuclear phosphoprotein bound to specific DNA sequences. The product of the p53 gene works as a transcription factor and in cells it takes the form of tetramer that, under normal conditions, stimulates an expression of various genes and thus plays an important role in the cell cycle and apoptosis. The expression of a normal, unmutated, so called wild-type p53 protein increases as a physiological response to various stimuli inducing cell stress. This results in holding the cell cycle in G1-S regulation point and during this resting period various cell analyzers assess the degree of DNA damage. If the defect is repairable p53 initiates the repair process of damaged DNA sequences; if the defects are rather serious p53 launches mechanisms of apoptosis. This control system is very important in preventing the transmission of defective genetic information to daughter cells. Therefore, p53 is sometimes described as "the guardian of the genome" (Kolář et al., 2003).

Apoptosis is a genetically determined mechanism irreversibly removing damaged cells from most types of tissues. It concerns a programmed cell death and it plays a focal role in tissue homeostasis. During apoptosis the important interlink p53 ensures an expression of specific genes, such as Bax, GADD45 and p21, which activate endonucleases. These enzymes then, under presence of Ca and Mg, degrade DNA to numerous oligonucleosomal fragments and cause disintegration of cell nucleus and destruction of the cell. Subsequently, the apoptotic residues are absorbed by the surrounding cells and degraded in lysosomes. The paradox is that despite p53 activating a large number of genes none of them are able to self-induce the cell apoptosis. Not even p53 is able, on its own, to determine the future destiny of a cell after DNA damage. In addition to factors inducing apoptosis the important products, on the contrary, selectively stimulate proliferation and thus inhibit the apoptosis. Such inhibitors include various growth factors, sex hormones and oncogene products. In this respect the most thoroughly studied is the effect of the bcl-2 oncogene (antiapoptotic gene), product of which concerns the bcl-2 protein (see chapter Bcl-2). Its abundance inhibits the destruction of a cell through apoptosis and supports cell proliferation. In tumours, apoptosis occurs spontaneously and its progress depends on the type of tumour. Considering it plays a crucial role in tissue homeostasis it is understandable that a great deal of attention has been paid to apoptosis (Wang et al., 2001).

The presence of a mutated p53 gene is conventionally proved by immunohistochemical staining. The life span of a wild-type, unmutated product of the p53 gene is short and therefore it is basically undetectable by the immunohistochemical staining. The gene damage caused by various types of mutations results in an increased expression of the mutated p53 protein with an altered function and it is therefore functionally defective and resistant to degradation. Its prolonged biological half-time allows for immunohistochemical detection of the p53 protein product (Battifora et al., 1994). It has been demonstrated that the increased expression of the mutated p53 protein and related strong immunohistochemical staining is primarily a result of so called "missense" mutations (substitution of a single nucleotide or point mutation in a DNA sequence may alter the coding triplet and cause the replacement of an amino acid in the gene product for a different one - therefore such mutations are called mutations changing the codon sense, "missense mutations", because they alter the sense of the codon by specifying a different amino acid . Another type of mutations concerns so called "nonsense mutations" resulting in the occurrence of a shortened protein). Alterations of p53 caused by the substitution of bases, deletion or insertion have been shown in approximately 20% of endometrial carcinomas. In general, p53 mutations are more frequent in poorly differentiated adenocarcinomas; papillary serous carcinomas demonstrate increased expression in up to 80% (Tashiro et al., 1997). Frequent studies demonstrate the correlation between an abnormally increased expression of p53 and aggressive histological types, advanced stage of disease and shorter survival time (Cherchi et al., 2001, Marková et al., 2010, Ohkouchi et al., 2002). It seems that the p53 gene mutations play an important role primarily in the late stages of endometrial carcinogenesis.

3.2.2 PTEN

The PTEN tumour suppressor gene means Phosphatase and TENsin homolog. Alternatively, it is sometimes identified as MMAC1 (**M**utated in **M**ultiple **A**dvanced **C**ancer). The gene is located on chromosome 10q23.3 and codes for protein of molecular weight 47 kD that works as a tumour suppressor. It regulates the interaction between the cell and intracellular matrix that are closely connected with apoptosis. For its correct function the co-operation with p53 and Rb signal pathways is necessary.

The PTEN gene protein demonstrates lipid phosphatase and protein phosphatase activity. Under the lipid phosphatase activity it negatively regulates the level of phosphatidylinositol (3,4,5)-trisphosphate and is able, partially in co-operation with the increased regulation of cyclin-dependent kinase inhibitor p27, to block the cell cycle in the G1/S stage. The protein phosphatase activity includes the regulation of functions of the main adhesion and signal receptor proteins, which mediate the cell migration and invasion, and also controls cytoskeletal organization, cell growth and apoptosis. Therefore, the combination of defects in both functions (lipid and protein phosphatase) may result in defective cell growth and possible escape from apoptosis as well as in possible abnormal cell spread and migration (Wu et al., 2003).

The PTEN gene mutations have been found in various types of human tumours. In germ cells these mutations are found in autosomal dominant Cowden syndrome defined by the occurrence of numerous hamartomas and the increased risk of breast and thyroid cancer. Somatic mutations have been identified in various types of malignant tumours, such as brain glioblastoma, skin melanoblastoma, breast or prostate carcinoma (Li et al., 1997). At present, the PTEN gene mutation is considered to be the most frequent gene alteration in endometrioid carcinoma. In sporadic endometrial carcinoma the mutations of this gene have been described in 30 to 50% of cases while the loss of heterozygosity of chromosome 10q23 occurs in about 40%. Considering that up to 55% of precancerous lesions of endometrial carcinoma show some alteration of the PTEN gene, the lost function of this gene may belong among the early stages in endometrial carcinogenesis (Mutter & Lin, 2000). In non-endometrioid types of carcinomas the PTEN gene mutations are, on the contrary, extremely rare. The responsible genetic alterations, if the expression and function of PTEN are lost, thus usually concern mutations; the loss of heterozygosity without mutation is less frequent. In approximately 20% of cases the cause for loss of expression has been determined to be methylation of promoter, out of which the majority concerns the clinically worse stages of endometrial carcinoma. The inactivation of the PTEN gene caused by mutation correlates with the early stage of disease and better survival. A five-year survival period in cases demonstrating PTEN mutations is found in about 80% of patients compared to a 50% survival chance in cases without mutation. Some authors have described the relationship between the microsatellite instability (MSI) (see below) and PTEN gene mutations. In approximately 50% of cases of endometrial carcinomas with positive MSI the PTEN gene mutations have been detected as short coding mononucleotide repeats resulting in a frameshift mutation. Therefore, the deficit in the mismatch repair system (see below) that represents the final step in acquiring the MSI phenotype may result in frameshift mutation of the PTEN gene and thus may represent the earliest step of the multistep progression of endometrial carcinogenesis. It seems that the detection of the altered PTEN gene expression could be used as a diagnostic marker of precancerous endometrial lesions (Mutter & Lin, 2000).

3.2.3 p21

The p21 is a tumour suppressor gene coding for p21 protein also known as CDKN1A (cyclin-dependent kinase inhibitor 1A) and is located on chromosome 6p21.2. The product of this gene takes an active part in a very complex process of cell cycle regulation. The p21 gene expression is strictly controlled by the p53 tumour suppressor gene which, through transcription activation of the p21 gene followed by an inhibition of cyclin-dependent kinases, stops the cycle in the G1 stage and prevents it from entering the S stage. Furthermore, the p21 protein co-operates with PCNA (proliferating cell nuclear antigen), inhibits the activity of a complex of CDK2 and CDK4 cyclins and thus plays the regulator role during the DNA replication in the S cycle stage. This gene thus represents, especially in co-operation with p53, an important factor in the process of cell growth control and its inactivation may potentially lead to tumorous spread (Gartel et al., 2005). It has also been demonstrated that the p21 expression may be reduced even without the direct effect of the p53 gene, which would be that the inactivation of the p21 gene may also include other mechanisms.

Compared to a normal endometrial tissue, the reduced expression of p21 has been described in the endometrial carcinoma. An univariate analysis of certain studies has shown that the loss of the p21 expression correlated with a shorter survival, however, a multivariate analysis has not demonstrated any prognostic impact (Salvesen et al., 1999).

3.2.4 p16

The p16 is a tumour suppressor gene coding for p16 protein also known as CDKN2A (cyclin-dependent kinase inhibitor 2A) and is located on chromosome 9p21.3. It also plays an important role in the regulation of the cell cycle and the p16 gene mutations increase the risk of developing numerous malignant diseases, in particular melanoma. The protein product of the p16 gene is able to bind itself to cyclin-dependent kinase CDK4 and inhibit catalytic activity of the SDK4-cyclin D complex which negatively affects the cell cycle.

In addition to melanoma, p16 gene mutations are also associated with an increased risk of developing other types of malignancies, such as carcinoma of the pancreas, stomach or oesophagus. In endometrial carcinomas the p16 gene alterations occur more rarely. However, the loss of the p16 protein expression has been identified in association with aggressive types of endometrial carcinomas, plus in connection with high proliferation activity of the Ki-67 marker. It seems that the degree of the p16 nuclear expression may be used as an independent prognostic factor in endometrial carcinomas (Salvesen et al., 2000).

3.2.5 Mismatch repair system genes

Under the hereditary breast and ovarian carcinoma syndrome it is also definitely necessary to include so called mismatch repair system genes MMR (MLH1, MSH2, MSH6, PMS1 and PMS2) among the tumour suppressor genes. The vast majority of patients carry so called Lynch syndrome, also known as HNPCC (hereditary nonpolyposis colorectal cancer). HNPCC is a familial cancer syndrome caused by mutations in one of five different genes for DNA repair responsible for the repair of DNA segments in which the correct pairing of bases has been disrupted - so called mismatch repair system genes. Genes for HNPCC are the prototype of tumour suppressor genes of the "caretaker" type. The probability of germline mutation of mismatch repair system genes being transmitted from parents to children is 50%, thus it is an autosomal dominant mode of inheritance. Same as for other tumour suppressor genes the autosomal dominant mode of inheritance is derived from the inheritance of one mutated allele and subsequent mutation or inactivation of the remaining normal allele in a somatic cell. At the cell level, the most apparent phenotypic manifestation concerns the enormous increase in point mutation and instability of DNA sequences containing simple repeats (see chapter Microsatellite instability). This instability known as "replication error positive" phenotype appears in cells that lack both copies of the gene for DNA mismatch with a frequency one hundred times higher (Lu & Broaddus, 2005, Nussbaum et al., 2004).

The lifelong risk of developing endometrial carcinoma is between 27 and 71% and the risk of colorectal carcinoma between 24 and 52%. The above risks depend on the gene in which the respective hereditary defect is localised; the crucial role in carcinogenesis of endometrial carcinoma is probably played by the inactivation of the MSH2/MSH6 complex. In terms of other possible malignancies, there is an increased risk of ovarian carcinoma (3-13%). HNPCC is also associated with an increased risk of stomach cancer (2-13 %), urinary tract cancer (1-12%), hepatobiliary tract cancer (2%) and brain tumours (1-4%). Carcinoma of the small intestine is considered to be a very sensitive indicator of hereditary disposition as it is very rare in the general population (the lifelong risk for an individual with disposition is 4 to 7%, which is 25 to 100 times higher compared to the general population) (Vasen et al., 2007). The risk of breast cancer may be slightly increased.

In patients with HNPCC the endometrioid carcinoma is to a certain point similar to the type I carcinoma as in the vast majority of cases it is diagnosed in stage I (78%), occurs earlier in life (median age is 40 years), shows endometrioid histology (92%) and often a higher grading. Under the Lynch syndrome tumour duplicity with colorectal carcinoma is very frequent (up to 61%) while in about 50% of these patients the first diagnosis is gynaecological. In molecular analysis of tumours, in addition to microsatellite instability, mutations and inactivation of the PTEN tumour suppressor gene are found (in up to 90% of cases). In terms of prognosis, endometrial carcinomas in women with MMR system gene mutations are not different from the same-stage tumours in women without the hereditary mutation (Zhou et al., 2002).

3.3 Microsatellite instability

Under the organization of the human genome structure we differentiate between the DNA coding sequences, which take up less than 1.5% of the genome, and noncoding sequences, which take up the remaining 98.5% of the total DNA. About one half of this noncoding DNA consists of various types of repetitive sequences, i.e. DNA sections of various length that appear in many copies at various places of the genome. Most of them are products of reverse transcription and thus they have a crucial effect on the structure of the genome in

humans and other organisms. The importance of the repetitive sequences probably lies in maintaining the chromosomal structure and apparently they also play an important role in the evolution of genes and genomes (Venter et al., 2001).
Microsatellite DNA refers to sections with repeats of 2 to 5 nucleotides occurring in various places of the genome. They are highly polymorphous and, simultaneously, they represent the most frequent form of repetitive DNA. They are specific for each individual, which provides a basis for precise identification used in forensic medicine. Thanks to its repetitive structure the microsatellites are susceptible to errors in replication. Mutations in these short sequences, known as microsatellite instability (MSI), are usually repaired by a protein system of various genes that are able to replace the incorrect bases in DNA. The most well-known include MLH1, MSH2 or MSH6, which are genes of the mismatch repair system (MMR). These genes may be inactivated by various mechanisms, in particular by mutation or methylation. MSI occurs in up to 90% of hereditary colorectal carcinoma but it has also been detected in sporadic tumours (Lynch et al., 1996). The majority of sporadic endometrial carcinomas do not show mutations in MMR genes; the likely cause of MSI in this type of tumour concerns hypermethylation of the MLH1 promoter resulting in epigenetic inactivation of the MLH1 gene. MSI has been found in about 30% of endometrial carcinomas, especially in endometrioid types I, and is associated with a favourable prognosis. Although the majority of studies have not demonstrated the correlation between MSI and age, grading, clinical stage and depth of myometrial invasion, a five-year survival in patients with endometrial carcinoma with positive MSI was by about 20% better than in patients without MSI. On the top of that the endometrial carcinomas with MSI more frequently show mutations in the PTEN gene and a less frequently increased expression of p53, which is a typical abnormality for nonendometrioid types of tumours (Maxwell et al., 2001).

3.4 Loss of heterozygosity (LOH)

Each chromosome carries a different set of genes linearly placed in chromosomal DNA. Homologous chromosomes carry paired genetic information, i.e. the same genes in the same sequence. In any specific locus, however, there may be two identical or slightly different forms of the same gene, i.e. every gene in our chromosomes is present in two forms, called alleles (one chromosome of each chromosomal pair is inherited from the father, the other from the mother). If one parental allele is lost, an effect called hemizygosity occurs. When analysing a tumour such a gene deficit is manifested as a loss of heterozygosity - LOH. In human solid tumours this loss of heterozygosity also usually means the loss of the tumour suppressor gene. LOH thus represents, according to the two-hit theory, the second hit to the remaining normal allele. It may result from interstitial deletion, somatic recombination or loss of the entire chromosome.
LOH has been described in many tumours, hereditary as well as sporadic (e.g. retinoblastoma, breast or colorectal carcinoma) and it is often considered to be the evidence of the tumour suppressor gene existence despite the gene has not been found yet. The studies of LOH while focusing on specific spots in the genome that could contain tumour suppressor genes associated with endometrial carcinoma have been carried out by several authors. In relation to endometrial carcinoma LOH has thus been demonstrated on many chromosomes, but the locuses on chromosomes 3p, 10q, 17p and 18q seem rather specific.

Numerous losses of heterozygosity are typical for nonendometrioid carcinomas (Albertson et al., 2003, Tashiro et al., 1997).

3.5 Aneuploidy

A certain degree of genetic instability that may, as a result of defects in mitotic segregation or recombination during cell division, lead to significant changes in the genome is typical for the genetic material in tumour cells. Normal somatic cells with 46 chromosomes (23 pairs) are called diploid cells, while extra or missing chromosomes are identified as aneuploidy. Chromosomal instability causing structural or numeric aberrations occurs in early as well as later and more invasive stage of tumour development and is typical for various types of malignant tumours. These cytogenetic changes indicate that defects in genes associated with maintaining chromosomal stability and integrity and assuring the exact mitotic segregation represent a significant element of tumour progression (Nussbaum et al., 2004).

In endometrial carcinoma the aneuploid changes occur in 25 - 30% of cases. According to a number of studies approximately 67% of endometrioid carcinomas are diploid, whereas about 55% of nonendometrioid carcinomas demonstrate aneuploid changes (Mutter & Baak, 2000). Diploid tumours are usually well differentiated tumours with only surface invasion to myometrium and are associated with longer survival than aneuploid tumours. Aneuploid tumours are in general associated with a poorer prognosis, higher number of recurrences and shorter disease free survival. The percentage of disease free survival for tumours in stage I, which is 94%, versus 64% in aneuploid tumours shows a clear difference. The important fact remains that in the vast majority of studies the ploidity is mentioned as independent prognostic factor (Pradhan et al., 2006, Suehiro et al., 2008).

3.6 Other prognostic markers

3.6.1 Ki-67

One of the most well-known markers of cell proliferation includes the Ki-67 protein, also known as MKI67. The respective gene (MKI67) coding for this protein is located on chromosome 10q25. The expression of the Ki-67 human protein is strictly associated with cell proliferation. During interphase Ki-67 can be easily detected within the cell nucleus, whereas in mitosis most of the protein is relocated to the surface of the chromosomes. The Ki-67 protein is present during all active phases of the cell cycle (G1, S, G2 and mitosis), but its expression is basically absent from resting cells (G0). That is the reason why Ki-67 can be identified as an excellent marker to determine the growth fraction of a given cell population. This growth fraction of Ki-67-positive tumour cells (Ki-67 index) is often correlated with clinical stage of various malignant diseases. The best-studied examples in this context are prostatic and breast carcinomas. For these types of tumours the prognostic value for survival and tumour recurrence have repeatedly been proven in uni- and multivariate analyses.

MIB-1 is a commonly used monoclonal antibody that detects the Ki-67 antigen. One of its primary advantages is that it can be used on formalin-fixed paraffin-embedded sections, which is the reason why it has essentially supplanted the original Ki-67 antibody for clinical use. Recently the use of the Ki-67 protein as proliferation markers in laboratory animals has been expended to embrace the preparation of new monoclonal antibodies prepared from rodents. Although the molecular level of the Ki-67 protein has been well-studied and its application as a proliferation marker is widely used, its functional meaning is still not fully clear. Nevertheless, there is obvious evidence that the Ki-67 protein expression is indispensable for the cell division process to be successful (Scholzen & Gerdes, 2000).

Most endometrial carcinomas demonstrate a low Ki-67 proliferation index with a favourable prognosis, while most serous and clearly cellular tumours demonstrate a high proliferation index with poor prognosis. The correlation with grading, stage of the disease and histopathological type of tumour has been confirmed by many studies (Ferrandina et al., 2005, Markova et al., 2010).

3.6.2 β-catenin

β-catenin is a submembranous protein that is encoded by the CTNNB1 gene located on chromosome 3p21. β-catenin is a part of a complex of proteins that constitute adherens junctions which are necessary for the creation and maintenance of epithelial cell layers by regulating the cell growth and adhesion between cells. Therefore, it takes part in maintaining tissue architecture. It is known that β-catenin is able to bind to various proteins. For example, it creates complexes with cadherines, which are transmembrane proteins functioning as transcription factors, so it plays an important role in regulating transcription. It is also known that it represents an integral component of the Wnt signal pathway, which is a network of proteins with a significant role in embryogenesis and tumorigenesis (Bullions & Levine, 1998).

Under defects of the above functions β-catenin can function as an oncogene. An increased level of β-catenin and mutations of the CTNNB1 gene have been described in various tumours - basal cell carcinoma, colorectal carcinoma, medulloblastoma or ovarian carcinoma. In endometrial carcinoma the nuclear accumulation of β-catenin and, simultaneously, mutations of its CTNNB1 gene have been described in may studies. The nuclear β-catenin has been identified in 16 to 38% of endometrial carcinomas, while its expression was significantly higher in the endometrioid (type I) (31 - 47%) than in nonmetrioid (type II) (0 - 3%) carcinoma. Mutations of CNNTB1 in endometrioid carcinoma have been described in 15 to 25%, while in nonendometrioid carcinoma none has been identified. Accumulation of β-catenin in cell nucleus has been found in less aggressive tumours with low metastasizing potential and, similarly, mutations of CNNTB1 are associated with well differentiated carcinomas (Machin et al., 2002, Scholten et al., 2003).

3.6.3 Steroid receptors

Endometrium is the target tissue of steroid hormones produced by ovaries. Oestrogen (ER) and progesterone (PR) receptors are present in both epithelial and stromal endometrial cells. It is generally known that ovarian steroids, oestrogen and progesterone, have the critical importance for regulating the growth and differentiation in endometrial cells. A normal course of the menstrual cycle (proliferation, differentiation and degeneration of endometrium) reflects cyclic changes in sex steroid levels. The proliferation stage of the cycle is mostly under the influence of oestrogens that stimulate proliferation of epithelial and stromal endometrial components, whereas during the secretory stage the main function of progesterone is glandular differentiation and glycogenesis with inhibition of oestrogen-mediated proliferation. Just as the ovarian steroids play an indispensable role in normal endometrium, they also significantly influence the development of endometrial carcinoma (Graham & Clarke, 1997).

ER and PR belong among a group of nuclear receptors with typically immunohistochemically detectable cyclic changes in their expression based on the cycle stage. After their activation they bind to specific target places in DNA where they modulate an expression of respective genes. In addition to this direct activation of target genes an indirect mechanism of their effect via relation to transcription factors, such as AP-1 (c-fos, c-jun) or NF-κB, has been described (Oehler et al., 2000).

Oestrogen receptors (ER) belong among the group of receptors subject to 17β-estradiol activation. ER primarily function as a transcription factor regulating the expression of other genes. Two subtypes of ER, ERα and ERβ, have recently been described; each of them is encoded by a different gene. The ESR1 gene for ERα is located on chromosome 6q24-q27, the ESR2 gene for ERβ on chromosome 14q21-q22. ER play an important role in the development of various malignancies, primarily in breast cancer (an increased expression is indicated in about 70% of cases) cancer of the ovaries, colon, prostate and, of course, endometrial carcinoma. While ERα is the dominant receptor in endometrium and participates primarily in increased proliferation, ERβ's effect is anti-proliferating and it apparently modulates the ERα function. The imbalance between the expression of ERα and ERβ is considered to be the critical moment in oestrogen-dependent carcinogenesis (type I). In endometrial carcinoma a decreasing level of the ERα mRNA expression and protein has been described, together with dedifferentiation of this tumour from grade 1 to grade 3. Under the unchanged expression of ERβ the ERα/ERβ ratio decreases (Jazaeri et al., 2001). In addition to the changed ratio of ER isoforms, incorrectly transcribed proteins derived from ERα or ERβ take part in endometrial carcinogenesis. For example, they include 5 ERα, which has been described in endometrial carcinoma but has not been detected in normal endometrium, or ER βcx with a dominant negative effect on ERα (Skrzypczak et al., 2004).

The progesterone receptor (PR), also known as NR3C3 (nuclear receptor subfamily 3, group C, member 3), is an intracellular receptor able to specifically bind progesterone.

PR is encoded by one PGR gene located on chromosome 11q22. It also exists in two isoforms differing by their molecular weight: PR-A and PR-B. One of the main functions of PR-A in endometrium is down-regulation of oestrogen activity via ERα inhibition. On the other hand, PR-B works as an oestrogen agonist in endometrial cells. Imbalances in PR-A/PR-B ratio are similarly considered to be a critical moment in the development of endometrial carcinoma (type I) (Arnett-Mansfield et al. 2001).

A number of studies have demonstrated that the presence and quantity of these steroid receptors correlate with the stage of tumour, grading and survival. The absence of steroid receptors is seen as a negative prognostic factor of aggressive growth and poor prognosis (Ferrandina et al., 2005, Jazaeri et al., 2001, Pilka et al., 2008). Nevertheless, the mechanisms of the loss of their expression in endometrial tumours is not fully known.

3.6.4 Growth factors

Steroid hormones regulate a number of growth factors that apparently participate in the paracrine and autocrine regulation of endometrial proliferation. They primarily include epidermal growth factor (EGF) and transforming growth factor alpha (TGF- α), which influence the endometrial cells through an EGF receptor. Both growth factors and their receptor stimulate cell growth in endometrial carcinoma in vitro. Other growth factors involved in endometrial carcinogenesis (type I) include transforming growth factor beta (TGF- β), basic fibroblast growth factor (bFGF) and insulin-like growth factor I(IGF-I) (Myeroff et al., 1995).

3.6.5 Matrix metalloproteinase

Matrix metalloproteinase belongs among the family of enzymes of zinc-dependent endopeptidases that are capable of degrading extracellular matrix. So far, more than 25 subtypes of these enzymes have been identified; based on their structure they are further classified into 8 different classes and their production is induced by an inflammatory or tumorous process (Nagase et al., 1999). One of the important members of the metalloproteinase family with an epithelial expression concerns MMP-7 (matrilysin-1), expression of which has been detected in both normal and malign epithelial cells. Only a limited number of studies focused on the MMP-7 expression in endometrial carcinoma has been published. In his study Ueno et al. demonstrated an increased expression of MMP-7 correlating with the worse clinical stage of the disease and presence of lymphatic metastases (Ueno et al., 1999). A similar trend is also described in the study carried out by (Graesslin et al. 2006, Wang et al., 2005). Markova et al. describes a significant relation between age and MMP-7 as in patients older than 65 the expression of MMP-7 was significantly lower (Markova et al., 2010).

Another member of the matrilysin enzymes subfamily is identified as MMP-26 (matrilysin-2). Likewise, MMP-26 is also generated in various tissues, both normal and malignant, including endometrial carcinoma. The outcomes of studies carried out by various authors indicate that despite MMP-26 belonging among the same subfamily of metalloproteinases as MMP-7, its function may apparently be different. It is known that the expression of MMP-26 specifically fluctuates during the menstrual cycle. The detection of high levels in the middle of the cycle and in hyperplastic endometrium, and, on the other hand, low levels in the late stage of the cycle and endometrial carcinoma indicate the correlation with oestrogen receptors. Isaka et al. and Pilka et al. demonstrated a significantly reduced expression of MMP-26 in endometrial carcinoma, which goes against the results of study carried out by Tunuguntla et al., who describes an increased immunohistochemical expression of MMP-26 in low-differentiated endometrial carcinoma (Isaka et al., 2003, Pilka et al., 2004, Tunuguntla et al., 2003).

4. Conclusion

The efficient treatment of malignancies requires an early and accurate diagnosis enabling to optimize therapy and minimize adverse effects. Early diagnosis of cancer, together with individual "custom-made" therapy, may reduce mortality and improve the prospects and quality of the patient's life. Gynaecological malignant tumours represent a group of diseases where the prognosis depends on subtle genomic, epigenetic and proteomic changes. The application of molecular biology techniques, including analysis of methylation and acetylation, and preoteomic techniques have become an important tool not only in basic research but also when determining the appropriate therapy.

The significance of various immunohistochemical parameters for the prognosis in patients suffering from endometrial carcinoma has not been unambiguously determined yet. The aim is, by applying the information acquired based on the expression of tumour biomarkers, to limit the radicalism in surgical and radiation therapy. The future objective is to further classify the subtypes of endometrial carcinoma based on their genetic alterations, in particular those that are significant in terms of prognosis. It is probable that future histological classifications will be based more on a molecular basis. In addition to clinical pathological factors, the molecular biological prognostic factor may improve the characteristics of tumours and provide a more accurate definition of their clinical behaviour. Although these factors will apparently be more important in managing the endometrial carcinoma treatment in the near future, any practical diagnostic and therapeutic application of biological factors will require more detailed studies.

5. References

Adam, Z., Kalvodová, L., Nový, F. et al. (2008). *Slovníček odborných pojmů.* Česká onkologická společnost ČLS J.E.Purkyně, Available from: www.linkos.cz/pacienti/slovnicek.php

Albertson, D. G., Collins, C., McCormick, F., et al. (2003). Chromosome aberrations in solid tumors. *Nature Genetics*, Vol. 34, pp.369-376

Arnett-Mansfield, R.L., deFazio, A., Wain, G. V., et al. (2001). Relative expression of progesterone receptors A and B in endometrioid cancers of the endometrium. *Cancer Research*, Vol. 61, pp. 4576-4582

Battifora, H. (1994). p53 immunohisochemistry: a word of caution. *Human Pathology*, Vol. 25, pp. 435-437

Bullions, L. C. & Levine, A. J. (1998). The role of beta-catenin in cell adhesion, signal transduction, and cancer. *Current Opinion in Oncology*, Vol. 10, pp.81-87

Cristofano, A.D. & Ellenson, L.H. (2007). Endometrial carcinoma. *Annual Review of Pathology*, Vol. 2, pp. 57–85

Erdem, O., Erdem, M., Dursum, A. et al. (2003). Angiogenesis, p53 and bcl-2 expression as prognostic indicators in endometrial cancer: Comparison with traditional clinicopathological variables. *Interational Journal of Gynecologic Pathology*, Vol. 22, pp.254-260

Ferrandina, G., Ranelletti, F. O., Gallotta, V., et al. (2005). Expression of cyclooxygenase-2 (COX-2), receptors for estrogen (ER), and progesterone (PR), p53, ki67, and neu protein in endometrial cancer. *Gynecologic Oncology*, Vol. 98. pp.383-389.

Gartel, A.L. & Radhakrishnan, S.K. (2005). Lost in transcription: p21 repression, mechanisms, and consequences. *Cancer Research*, Vol.65, No.10, pp. 3980-3985

Geisler, J. P., Geisler, H. E., Manahan, K. J., et al. (2004). Nuclear and cytoplasmic c-myc staining in endometrial carcinoma and their relationship to survival. *International Journal of Gynecological Cancer*, Vol. 14, pp.133-137

Glantz, L.A., Gilmore, J.H., Lieberman, J.A. et al. (2006). Apoptotic mechanisms and the synaptic pathology of schizophrenia. *Schizophrenia Research*, Vol. 81, No. 1, pp. 47-63

Graesslin, O., Cortez, A., Uzan, C. et al. (2006). Endometrial tumor invasiveness is related to metalloproteinase 2 and tissue inhibitor of metalloproteinase 2 expressions. *International Journal of Gynecological Cancer,* Vol. 16, pp.1911-1917

Graham, J.D. & Clarke, C.L. (1997). Physiological action of progesterone in target tissues. *Endocrine Review Journal,* Vol. 18, pp.502-519

Hudis, C.A. (2007). Trastuzumab - mechanism of action and use in clinical practise. *The New England Journal of Medicine* Vol. 35, No. 1, pp. 39-5

Chen, Y., Sato, M., Fujimura, S., et al. (1999). Expression of Bcl-2, Bax, and p53 proteins in carcinogenesis of squamous cell lung cancer. *Anticancer Research,* Vol. 19, No.2B, pp.1351-1356

Cherchi, P. L., Marras, V., Capobianco, G., et al. (2001). Prognostic value of p53, c-erb-B2 and MIB-1 in endometrial carcinoma. *European Journal of Gynaecological Oncology,* Vol. 22, pp.451-453

Isaka, K., Nishi, H., Nakai, H et al. (2003). Matrix metalloproteinase-26 is expressed in human endometrium but not in endometrial cancer. *Cancer,* Vol. 7, No.1, pp. 79-89

Jazaeri, A.A., Nunes, K. J., Dalton, M. S., et al. (2001). Well-differentiated endometrial adenocarcinomas and poorly differentiated mixed mullerian tumors have altered ER and PR isoform expression. *Oncogene,* Vol. 20, pp.6965-6969

Kakar, S., Puangsuvan, N., Stevens, J.M. et al. (2000). HER-2/neu assessment in breast cancer by immunohistochemistry and fluorescence in situ hybridization: comparison of results and correlation with survival. *Molecular Diagnosis,* Vol. 5, No. 3, pp.199-207

Knudson, A.G. (1971). Mutation and cancer: statistical study of retinoblastoma. *Proceedings of the National Academy of Sciences of the USA,* Vol. 68, pp. 820-823

Kolář, Z. et al. (2003). *Molekulární patologie nádorů,* (1.) , Epava, ISBN 80-86297-15-2, Olomouc

Lagarda, H., Catasus, L., Arguelles, R., et al. (2001). K-ras mutations in endometrial carcinomas with microsatellite instability. *Journal of Pathology,* Vol. 193, pp.193-199

Li, A., Ojogho, O. & Escher, A. (2006). Saving death: apoptosis for intervention in transplantation and autoimmunity. *Clinical and Developmental Immunology,* Vol.13, No.2-4, pp. 273-282

Li, J., Yen, C., Liaw, D. et al. (1997). PTEN, a putative protein tyrosine phosphatase gene mutated in human brain, breast, and prostate cancer. *Science,* Vol. 275, pp. 1943-1947

Lu, K.H. & Broaddus, R.R. (2005). Gynecologic cancers in Lynch syndrome/HNPCC. *Familial Cancer,* Vol. 4, p.249

Lynch, H.T., Smyrk, T. & Lynch, J.F. (1996). Overview of natural history, pathology, molecular genetics and management of HNPCC (Lynch syndrome). *International Journal of Cancer,* Vol. 69, pp. 38-43 Machin, P., Catasus, L., Pons, C., et al. (2002). CTNNB1 mutations and beta-catenin expression in endometrial carcinomas. *Human Pathology,* Vol. 33, pp.206-212

Mariani A., Sebo T.J., Webb M.J. et al. (2003). Molecular and histopathologic predictors of distant failure in endometrial cancer. *Cancer detection and prevention*, Vol. 27, No. 6, pp. 434-441

Markova I., Duskova M., Lubusky M. et al. (2010). Selected immunohistochemical prognostic factors in endometrial cancer. *International Journal of Gynecogical Cancer*, Vol. 20, No. 4, pp. 576-582

Mattias-Guiu, X., Catasus, L., Bussaglia, E. et al. (2001). Molecular pathology of endometrial hyperplasia and carcinoma. *Human Pathology*, Vol. 32, pp. 569-577 Maxwell, G.L., Risinger, J.I., Alvarez, A.A. et al. (2001). Favorable survival associated with microsatellite instability in endometroid endometrial cancers. *Obstetrics and Gynecology*, Vol. 97, pp. 417-422

Morrison, C., Zanagnolo, V., Ramirez, N. et al. (2006). HER-2 is an independent prognostic factor in endometrial cancer: association with outcome in a large cohort of surgically staged patients. *Journal of Clinical Oncology*, Vol. 24, No.15, pp. 2376-2385

Mutter, G. L., Baak, J. P., Crum, C. P., et al. (2000). Endometrial precancer diagnosis by histopathology, clonal analysis, and computerized morphometry. *Journal of Pathology*, Vol. 190, pp.462-469

Mutter, G.L., Lin, M.C., Fitzerald, J.T. et al. (2000). Altered PTEN expression as a diagnostic marker for the earliest endometrial precancers. *Journal of the National Cancer Institute*, Vol. 92, pp.924-930

Myeroff, L. L., Parsons, R., Kim, S. J., et al . (1995). Atransforming growth factor beta receptor type II gene mutation common in colon and gastric but rare in endometrial cancers with microsatellite instability. *Cancer Research*, Vol. 55, pp.5545-5547

Nagase, H. & Woessner, J.F.jr. (1999). Matrix metalloproteinases. *Journal of Biological Chemistry*, Vol. 274, pp. 21491-21494

Nussbaum, R.L., McInnes, .R. & Willard, H.F. (2004). *Thompson and Thompson Klinická genetika* (6.), pp.301-302, Triton, ISBN 80-7254-475-6, Praha

Oehler, M. K., Rees, M. C. & Bicknell, R. (2000). Steroids and the endometrium. *Current Medicinal Chemistry*, Vol. 7, pp.543-560

Ohkouchi T., Sakuragi, N., Watari, H. et al. (2002). Prognostic significance of Bcl-2, p53 overexpression, and lymph node metastasis in surgically staged endometrial carcinoma. *American Journal of Obstetrics and Gynecology*, Vol. 187, No. 2, pp.353-359

Pilka R., Míčková I., Lubušký M. et al. (2008). Exprese p53, Ki-67, bcl-2, c-erb-2, estrogenového, aprogesteronového receptoru vendometriálním karcinomu. *Česká Gynekologie*, Vol. 73, No. 4, pp. 222-227

Pilka, R., Norata, G.D., Domanski, H. et al. (2004). Matrix metalloproteinase-26 (matrilysin-2)expression is high in endometrial hyperplasia and decreases with loss of histological differetiation in endometrial cancer. *Gynecological Oncology*, Vol. 94, No. 3, pp. 661-670

Popescu, R.A., Lohri, A., de Kant, E. et al. (1998). Bcl-2 expression is reciprocal to p53 and c-myc expression in metastatic human colorectal cancer. *European Journal of Cancer*, Vol. 34, pp. 1268-1273

Pradhan, M., Abeler, M.V., Danielsen, H.E et al. (2006). Image cytometry DNA ploidy correlates with histological subtypes in endometrial carcinomas. *Modern Pathology*, Vol. 19, pp.250-256

Ruddon, R.W. (2007). *Cancer Biology* (4.), pp.61-96, NY: Oxford University Press, New York

Salvesen, H. B., Iversen & O. E.Akslen, L. A.(1999). Prognostic significance of angiogenesis and Ki-67, p53 and p21 expression: apopulation-based endometrial carcinoma study. *Journal of Clinical Oncology*, Vol. 17, pp.1382-1390

Salvesen, H.B., Das, S., Akslen, L.A. et al. (2000). Loss of nuclear p16 protein expression is not associated with promoter methylation but defines a subgroup of aggressive endometrial carinomas with poor prognosis. *Clinical Cancer Research*, Vol. 6, pp.153-159

Santin, A.D., Bellone, S., Roman, J.J.et al. (2008). Trastuzumab treatment in patients with advanced or recurrent endometrial carcinoma overexpressing HER2/neu. *International Journal of Gynecology and Obsterics.*, Vol. 102, No. 2, pp. 128-131

Scholten, A.N., Creutzberg, C. L., van den Broek, L. J., et al. (2003). Nuclear beta-catenin is amolecular feature of type Iendometrial carcinoma. *Journal of Pathology*, Vol. 201, pp.460-465

Scholzen, T. & Gerdes, J. (2000). The Ki-67 protein: from the known and the unknown. *Journal of Cellular Physiology*, Vol. 183, No.3, pp. 311-322

Skrzypczak, M., Bieche, I., Szymczak, S., et al. (2004). Evaluation of mRNA expression of estrogen receptor beta and its isoforms in human normal and neoplastic endometrium. *International Journal of Cancer*, Vol. 110, pp.783-787

Suehiro, Y., Okada, Tos., Okada, Tak. et al. (2008). Aneuploidy predicts outcome in patients with endometrial carcinoma and is related to lack of CDH13 hypermetylation. *Clinical Cancer Research*, Vol. 14, pp. 3354-3361

Tashiro, H., Isacson, C., Levine, R., et al. (1997). p53 gene mutations are common in uterine serous carcinoma and occur early in their pathogenesis. *American Journal of Pathology*, Vol. 150, pp.177-185

Tunuguntla, R, Ripley, D, Sang, QX et al. (2003). Expression of matrix metalloproteinase-26 and tissue inhibitors of metalloproteinases TIMP-3 and-4 in benign endometrium and endometrial cancer small star, filled. *Gynecological Oncology*, Vol. 89, No. 3, pp. 453-459

Ueno H., Yamashita, K., Azumano, I. et al. (1999). Enhanced production and activation of matrix metalloproteinase7 (matrilysin) in human endometrial carcinomas. *International Journal of Cancer*, Vol. 84, No. 5, pp. 470-477

Vasen, H.F.A, Moslein, G., Alonso, A. et al. (2007). Guidelines for the clinical management of Lynch syndrome (hereditary non-polyposis cancer). *Journal of Medical Genetics*, Vol. 44, pp.353-362

Venter, J.C., Adams, M.D., Myers, E.W. et al. (2001). The sequence of human genome. *Science*, Vol. 291, pp. 1304-1351

Wang, F.Q., So, J., Reierstad, S. et al. (2005). Matrilysin(MMP-7) promotes invasion of ovarian cancer cells by activation of progelatinase. *International Journal of Cancer*, Vol. 114, pp. 19-31

Wang, J.Y.J. (2001). DNA damage and apoptosis. *Cell death differentiation journal*, Vol .8, pp.1047-1048

Wu, H., Goel, V. & Haluska, F.G. (2003). PTEN signaling pathways in melanoma. *Oncogene*, Vol. 22, pp.3113-3122

Zhou, X.P., Kuismanen, S., Nystrom-Lathi, M.et al. (2002). Distinct PTEN mutational spectra in hereditary non-polyposis colon cancer syndrome-related endometrial carcinomas compared to sporadic microsatellite unstable tumors. *Human Molecular Genetics*, Vol. 11, pp. 445-450

2

The Role of ErbB Receptors in Endometrial Cancer

Adonakis Georgios and Androutsopoulos Georgios
Department of Obstetrics and Gynecology, University of Patras, Medical School
Greece

1. Introduction

Endometrial cancer (EC) is the most common malignancy of the female genital tract. Overall, about 2% to 3% of women develop EC during their lifetime [Jemal et al., 2006]. EC is a malignancy that occurs primarily in postmenopausal women.

Based on clinical and pathological features, EC is classified into 2 types [Bokhman, 1983]. Type I EC, represents the majority of sporadic EC cases (70-80%), is usually well differentiated and endometrioid in histology. Type II EC, represents the minority of sporadic EC cases (10-20%), is poorly differentiated and usually papillary serous or clear cell in histology [Bokhman, 1983; Lax, 2004; Doll et al., 2008].

The Epidermal Growth Factor system (EGF system) is present in human organs and play important role in embryogenesis and postnatal development [Casalini et al., 2004; Uberall et al., 2008].

Dysregulation of the EGF signaling network is implicated in various disorders [Marmor et al., 2004; Uberall et al., 2008]. In cancer, the EGF system contributes in proliferation, transformation, angiogenesis, migration and invasion [Holbro et al., 2003].

2. Epidermal growth factor system

2.1 Receptors and ligands

The EGF system is present in human organs and play important role in cell proliferation, differentiation and apoptosis during embryogenesis and postnatal development [Casalini et al., 2004; Uberall et al., 2008].

The EGF system has four receptors: epidermal growth factor receptor (EGFR) (also known as ErbB-1, HER1), ErbB-2 (also called HER2, Neu), ErbB-3 (also called HER3) and ErbB-4 (also called HER4)] [Holbro et al., 2003; Yarden, 2001a; Yarden & Sliwkowski, 2001b].

ErbB receptors belong to subclass I of the superfamily of Receptor Tyrosine Kinases (RTKs) [Holbro et al., 2003; Uberall et al., 2008]. They are trans-membrane glycoproteins with an extracellular region containing two ligand-binding domains, an extracellular juxtamembrane region, a hydrophobic transmembrane domain and an intracellular domain with tyrosine kinase activity [Riese et al., 2007; Yarden, 2001a; Yarden & Sliwkowski, 2001b]. They catalyze the transfer of the γ phosphate of ATP to hydroxyl groups of tyrosines in target proteins [Hunter, 1998]. ErbB-3 lacks intrinsic tyrosine kinase activity [Mass, 2004].

The extracellular region of ErbB receptors has 4 subdomains (I-IV). Subdomains I and III (also called L1 and L2) are important for ligand binding. Subdomain II (also called S1) is important for dimerization between two receptors [Ogiso et al., 2002].

The EGF system has numerous ligands. According to their affinity for one or more ErbB receptors, they divided into three groups:

1. The first group includes ligands with binding specificity for EGFR: EGF, transforming growth factor-a (TGF-a) and amphiregulin (AR) [Yarden, 2001a; Yarden & Sliwkowski, 2001b; Holbro et al., 2003; Normanno et al., 2003;].
2. The second group includes ligands with dual binding specificity for EGFR and ErbB4: betacellulin (BTC), heparin-binding growth factor (HB-EGF) and epiregulin (EPR) [Yarden, 2001a; Yarden & Sliwkowski, 2001b; Holbro et al., 2003; Normanno et al., 2003;].
3. The third group includes ligands with binding specificity for ErbB-3 and ErbB-4: neuregulins (NRGs) or heregulins (HRGs). They divided in two subgroups based on their ability to bind ErbB-3 and ErbB-4 (NRG-1 and NRG-2) or only ErbB-4 (NRG-3 and NRG-4) [Zhang et al., 1997; Harari et al., 1999; Yarden, 2001a; Yarden & Sliwkowski, 2001b; Holbro et al., 2003; Normanno et al., 2003].

The ligands for ErbB receptors bind to the extracellular domain, resulting in receptor activation by homodimer and/or heterodimer formation and the subsequent transphosphorylation of tyrosine residues in the cytoplasmic region [Alroy & Yarden, 1997; Yarden, 2001a; Yarden & Sliwkowski, 2001b ; Holbro et al., 2003]. No direct ligand for ErbB-2 has been described [Holbro et al., 2003].

2.2 ErbB receptors homodimerization and heterodimerization

The extracellular region of EGFR, ErbB-3 and ErbB-4 has two distinct conformations:

1. The closed conformation (inactive), has intramolecular interactions between subdomains II and IV [Ferguson et al., 2003; Dawson et al., 2005; Riese et al., 2007].
2. The open conformation (active), where subdomains I and III form a ligand-binding pocket that permits interactions between a single ligand and subdomains I and III [Ferguson et al., 2003; Dawson et al., 2005; Riese et al., 2007].

In the absence of ligand binding, the extracellular region of EGFR, ErbB-3 and ErbB-4 has equilibrium between closed and open conformation [Ferguson et al., 2003; Dawson et al., 2005; Ozcan et al., 2006; Riese et al., 2007]. This equilibrium favours the closed conformation [Ozcan et al., 2006; Riese et al., 2007].

Ligand binding stabilizes extracellular region in the open conformation and leads to the formation of both homodimeric and heterodimeric ErbB receptor complexes [Olayioye et al., 2000; Dawson et al., 2005; Ozcan et al., 2006; Riese et al., 2007]. The dimeric formation triggers receptor activation by an allosteric mechanism [Zhang et al., 2006]. That leads to intracellular kinase activation and initiation of downstream signaling pathways [Qian et al., 1994; Olayioye et al., 2000; Yarden & Sliwkowski, 2001b].

The extracellular region of ErbB-2 has a conformation not suitable for ligand binding [Garrett et al., 2003]. However, this conformation allows extension of the receptor dimerization arm in subdomain II [Burgess et al., 2003; Garrett et al., 2003; Riese et al., 2007]. This suggests that ErbB-2 is capable for ligand independent dimerization and signaling [Riese et al., 2007]. ErbB-2 heterodimerizes with other ErbB receptors and it is their preferred heterodimerization partner [Hynes & Stern, 1994; Graus-Porta et al., 1997; Olayioye et al.,

2000; Yarden & Sliwkowski, 2001b; Garrett et al., 2003]. At elevated expression levels ErbB-2 homodimerizes [Garrett et al., 2003].

ErbB-3 lacks intrinsic tyrosine kinase activity and therefore can initiate signaling only in association with another ErbB receptor, usually ErbB-2 [Mass, 2004].

Although both homodimerization and heterodimerization result in activation of the EGF system network, heterodimers are more potent and mitogenic [Marmor et al., 2004]. ErbB-2 and ErbB-3 heterodimer is the most transforming and mitogenic receptor complex and increases cell motility on stimulation with a ligand [Alimandi et al., 1995; Wallasch et al., 1995; Yarden & Sliwkowski, 2001].

The dimerization of ErbB receptors represents the fundamental mechanism that drives transformation [Zhang et al., 2007].

2.3 ErbB receptors signaling

Dimerization of ErbB receptors leads to intracellular kinase activation [Olayioye et al., 2000; Qian et al., 1994; Yarden & Sliwkowski, 2001b]. As a result, a number of tyrosine residues in the COOH-terminal portion of ErbB receptors become phosphorylated [Burgess et al., 2003; Holbro et al., 2003; Zhang et al., 2007]. These phosphorylated tyrosine residues function as docking sites for cytoplasmic proteins containing Src homology 2 (SH2) and phosphotyrosine binding (PTB) domains [Songyang et al., 1993; Marmor et al., 2004; Yarden & Sliwkowski, 2001b; Zhang et al., 2007]. Recruitment of proteins initiates intracellular signaling via several pathways:

2.3.1 Ras / Raf / mitogen-activated protein kinase (MAPK) pathway

The Ras / Raf / mitogen-activated protein kinase (MAPK) pathway regulates cell proliferation and survival [Scaltriti & Baselga, 2006]. Following ErbB phosphorylation, the complex of Grb2 and Sos adaptor proteins binds directly or indirectly (through Shc adaptor protein) to specific intracellular ErbB docking sites [Lowenstein et al., 1992; Batzer et al., 1994].

This interaction results in conformational modification of Sos, leading to recruitment of Ras-GDP and subsequent Ras activation (Ras-GTP) [Hallberg et al., 1994]. Ras-GTP activates Raf-1 and, through intermediate steps, phosphorylates MAPK-1 and MAPK-2 [Hallberg et al., 1994; Liebmann, 2001]. Activated MAPKs phosphorylate and regulate specific intranuclear transcription factors involved in cell migration and proliferation [Hill & Treisman, 1995; Scaltriti & Baselga, 2006 Gaestel, 2006].

2.3.2 Phosphatidylinositol 3-kinase (PI3K) / Akt pathway

The Phosphatidylinositol 3-kinase (PI3K) / Akt pathway regulates cell growth, apoptosis, tumor invasion, migration and resistance to chemotherapy [Vivanco & Sawyers, 2002; Shaw & Cantley, 2006].

PI3K is a dimeric enzyme that composed of a regulatory p85 subunit and a catalytic p110 subunit [Vivanco & Sawyers, 2002]. The regulatory p85 subunit, is responsible of the anchorage to ErbB receptor specific docking sites, through interaction of its Src homology domain 2 (SH2) with phosphotyrosine residues [Yu et al, 1998a; Yu et al., 1998b]. The catalytic p110 subunit, catalyze the phosphorylation of phosphatidylinositol 4, 5 diphosphate at the 3′ position [Vivanco & Sawyers, 2002]. Phosphatidylinositol 3, 4, 5 triphosphate, phosphorylates and activates the protein serine/threonine kinase Akt [Stokoe et al., 1997; Vivanco & Sawyers, 2002].

ErbB receptor specific docking sites for p85 subunit are present on ErbB-3 and absent on EGFR [Carpenter et al., 1993; Yarden & Sliwkowski, 2001b]. EGFR dependent PI3K activation occurs through dimerization of EGFR with ErbB-3 or through the docking protein Gab-1 [Mattoon et al., 2004; Scaltriti & Baselga, 2006].

2.3.3 Signal transducers and activators of transcription (STAT) pathway

Signal transducers and activators of transcription (STAT) pathway regulates oncogenesis and tumor progression [Bromberg, 2002].

STAT proteins interact with phosphotyrosine residues via their Src homology domain 2 (SH2) and, on dimerization, translocate to the nucleus and induce the expression of specific target genes [Haura et al., 2005; Yu et al., 2004; Zhong et al., 1994]. Constitutive activation of STAT proteins (especially STAT-3 and STAT-5) is present in various primary cancers [Bromberg, 2002; Haura et al., 2005].

EGFR regulate STAT pathway through a Janus kinase (JAK) or a JAK independent mechanism [Kloth et al., 2003; Andl et al., 2004]. Augmented activity of EGFR and ErbB-2, promote persistent STAT-3 activation and subsequently induce oncogenesis and tumor progression [Bromberg, 2002].

2.3.4 Src kinase pathway

The Src kinase pathway regulates cell proliferation, migration, adhesion, angiogenesis, and immune function.

Src is a member of a 10 gene family (FYN, YES, BLK, FRK, FGR, HCK, LCK, LYN, SRMS) of non-RTKs. It is located in the cytoplasm and cross-connected with other signaling pathways, such as PI3K and STAT pathway [Yeatman, 2004; Summy & Gallick, 2006;].

Although Src functions independently, it may interact with RTKs such as EGFR. The interaction between Src and EGFR may enhance ErbB signaling and may be involved in resistance to EGFR targeted therapy [Jorissen et al., 2003; Leu & Maa, 2003].

2.3.5 Phospholipase Cγ / protein kinase C pathway

Phospholipase Cγ (PLCγ) interacts directly with activated EGFR and ErbB-2 and hydrolyses phosphatidylinositol 4, 5 diphosphate to inositol 1, 3, 5 triphosphate (IP3) and 1, 2 diacylglycerol (DAG) [Chattopadhyay et al., 1999; Patterson et al., 2005].

IP3 is important for intracellular calcium release. DAG is cofactor in protein kinase C (PKC) activation. Activated PKC activates MAPK and c-Jun NH2-terminal kinase [Schönwasser et al., 1998; McClellan et al., 1999].

3. ErbB receptors and cancer

3.1 The role of epidermal growth factor system in carcinogenesis

Dysregulation of the EGF system signaling network is implicated in cancer, diabetes, autoimmune, inflammatory, cardiovascular and nervous system disorders [Marmor et al., 2004; Uberall et al., 2008].

Loss of control of the cell functions mediated by the EGF system signaling network is a hallmark of oncogenesis, in which the balance between cell proliferation and differentiation is disturbed. Several types of human cancers associated with dysregulation of the EGF system signaling network [Uberall et al., 2008].

The EGF system signaling network in cancer becomes hyperactivated with a range of mechanisms (ligand overproduction, receptor overproduction, constitutive receptor activation) [Marmor et al., 2004; Salomon et al, 1995; Yarden & Sliwkowski, 2001b]. It is also contributes in proliferation, transformation, angiogenesis, migration and invasion [Holbro et al., 2003].

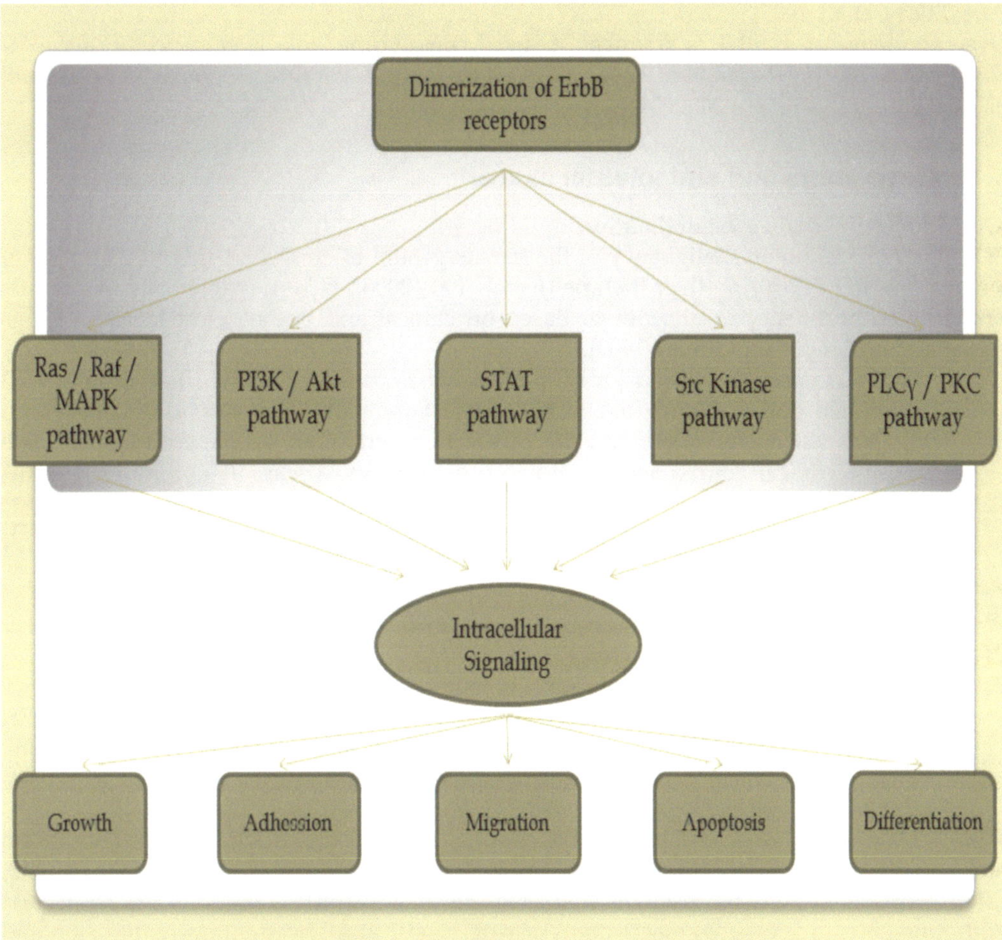

Fig. 1. ErbB receptors signalling.

3.2 Expression of ErbB receptors in cancer

Overexpression and structural alterations of EGFR are frequent in head, neck, esophageal, breast, lung, gastric, liver, kidney, colorectal, prostate, bladder and ovarian cancer [Moscatello et al., 1995; Yarden & Sliwkowski, 2001b; Uberall et al., 2008]. They associated with higher grade, disease progression, poor survival and resistance to radiotherapy and chemotherapy [Yarden & Sliwkowski, 2001b; Lurje & Lenz, 2009].

Overexpression of ErbB-2 is frequent in head, neck, breast, lung, pancreatic, esophageal, liver, colorectal, prostate, bladder, ovarian, endometrial and cervical cancer [Odicino et al.; Ross & Fletcher, 1998; Yarden & Sliwkowski, 2001b; Uberall et al., 2008]. It is an indicator of a more aggressive clinical behavior [Ross & Fletcher, 1998; Yarden & Sliwkowski, 2001b; Odicino et al., 2008].

Overexpression of ErbB-3 is frequent in head, neck, breast, gastric, liver, colorectal, prostate and ovarian cancer [Yarden & Sliwkowski, 2001b; Uberall et al., 2008]. Although ErbB-3 overexpression related with ErbB-2 positivity and lymph node involvement, a definitive relationship with survival has not been established [Lemoine et al., 1992; Gasparini et al., 1994; Bièche et al., 2003].

Overexpression of ErbB-4 is frequent in head, neck, lung and liver cancer [Yarden & Sliwkowski, 2001b; Uberall et al., 2008]. It is related with favorable prognosis in breast and bladder cancer [Suo et al., 2002; Memon et al., 2004; Barnes et al., 2005].

4. ErbB receptors and endometrial cancer

4.1 Endometrial cancer classification

EC is the most common malignancy of the female genital tract. Overall, about 2% to 3% of women develop EC during their lifetime [Jemal et al., 2006]. EC is a malignancy that occurs primarily in postmenopausal women. Based on clinical and pathological features, EC is classified into 2 types [Bokhman, 1983]:

1. Type I EC, represents the majority of sporadic EC cases (70-80%). It is usually well differentiated and endometrioid in histology [Bokhman, 1983; Lax, 2004 Doll et al., 2008]. It is estrogen-related, usually arises from endometrial hyperplasia, has less aggressive clinical course and favorable prognosis [Bokhman, 1983; Sherman et al., 1997; Doll et al., 2008]. Type I EC overexpress genes hormonally regulated during the menstrual cycle and involved in endometrial homeostasis (MGB2, LTF, END1, MMP11) [Moreno-Bueno et al., 2003; Risinger et al., 2003]. It is also associated with defects in DNA mismatch repair, microsatelite instability MLH1/MSH6 and specific mutations in PTEN, K-ras and β-catenin genes [Basil et al., 2000; Lax et al., 2000; Lax, 2004; Hecht & Mutter, 2006; Bansal et al., 2009].
2. Type II EC, represents the minority of sporadic EC cases (10-20%). It is poorly differentiated and usually papillary serous or clear cell in histology [Bokhman, 1983; Lax, 2004 Doll et al., 2008]. It is not estrogen-related, arises from atrophic endometrium, has aggressive clinical course and propensity for early spread and poor prognosis [Bokhman, 1983; Abeler & Kjorstad, 1991; Goff et al, 1994].

Type II EC overexpress genes involved in the regulation of the mitotic spindle checkpoint and associated with aneuploidy and aggressive clinical behavior (STK15, BUB1, CCNB2) [Moreno-Bueno et al., 2003; Risinger et al., 2003 Hecht & Mutter, 2006]. It is also associated with mutations in p53 gene, inactivation of p16, ErbB-2 amplification/overexpression and decreased expression of E-cadherin [Hetzel et al., 1992; Tashiro et al. 1997; Lax et al., 2000; Holcomb et al., 2002; Lax, 2004; Santin et al., 2005; Hecht & Mutter, 2006; Grushko et al., 2008; Bansal et al., 2009].

4.2 Expression and clinical significance of ErbB receptors in endometrial cancer

Due to the inactive status of postmenopausal endometrium, it is expectable to find significantly higher expression of the 4 ErbB receptors in EC tissue [Ejskjaer et al., 2007].

EGFR, in endometrium, is localized to the basal part of surface epithelial cells, only in stromal cells, or both to epithelial and stromal cells [Bigsby et al., 1992; Wang et al., 1994; Imai et al., 1995; Möller et al., 2001; Ejskjaer et al., 2005]. It is primarily located to the cell membrane but also to the cytoplasm [Nyholm et al., 1993; Reinartz et al., 1994; Khalifa et al., 1994; Niikura et al., 1996; Ejskjaer et al., 2007].

In unselected patients with EC, it has been reported EGFR expression in 43–67% of cases [Reinartz et al., 1994; Khalifa et al., 1994; Scambia et al, 1994; Niikura et al., 1996; Androutsopoulos et al., 2006; Adonakis et al., 2008]. In patients with type I EC, it has been reported EGFR expression in 46% of cases. In patients with type II EC, it has been reported EGFR expression in 34% of cases [Konecny et al., 2009].

Although the clinical significance of EGFR has not been studied well in EC, it may have a dual role. EGFR overexpression did not affect disease progression in type I EC, although affects disease progression in type II EC. EGFR overexpression in type II EC associated with high grade and adverse clinical outcome [Konecny et al., 2009].

ErbB-2, in endometrium, is localized baso-laterally in the glands and surface epithelial cells [Bigsby et al., 1992; Wang et al., 1994; Miturski et al., 1998; Ejskjaer et al., 2005]. It is located to the cell membrane [Reinartz et al., 1994; Khalifa et al., 1994; Ejskjaer et al., 2007; Odicino et al., 2008].

In unselected patients with EC, ErbB-2 amplification/overexpression represents a rare event. In patients with type I EC, it has been reported ErbB-2 receptor overexpression in 8% of cases and ErbB-2 gene amplification in 1.4-3% of cases [Morrison et al., 2006; Konecny et al., 2009].

Although, ErbB-2 amplification/overexpression is more common in patients with type II EC, the exact frequency remains controversial. In patients with papillary serous EC, it has been reported ErbB-2 receptor overexpression in 18%-80% of cases and ErbB-2 gene amplification in 17-47% of cases [Santin et al., 2005; Morrison et al., 2006; Slomovitz et al., 2008; Grushko et al., 2008; Konecny et al., 2009;]. In patients with clear cell EC, it has been reported ErbB-2 receptor overexpression in 33% of cases and ErbB-2 gene amplification in 16-50% of cases [Morrison et al., 2006; Grushko et al., 2008; Konecny et al., 2009]. ErbB-2 overexpression especially in type II EC, is an indicator of a highly aggressive disease and a poor overall survival [Lukes et al., 1992; Santin et al., 2005; Morrison et al., 2006; Odicino et al., 2008].

ErbB-3, in endometrium, is localized to surface epithelial cells [Prigent et al., 1992; Srinivasan et al., 1999 Ejskjaer et al., 2005]. It is located to the cytoplasm, with membrane staining in a minority of samples [Srinivasan et al., 1999; Ejskjaer et al., 2007].

The clinical significance of ErbB-3 has not been studied well in EC [Srinivasan et al., 1999; Androutsopoulos et al., 2006; Ejskjaer et al., 2007; Adonakis et al., 2008].

ErbB-4, in endometrium, is localized to epithelial and stromal cells [Srinivasan et al., 1999; Chobotova et al., 2005; Ejskjaer et al., 2005]. It is located to the cytoplasm, with membrane staining in a minority of samples [Srinivasan et al., 1999; Ejskjaer et al., 2007;].

The clinical significance of ErbB-4 has not been studied well in EC [Srinivasan et al., 1999; Androutsopoulos et al., 2006; Ejskjaer et al., 2007; Adonakis et al., 2008].

4.3 Endometrial cancer and ErbB-targeted therapies

EGFR and ErbB-2 as targets for cancer therapy have been investigated for over 20 years. Two major classes of ErbB-targeted therapies have been developed.

4.3.1 Anti-ErbB monoclonal antibodies (MoAbs)

1. Anti-EGFR MoAbs (cetuximab, panitumumab) bind to the extracellular domain of EGFR and prevent ligand binding and ligand dependent receptor activation.
2. Anti-ErbB-2 MoAb (trastuzumab) binds to the extracellular domain of ErbB-2 and interferes with ligand independent receptor activation, but the exact mechanism of action is still subject of ongoing debate [Baselga & Arteaga, 2005; Lurje & Lenz, 2009].

3. There is a new class of Anti-ErbB MoAb (pertuzumab) that prevent receptor heterodimerization [Baselga & Arteaga, 2005].

4.3.2 ErbB-specific tyrosine kinase inhibitors (TKIs)

TKI block the binding of adenosine triphosphate to the intracellular domain of EGFR (gefitinib, erlotinib) or EGFR and ErbB-2 (lapatinib) and blocks ErbB activity and subsequent intracellular signaling [Baselga & Arteaga, 2005; Lurje & Lenz, 2009].

4.3.3 Effectiveness of ErbB-targeted therapies

Overall response rate to these drugs is modest, unless they are associated with chemotherapy or radiotherapy [Baselga & Arteaga, 2005]. ErbB-targeted therapies have not been clinically tested in type II EC [Konecny et al., 2009]. Preclinical data suggest that ErbB-targeted therapies may be clinically active in well-defined subgroups of type II EC patients with EGFR and ErbB-2 overexpression [Villella et al., 2006; Jewell et al., 2006; Konecny et al., 2008; Santin et al., 2008; Vandenput et al., 2009; El-Sahwi et al., 2010;].

The role of ErbB-targeted therapies in EC should be further investigated in clinical trials to evaluate their therapeutic efficacy [Odicino et al., 2008; Oza et al., 2008; Santin et al., 2008; Konecny et al., 2009; Fleming et al., 2010; Santin, 2010]. Also, further studies into the molecular pathways of EC development and progression, will increase our knowledge of this disease and will lead to the discovery of new generation molecules with higher therapeutic efficacy.

5. Conclusion

Additional studies into the molecular pathways of EC development and progression, will increase our knowledge of this disease and will lead to the discovery of new generation molecules with higher therapeutic efficacy.

6. References

Abeler, VM. & Kjorstad, KE. (1991). Clear cell carcinoma of the endometrium: a histopathological and clinical study of 97 cases. Gynecol Oncol 40(3):207-217.

Adonakis, G., Androutsopoulos, G., Koumoundourou, D., Liava, A., Ravazoula, P. & Kourounis, G. (2008). Expression of the epidermal growth factor system in endometrial cancer. Eur J Gynaecol Oncol 29(5):450-454.

Alimandi, M., Romano, A., Curia, MC., Muraro, R., Fedi, P., Aaronson, SA., Di Fiore, PP. & Kraus, MH. (1995). Cooperative signaling of ErbB3 and ErbB2 in neoplastic transformation and human mammary carcinomas. Oncogene 10(9):1813-1821.

Alroy, I. & Yarden, Y. (1997). The ErbB signaling network in embryogenesis and oncogenesis: signal diversification through combinatorial ligand-receptor interactions. FEBS Lett 410(1):83-86.

Andl, CD., Mizushima, T., Oyama, K., Bowser, M., Nakagawa, H. & Rustgi, AK. (2004) EGFR-induced cell migration is mediated predominantly by the JAK-STAT pathway in primary esophageal keratinocytes. Am J Physiol Gastrointest Liver Physiol 287(6):G1227-G1237.

Androutsopoulos, G., Adonakis, G., Gkermpesi, M., Gkogkos, P., Ravazoula, P. & Kourounis, G. (2006). Expression of the epidermal growth factor system in endometrial cancer after adjuvant tamoxifen treatment for breast cancer. Eur J Gynaecol Oncol 27(5):490-494.

Bansal, N., Yendluri, V. & Wenham, RM. (2009). The molecular biology of endometrial cancers and the implications for pathogenesis, classification, and targeted therapies. Cancer Control 16(1):8-13.

Barnes, NL., Khavari, S., Boland, GP., Cramer, A., Knox, WF. & Bundred, NJ. (2005). Absence of HER4 expression predicts recurrence of ductal carcinoma in situ of the breast. Clin Cancer Res 11(6):2163-2168.

Baselga, J. & Arteaga, CL. (2005). Critical update and emerging trends in epidermal growth factor receptor targeting in cancer. J Clin Oncol 23(11):2445-2459.

Basil, JB., Goodfellow, PJ., Rader, JS., Mutch, DG. & Herzog, TJ. (2000). Clinical significance of microsatellite instability in endometrial carcinoma. Cancer 89(8):1758-1764.

Batzer, AG., Rotin, D., Ureña, JM., Skolnik, EY. & Schlessinger, J. (1994). Hierarchy of binding sites for Grb2 and Shc on the epidermal growth factor receptor. Mol Cell Biol 14(8):5192-5201.

Bièche, I., Onody, P., Tozlu, S., Driouch, K., Vidaud, M. 7 Lidereau, R. (2003). Prognostic value of ERBB family mRNA expression in breast carcinomas. Int J Cancer 106(5):758-765.

Bigsby, RM., Li, AX., Bomalaski, J., Stehman, FB., Look, KY. & Sutton, GP. (1992). Immunohistochemical study of HER-2/neu, epidermal growth factor receptor, and steroid receptor expression in normal and malignant endometrium. Obstet Gynecol 79(1):95-100.

Bokhman JV. (1983). Two pathogenetic types of endometrial carcinoma. Gynecol Oncol 15(1):10-17.

Bromberg, J. (2002). Stat proteins and oncogenesis. J Clin Invest 109(9):1139-1142.

Burgess, AW., Cho, HS., Eigenbrot, C., Ferguson, KM., Garrett, TP., Leahy, DJ., Lemmon, MA., Sliwkowski, MX., Ward, CW. & Yokoyama, S. (2003). An open-and-shut case? Recent insights into the activation of EGF/ErbB receptors. Mol Cell 12(3):541-552.

Casalini, P., Iorio, MV., Galmozzi, E. & Ménard, S. (2004). Role of HER receptors family in development and differentiation. J Cell Physiol 200(3):343-350.

Carpenter, CL., Auger, KR., Chanudhuri, M., Yoakim, M., Schaffhausen, B., Shoelson, S. & Cantley, LC. (1993). Phosphoinositide 3-kinase is activated by phosphopeptides that bind to the SH2 domains of the 85-kDa subunit. J Biol Chem 268(13):9478-9483.

Chattopadhyay, A., Vecchi, M., Ji, Q., Mernaugh, R. & Carpenter, G. (1999). The role of individual SH2 domains in mediating association of phospholipase C-gamma1 with the activated EGF receptor. J Biol Chem 274(37):26091-26097.

Chobotova, K., Karpovich, N., Carver, J., Manek, S., Gullick, WJ., Barlow, DH. & Mardon, HJ. (2005). Heparin-binding epidermal growth factor and its receptors mediate decidualization and potentiate survival of human endometrial stromal cells. J Clin Endocrinol Metab 90(2):913-919.

Dawson, JP., Berger, MB., Lin, CC., Schlessinger, J., Lemmon, MA. & Ferguson, KM. (2005). Epidermal growth factor receptor dimerization and activation require ligand-induced conformational changes in the dimer interface. Mol Cell Biol 25(17):7734-7742.

Doll, A., Abal, M., Rigau, M., Monge, M., Gonzalez, M., Demajo, S., Colás, E., Llauradó, M., Alazzouzi, H., Planagumá, J., Lohmann, MA., Garcia, J., Castellvi, S., Ramon y Caja,l J., Gil-Moreno, A., Xercavins, J., Alameda, F. & Reventós J. (2008). Novel molecular profiles of endometrial cancer-new light through old windows. J Steroid Biochem Mol Biol 108(3-5):221-229.

Ejskjaer, K., Sørensen, BS., Poulsen, SS., Mogensen, O., Forman, A. & Nexø, E. (2005). Expression of the epidermal growth factor system in human endometrium during the menstrual cycle. Mol Hum Reprod 11(8):543-551.

Ejskjaer, K., Sørensen, BS., Poulsen, SS., Forman, A., Nexø, E. & Mogensen, O. (2007). Expression of the epidermal growth factor system in endometrioid endometrial cancer. Gynecol Oncol 104(1):158-167.

El-Sahwi, K., Bellone, S., Cocco, E., Cargnelutti, M., Casagrande, F., Bellone, M., Abu-Khalaf, M., Buza, N., Tavassoli, FA., Hui, P., Silasi, DA., Azodi, M., Schwartz, PE., Rutherford, TJ., Pecorelli, S. & Santin AD. (2010). In vitro activity of pertuzumab in combination with trastuzumab in uterine serous papillary adenocarcinoma. Br J Cancer 102(1):134-143.

Ferguson, KM., Berger, MB., Mendrola, JM., Cho, HS., Leahy, DJ. & Lemmon, MA. (2003). EGF activates its receptor by removing interactions that autoinhibit ectodomain dimerization. Mol Cell 11(2):507-517.

Fleming, GF., Sill, MW., Darcy, KM., McMeekin, DS., Thigpen, JT., Adler, LM., Berek, JS., Chapman, JA., DiSilvestro, PA., Horowitz, IR. & Fiorica, JV. (2010). Phase II trial of trastuzumab in women with advanced or recurrent, HER2-positive endometrial carcinoma: a Gynecologic Oncology Group study. Gynecol Oncol 116(1):15-20.

Garrett, TP., McKern, NM., Lou, M., Elleman, TC., Adams, TE., Lovrecz, GO., Kofler, M., Jorissen, RN., Nice, EC., Burgess, AW. & Ward, CW. (2003). The crystal structure of a truncated ErbB2 ectodomain reveals an active conformation, poised to interact with other ErbB receptors. Mol Cell 11(2):495-505.

Gaestel, M. (2006). MAPKAP kinases - MKs - two's company, three's a crowd. Nat Rev Mol Cell Biol 7(2):120-130.

Gasparini, G., Gullick, WJ., Maluta, S., Dalla Palma, P., Caffo, O., Leonardi, E., Boracchi, P., Pozza, F., Lemoine, NR. & Bevilacqua, P. (1994). c-erbB-3 and c-erbB-2 protein expression in node-negative breast carcinoma--an immunocytochemical study. Eur J Cancer 30A(1):16-22.

Goff, BA., Kato, D., Schmidt, RA., Ek, M., Ferry, JA., Muntz, HG., Cain, JM., Tamimi, HK., Figge, DC. & Greer, BE. (1994). Uterine papillary serous carcinoma: patterns of metastatic spread. Gynecol Oncol 54(3):264-268.

Graus-Porta, D., Beerli, RR., Daly, JM. & Hynes, NE. (1997). ErbB-2, the preferred heterodimerization partner of all ErbB receptors, is a mediator of lateral signaling. EMBO J 16(7):1647-1655.

Grushko, TA., Filiaci, VL., Mundt, AJ., Ridderstrale, K., Olopade, OI., Fleming, GF. & Gynecologic Oncology Group. (2008). An exploratory analysis of HER-2 amplification and overexpression in advanced endometrial carcinoma: a Gynecologic Oncology Group study. Gynecol Oncol 108(1):3-9.

Hallberg, B., Rayter, SI. & Downward, J. (1994). Interaction of Ras and Raf in intact mammalian cells upon extracellular stimulation. J Biol Chem 269(6):3913-3916.

Harari, D., Tzahar, E., Romano, J., Shelly, M., Pierce, JH., Andrews, GC. & Yarden, Y. (1999). Neuregulin-4: a novel growth factor that acts through the ErbB-4 receptor tyrosine kinase. Oncogene 18(17):2681-2689.

Haura, EB., Turkson, J. & Jove, R. (2005). Mechanisms of disease: Insights into the emerging role of signal transducers and activators of transcription in cancer. Nat Clin Pract Oncol 2(6):315-324.

Hecht, JL. & Mutter, GL. (2006). Molecular and pathologic aspects of endometrial carcinogenesis. J Clin Oncol 24(29):4783-4791.

Hetzel, DJ., Wilson, TO., Keeney, GL., Roche, PC., Cha, SS. & Podratz, KC. (1992). HER-2/neu expression: a major prognostic factor in endometrial cancer. Gynecol Oncol 47(2):179-185.

Hill, CS. & Treisman, R. (1995). Transcriptional regulation by extracellular signals: mechanisms and specificity. Cell 80(2):199-211.

Holbro, T., Civenni, G. & Hynes, NE. (2003). The ErbB receptors and their role in cancer progression. Exp Cell Res 284(1):99-110.

Holcomb, K., Delatorre, R., Pedemonte, B., McLeod, C., Anderson, L. & Chambers, J. (2002). E-cadherin expression in endometrioid, papillary serous, and clear cell carcinoma of the endometrium. Obstet Gynecol 100(6):1290-1295.

Hunter, T. (1998). The Croonian Lecture 1997. The phosphorylation of proteins on tyrosine: its role in cell growth and disease. Philos Trans R Soc Lond B Biol Sci 353(1368):583-605.

Hynes, NE. & Stern, DF. (1994). The biology of erbB-2/neu/HER-2 and its role in cancer. Biochim Biophys Acta 1198(2-3):165-184.

Imai, T., Kurachi, H., Adachi, K., Adachi, H., Yoshimoto, Y., Homma, H., Tadokoro, C., Takeda, S., Yamaguchi, M., Sakata, M., Sakoyama, Y. & Miyake, A. (1995). Changes in epidermal growth factor receptor and the levels of its ligands during menstrual cycle in human endometrium. Biol Reprod 52(4):928-938.

Jemal, A., Siegel, R., Ward, E., Murray, T., Xu, J., Smigal, C. & Thun MJ. (2006). Cancer statistics, 2006. CA Cancer J Clin 56(2):106-130.

Jewell, E., Secord, AA., Brotherton, T. & Berchuck, A. (2006). Use of trastuzumab in the treatment of metastatic endometrial cancer. Int J Gynecol Cancer 16(3):1370-1373.

Jorissen, RN., Walker, F., Pouliot, N., Garrett, TP., Ward, CW. & Burgess, AW. (2003). Epidermal growth factor receptor: mechanisms of activation and signalling. Exp Cell Res 284(1):31-53.

Khalifa, MA., Mannel, RS., Haraway, SD., Walker, J. & Min, KW. (1994). Expression of EGFR, HER-2/neu, P53, and PCNA in endometrioid, serous papillary, and clear cell endometrial adenocarcinomas. Gynecol Oncol 53(1):84-92.

Kloth, MT., Laughlin, KK., Biscardi, JS., Boerner, JL., Parsons, SJ. & Silva, CM. (2003). STAT5b, a Mediator of Synergism between c-Src and the Epidermal Growth Factor Receptor. J Biol Chem 278(3):1671-1679.

Konecny, GE., Venkatesan, N., Yang, G., Dering, J., Ginther, C., Finn, R., Rahmeh, M., Fejzo, MS., Toft, D., Jiang, SW., Slamon, DJ. & Podratz KC. (2008). Activity of lapatinib a novel HER2 and EGFR dual kinase inhibitor in human endometrial cancer cells. Br J Cancer 98(6):1076-1084.

Konecny, GE., Santos, L., Winterhoff, B., Hatmal, M., Keeney, GL., Mariani, A., Jone, M., Neuper, C., Thomas, B., Muderspach, L., Riehle, D., Wang, HJ., Dowdy, S., Podratz,

KC. & Press, MF. (2009). HER2 gene amplification and EGFR expression in a large cohort of surgically staged patients with nonendometrioid (type II) endometrial cancer. Br J Cancer 100(1):89-95.

Lax, SF., Kendall, B., Tashiro, H., Slebos, RJ. & Hedrick, L. (2000). The frequency of p53, K-ras mutations, and microsatellite instability differs in uterine endometrioid and serous carcinoma: evidence of distinct molecular genetic pathways. Cancer 88(4):814-824.

Lax, SF. (2004). Molecular genetic pathways in various types of endometrial carcinoma: from a phenotypical to a molecular-based classification. Virchows Arch 444(3):213-223.

Lemoine, NR., Barnes, DM., Hollywood, DP., Hughes, CM., Smith, P., Dublin, E., Prigent, SA., Gullick, WJ. & Hurst, HC. (1992). Expression of the ERBB3 gene product in breast cancer. Br J Cancer 66(6):1116-1121.

Leu, TH. & Maa, MC. (2003). Functional implication of the interaction between EGF receptor and c-Src. Front Biosci 8:s28-38.

Liebmann, C. (2001). Regulation of MAP kinase activity by peptide receptor signalling pathway: paradigms of multiplicity. Cell Signal 13(11):777-785.

Lowenstein, EJ., Daly, RJ., Batzer, AG., Li, W., Margolis, B., Lammers, R., Ullrich, A., Skolnik, EY., Bar-Sagi, D. & Schlessinger, J. (1992). The SH2 and SH3 domain-containing protein GRB2 links receptor tyrosine kinases to ras signaling. Cell 70(3):431-442.

Lukes, AS., Kohler, MF., Pieper, CF., Kerns, BJ., Bentley, R., Rodriguez, GC., Soper, JT., Clarke-Pearson, DL., Bast, RC Jr. & Berchuck, A. (1994). Multivariable analysis of DNA ploidy, p53, and HER-2/neu as prognostic factors in endometrial cancer. Cancer 73(9):2380-2385.

Lurje, G. & Lenz, HJ. (2009). EGFR signaling and drug discovery. Oncology 77(6):400-410.

Marmor, MD., Skaria, KB. & Yarden, Y. (2004). Signal transduction and oncogenesis by ErbB/HER receptors. Int J Radiat Oncol Biol Phys 58(3):903-913.

Mass, RD. (2004). The HER receptor family: a rich target for therapeutic development. Int J Radiat Oncol Biol Phys 58(3):932-940.

Mattoon, DR., Lamothe, B., Lax, I. & Schlessinger, J. (2004). The docking protein Gab1 is the primary mediator of EGF-stimulated activation of the PI-3K/Akt cell survival pathway. BMC Biol 2:24.

McClellan, M., Kievit, P., Auersperg, N. & Rodland, K. (1999). Regulation of proliferation and apoptosis by epidermal growth factor and protein kinase C in human ovarian surface epithelial cells. Exp Cell Res 246(2):471-479.

Memon, AA., Sorensen, BS., Melgard, P., Fokdal, L., Thykjaer, T. & Nexo, E. (2004). Expression of HER3, HER4 and their ligand heregulin-4 is associated with better survival in bladder cancer patients. Br J Cancer 91(12):2034-2041.

Miturski, R., Semczuk, A. & Jakowicki, JA. (1998). C-erbB-2 expression in human proliferative and hyperplastic endometrium. Int J Gynaecol Obstet 61(1):73-74.

Möller, B., Rasmussen, C., Lindblom, B. & Olovsson, M. (2001). Expression of the angiogenic growth factors VEGF, FGF-2, EGF and their receptors in normal human endometrium during the menstrual cycle. Mol Hum Reprod 7(1):65-72.

Moreno-Bueno, G., Sánchez-Estévez, C., Cassia, R., Rodríguez-Perales, S., Díaz-Uriarte, R., Domínguez, O., Hardisson, D., Andujar, M., Prat, J., Matias-Guiu, X., Cigudosa, JC. & Palacios, J. (2003). Differential gene expression profile in endometrioid and nonendometrioid endometrial carcinoma: STK15 is frequently overexpressed and amplified in nonendometrioid carcinomas. Cancer Res 63(18):5697-5702.

Morrison, C., Zanagnolo, V., Ramirez, N., Cohn, DE., Kelbick, N., Copeland, L., Maxwell, GL. & Fowler, JM. (2006). HER-2 is an independent prognostic factor in endometrial cancer: association with outcome in a large cohort of surgically staged patients. J Clin Oncol 24(15):2376-2385.

Moscatello, DK., Holgado-Madruga, M., Godwin, AK., Ramirez, G., Gunn, G., Zoltick, PW., Biegel, JA., Hayes, RL. & Wong, AJ. (1995). Frequent expression of a mutant epidermal growth factor receptor in multiple human tumors. Cancer Res 55(23):5536-5539.

Niikura, H., Sasano, H., Kaga, K., Sato, S. & Yajima, A. (1996). Expression of epidermal growth factor family proteins and epidermal growth factor receptor in human endometrium. Hum Pathol 27(3):282-289.

Normanno, N., Bianco, C., De Luca, A., Maiello, MR. & Salomon, DS. (2003). Target-based agents against ErbB receptors and their ligands: a novel approach to cancer treatment. Endocr Relat Cancer 10(1):1-21.

Nyholm, HC., Nielsen, AL. & Ottesen, B. (1993). Expression of epidermal growth factor receptors in human endometrial carcinoma. Int J Gynecol Pathol 12(3):241-245.

Odicino, FE., Bignotti, E., Rossi, E., Pasinetti, B., Tassi, RA., Donzelli, C., Falchetti, M., Fontana, P., Grigolato, PG. & Pecorelli, S. (2008). HER-2/neu overexpression and amplification in uterine serous papillary carcinoma: comparative analysis of immunohistochemistry, real-time reverse transcription-polymerase chain reaction, and fluorescence in situ hybridization. Int J Gynecol Cancer 18(1):14-21.

Ogiso, H., Ishitani, R., Nureki, O., Fukai, S., Yamanaka, M., Kim, JH., Saito, K., Sakamoto, A., Inoue, M., Shirouzu, M. & Yokoyama, S. (2002). Crystal structure of the complex of human epidermal growth factor and receptor extracellular domains. Cell 110(6):775-787.

Olayioye, MA., Neve, RM., Lane, HA. & Hynes, NE. (2000). The ErbB signaling network: receptor heterodimerization in development and cancer. EMBO J 19(13):3159-3167.

Oza, AM., Eisenhauer, EA., Elit, L., Cutz, JC., Sakurada, A., Tsao, MS., Hoskins, PJ., Biagi, J., Ghatage, P., Mazurka, J., Provencher, D., Dore, N., Dancey, J. & Fyles, A. (2008). Phase II study of erlotinib in recurrent or metastatic endometrial cancer: NCIC IND-148. J Clin Oncol 26(26):4319-4325.

Ozcan, F., Klein, P., Lemmon, MA., Lax, I. & Schlessinger, J. (2006). On the nature of low- and high-affinity EGF receptors on living cells. Proc Natl Acad Sci U S A 103(15):5735-5740.

Patterson, RL., van Rossum, DB., Nikolaidis, N., Gill, DL. & Snyder, SH. (2005). Phospholipase C-gamma: diverse roles in receptor-mediated calcium signaling. Trends Biochem Sci 30(12):688-697.

Prigent, SA., Lemoine, NR., Hughes, CM., Plowman, GD., Selden, C. & Gullick, WJ. (1992). Expression of the c-erbB-3 protein in normal human adult and fetal tissues. Oncogene 7(7):1273-1278.

Qian, X., LeVea, CM., Freeman, JK., Dougall, WC. & Greene, MI. (1994). Heterodimerization of epidermal growth factor receptor and wild-type or kinase-deficient Neu: a mechanism of interreceptor kinase activation and transphosphorylation. Proc Natl Acad Sci U S A 91(4):1500-1504.

Reinartz, JJ., George, E., Lindgren, BR. & Niehans, GA. (1994). Expression of p53, transforming growth factor alpha, epidermal growth factor receptor, and c-erbB-2 in endometrial carcinoma and correlation with survival and known predictors of survival. Hum Pathol 25(10):1075-1083.

Riese, DJ., Gallo, RM. & Settleman, J. (2007). Mutational activation of ErbB family receptor tyrosine kinases: insights into mechanisms of signal transduction and tumorigenesis. Bioessays 29(6):558-565.

Risinger, JI., Maxwell, GL., Chandramouli, GV., Jazaeri, A., Aprelikova, O., Patterson, T., Berchuck, A. & Barrett, JC. (2003). Microarray analysis reveals distinct gene expression profiles among different histologic types of endometrial cancer. Cancer Res 63(1):6-11.

Ross, JS. & Fletcher, JA. (1998). The HER-2/neu oncogene in breast cancer: prognostic factor, predictive factor, and target for therapy. Oncologist 3(4):237-252.

Salomon, DS., Brandt, R., Ciardiello, F. & Normanno, N. (1995). Epidermal growth factor-related peptides and their receptors in human malignancies. Crit Rev Oncol Hematol 19(3):183-232.

Santin, AD., Bellone, S., Van Stedum, S., Bushen, W., Palmieri, M., Siegel, ER., De Las Casas, LE., Roman, JJ., Burnett, A. & Pecorelli, S. (2005). Amplification of c-erbB2 oncogene: a major prognostic indicator in uterine serous papillary carcinoma. Cancer 104(7):1391-1397.

Santin, AD., Bellone, S., Roman, JJ., McKenney, JK. & Pecorelli, S. (2008). Trastuzumab treatment in patients with advanced or recurrent endometrial carcinoma overexpressing HER2/neu. Int J Gynaecol Obstet 102(2):128-131.

Santin, AD. (2010). Letter to the Editor referring to the manuscript entitled: "Phase II trial of trastuzumab in women with advanced or recurrent HER-positive endometrial carcinoma: a Gynecologic Oncology Group study" recently reported by Fleming et al., (Gynecol Oncol., 116;15-20;2010). Gynecol Oncol 118(1):95-96.

Scambia, G., Benedetti Panici, P., Ferrandina, G., Battaglia, F., Distefano, M., D'Andrea, G., De Vincenzo, R., Maneschi, F., Ranelletti, FO. & Mancuso, S. (1994). Significance of epidermal growth factor receptor expression in primary human endometrial cancer. Int J Cancer 56(1):26-30.

Scaltriti, M. & Baselga, J. (2006). The epidermal growth factor receptor pathway: a model for targeted therapy. Clin Cancer Res 2006;12(18):5268-5272.

Schönwasser, DC., Marais, RM., Marshall, CJ. & Parker, PJ. (1998). Activation of the mitogen-activated protein kinase/extracellular signal-regulated kinase pathway by conventional, novel, and atypical protein kinase C isotypes. Mol Cell Biol 18(2):790-798.

Shaw, RJ. & Cantley, LC. (2006). Ras, PI(3)K and mTOR signalling controls tumour cell growth. Nature 441(7092):424-430.

Sherman, ME., Sturgeon, S., Brinton, LA., Potischman, N., Kurman, RJ., Berman, ML., Mortel, R., Twiggs, LB., Barrett, RJ. & Wilbanks, GD. (1997). Risk factors and hormone levels in patients with serous and endometrioid uterine carcinomas. Mod Pathol 10(10):963-968.

Slomovitz, BM., Broaddus, RR., Burke, TW., Sneige, N., Soliman, PT., Wu, W., Sun, CC., Munsell, MF., Gershenson, DM. & Lu, KH. (2008). Her-2/neu overexpression and amplification in uterine papillary serous carcinoma. J Clin Oncol 22(15):3126-3132.

Songyang, Z., Shoelson, SE., Chaudhuri, M., Gish, G., Pawson, T., Haser, WG., King, F., Roberts, T., Ratnofsky, S., Lechleider, RJ., Neel, BG., Birge, RB., Fajardo, JE., Chou, MM., Hanafusa, H., Schaffhausen, B. & Cantley, LC. (1993). SH2 domains recognize specific phosphopeptide sequences. Cell 72(5):767-778.

Srinivasan, R., Benton, E., McCormick, F., Thomas, H. & Gullick, WJ. (1999). Expression of the c-erbB-3/HER-3 and c-erbB-4/HER-4 growth factor receptors and their ligands, neuregulin-1 alpha, neuregulin-1 beta, and betacellulin, in normal endometrium and endometrial cancer. Clin Cancer Res 5(10):2877-2883.

Stokoe, D., Stephens, LR., Copeland, T., Gaffney, PR., Reese, CB., Painter, GF., Holmes, AB., McCormick, F. & Hawkins, PT. (1997). Dual role of phosphatidylinositol-3,4,5-trisphosphate in the activation of protein kinase B. Science 277(5325):567-570.

Summy, JM. & Gallick, GE. (2006). Treatment for advanced tumors: SRC reclaims center stage. Clin Cancer Res 12(5):1398-1401.

Suo, Z., Risberg, B., Kalsson, MG., Willman, K., Tierens, A., Skovlund, E. & Nesland, JM. (2002). EGFR family expression in breast carcinomas. c-erbB-2 and c-erbB-4 receptors have different effects on survival. J Pathol 196(1):17-25.

Tashiro, H., Isacson, C., Levine, R., Kurman, RJ., Cho, KR. & Hedrick, L. (1997). p53 gene mutations are common in uterine serous carcinoma and occur early in their pathogenesis. Am J Pathol 150(1):177-185.

Uberall, I., Kolár, Z., Trojanec, R., Berkovcová, J., Hajdúch, M. (2008). The status and role of ErbB receptors in human cancer. Exp Mol Pathol 84(2):79-89.

Vandenput, I., Vanden Bempt, I., Leunen, K., Neven, P., Berteloot, P., Moerman, P., Vergote, I. & Amant, F. (2009). Limited clinical benefit from trastuzumab in recurrent endometrial cancer: two case reports. Gynecol Obstet Invest 67(1):46-48.

Villella, JA., Cohen, S., Smith, DH., Hibshoosh, H. & Hershman, D. (2006). HER-2/neu overexpression in uterine papillary serous cancers and its possible therapeutic implications. Int J Gynecol Cancer 16(5):1897-1902.

Vivanco, I. & Sawyers, CL. (2002). The phosphatidylinositol 3-Kinase AKT pathway in human cancer. Nat Rev Cancer 2(7):489-501.

Wallasch, C., Weiss, FU., Niederfellner, G., Jallal, B., Issing, W. & Ullrich, A. (1995). Heregulin-dependent regulation of HER2/neu oncogenic signaling by heterodimerization with HER3. EMBO J 14(17):4267-4275.

Wang, XN., Das, SK., Damm, D., Klagsbrun, M., Abraham, JA. & Dey, SK. (1994). Differential regulation of heparin-binding epidermal growth factor-like growth factor in the adult ovariectomized mouse uterus by progesterone and estrogen. Endocrinology 135(3):1264-1271.

Yarden, Y. (2001a). The EGFR family and its ligands in human cancer. signalling mechanisms and therapeutic opportunities. Eur J Cancer 37(Suppl 4):S3-S8.

Yarden, Y. & Sliwkowski, MX. (2001b). Untangling the ErbB signalling network. Nat Rev Mol Cell Biol 2(2):127-137.

Yeatman, TJ. (2004). A renaissance for SRC. Nat Rev Cancer 4(6):470-480.

Yu, J., Wjasow, C. & Backer, JM. (1998a) Regulation of the p85/p110 phosphatidylinositol 3-kinase. Distinct roles for the N-terminal and C-terminal SH2 domains. J Biol Chem 273:30199-30203.

Yu, J., Zhang, Y., McIlroy, J., Rordorf-Nikolic, T., Orr, GA. & Backer, JM. (1998b). Regulation of the p85/p110 phosphatidylinositol 3 -kinase: stabilization and inhibition of the p110 catalytic subunit by the p85 regulatory subunit. Mol Cell Biol 18:1379-1387.

Yu, H. & Jove, R. (2004). The STATs of cancer - new molecular targets come of age. Nat Rev Cancer 4:97-105.

Zhang, D., Sliwkowski, MX., Mark, M., Frantz, G., Akita, R., Sun, Y., Hillan, K., Crowley, C., Brush, J. & Godowski, PJ. (1997). Neuregulin-3 (NRG3): a novel neural tissue-enriched protein that binds and activates ErbB4. Proc Natl Acad Sci U S A 94(18):9562-9567.

Zhang, X., Gureasko, J., Shen, K., Cole, PA. & Kuriyan, J. (2006). An allosteric mechanism for activation of the kinase domain of epidermal growth factor receptor. Cell 125(6):1137-1149.

Zhang, H., Berezov, A., Wang, Q., Zhang, G., Drebin, J., Murali, R. & Greene, MI. (2007). ErbB receptors: from oncogenes to targeted cancer therapies. J Clin Invest 117:2051-2058.

Zhong, Z., Wen, Z. & Darnell, JE Jr. (1994). Stat3: a STAT family member activated by tyrosine phosphorylation in response to epidermal growth factor and interleukin-6. Science 264(5155):95-98.

3

Hereditary Endometrial Carcinoma

J. Salvador Saldivar
Texas Tech University Health Sciences Center
Department of Obstetrics & Gynecology,
Division of Gynecology Oncology, El Paso, Texas
USA

1. Introduction

Cancer of the uterine endometrium is the most common gynecologic malignancy diagnosed in women of the United States. It is estimated that in 2011, there will be 46,470 new endometrial cancers and 8,120 deaths due to this malignancy (American Cancer Society, 2011). The lifetime risk of developing endometrial cancer is approximately 3% in the general population. In Western countries, lifestyle changes and environmental factors play an important role in the carcinogenesis of endometrial cancer; however, there exist a proportion of cases in which an inherited predisposition increases this risk. In this chapter, hereditary nonpolyposis colorectal cancer syndrome or more commonly, Lynch Syndrome, will be reviewed and its association with endometrial cancer detailed.

2. Lynch syndrome: Definition and clinical features

Lynch syndrome (LS) or hereditary nonpolyposis colorectal cancer (HNPCC) is an autosomal-dominant hereditary cancer syndrome that predisposes carriers to multiple malignancies. It is caused by germline mutations in specific genes that participate in DNA mismatch repair (MMR), these include *MLH1, MSH2, MSH6, PMS2,* and most recently, *EPCAM* (Kupier et al., 2011; Lynch et al., 2003). As the name implies, colorectal cancer (CRC) traditionally has been perceived as the dominant malignancy with a lifetime risk of 43-48% for carriers, however, women with LS have an equal or greater lifetime risk of endometrial cancer (EC) (Stoffel et al., 2009). Further, in more than half of cases, women present with a gynecological cancer as their first or "sentinel" malignancy (Lu et al., 2005). For LS families, extracolonic cancers also include ovarian, stomach, upper urologic tract, small bowel, pancreas, hepato-biliary, brain (Turcot variant) and sebaceous adenomas/carcinomas (Muir-Torre variant) (Lynch et al., 2003). This predisposition for other cancers has led to the use of Lynch Syndrome instead of HNPCC. It is also important to distinguish between Lynch I, in which colon cancer is the only contracted cancer, from Lynch II, where there exists other extracolonic cancers in the familial syndrome. In addition, some authors have reported a Lynch III as an appropriate name for identifying individuals with constitutively compromised MMR associated with biallelic mutations as seen with the Turcot and Muir-Torre variants (Felton et al., 2007).

2.1 Clinical characteristics

Current population estimates are that approximately 1 in 300 to 1 in 500 people carry a LS mutation making it similar in prevalence to Hereditary Breast and Ovarian cancer syndrome (Antoniou et al., 2000). These MMR mutations are inherited in an autosomal dominant manner and first-degree relatives have a 50% chance of inheriting the LS-related cancers (Hampel et al., 2005). Women who inherit LS-associated germline mutations have a greatly increased risk of developing a gynecologic cancer. Further, among women with LS who develop two primary cancers, over 50% are diagnosed with a gynecologic cancer before colon cancer (Lu et al., 2005). The range of risk for EC in women with LS is 27-71% compared with 3% in the general population and this risk varies with the specific MMR gene(s) involved, which will be discussed below (Koornstra et al., 2009).

The suspicion of a LS mutation should be raised among women diagnosed with EC at younger ages. The mean age range of EC in women with LS is 46 to 54 years, compared to 60 years in sporadic EC (Boks et al., 2002; Hampel et al., 2006). In a study by Lu et al., of 100 women with EC under age 50, 9 (9%) were found to have identifiable mutations in the MMR genes *MLH1, MSH2* and *MSH6* (Lu et al., 2007). In another study that included 69 women with LS, EC was diagnosed under the age 40 in 18% of their cohort (Schmeler et al., 2006).

Currently, there is no evidence to suggest that LS-associated EC portends a better or worse prognosis in patients when compared to sporadic EC. In fact, the majority of LS endometrial cancers are diagnosed in early stages, and like their sporadic counterparts, carry a favorable prognosis (Boks et al., 2002; Vasen et al., 1994). A case-control study of 50 women with LS-associated EC matched to 100 controls with sporadic EC for age and stage, found similar 5-year cumulative survival rates, 88% vs. 82%, respectively (P=0.59) (Boks et al., 2002). In another series of 125 women with clinically defined HNPCC, the overall survival rate for patients diagnosed with EC was high, with only 12% of patients succumbing to their disease (Vasen et al., 1994). A large study comparing the pathological features of sporadic EC to that of 50 patients with LS found that 78% were diagnosed as stage I, 10% were stage II, and 12% were stage III/IV in the LS cohort. Deep myometrial involvement was noted in 26% of cases, while lymphvascular space involvement was seen in 24%. However, when the LS cases were compared to the sporadic EC cases, stage, myometrial invasion, and lymphvascular space involvement were not statistically significantly different (Broaddus et al., 2006).

2.2 Histopathologic characteristics

Like sporadic endometrial cancer, the majority of LS-associated histology is of the endometrioid variety. However, studies evaluating the histologies of endometrial tumors in patients with LS have reported a wide variety of non-endometrioid types, including papillary serous carcinoma, clear cell carcinoma, malignant mixed Mullerian and neuroendocrine tumors (Broaddus et al., 2006; Carcangiu et al., 2010). For example, a small study of six LS-related endometrial cancers found significantly more often, poorly differentiated (83% versus 27%), presence of a Crohn-like lymphoid reaction (100% versus 13%), lymphangio-invasive growth (67% versus 0%), and high number of tumor-infiltrating lymphocytes (100% versus 36%), when compared with sporadic ECs (van den Bos et al., 2004). As mentioned previously, there is no evidence of a significant survival advantage or disadvantage associated with LS-related endometrial cancer (Boks et al., 2002).

Conversely, tumor location appears to differ between sporadic and LS-associated endometrial cancer. Although the majority is commonly found in the uterine corpus, endometrial cancer in the lower uterine segment (LUS) appears to have a strong association with Lynch syndrome. One study that included over 1000 patients with EC, found the prevalence of LS in patients with LUS tumors (10 of 35 or 29%) to be much greater than that of the general EC patient population (Westin et al., 2008). On the basis of this finding, the authors recommend that LS should be considered in all women with LUS tumors.

3. Lynch syndrome: Mechanisms of carcinogenesis

Six variants of the mismatch repair gene (MMR) have been cloned: *MSH2* (MutS homolog 2, chromosome 2p16), *MLH1* (MutL homolog 1, chromosome 3p21), *MSH3* (MutS homolog 3, interacts with *MLH1*), *MSH6* (MutS homolog 6, chromosome 2p16), *PMS1* (postmeiotic segregation 1, chromosome 2q31) and *PMS2* (postmeiotic segregation 2, chromosome 7p22) (Koessler et al., 2008). However, germline mutation analysis in four of these DNA-MMR genes (*MLH1, MSH2, MSH6,* and *PMS2*) is confirmatory diagnosis for LS (Hampel et al., 2005). A fifth and most recently identified gene, *EPCAM* (previously TACSTD1), is not a mismatch repair gene; however, large deletions in the 3′ end in the upstream *EPCAM* gene affect *MSH2*. This occurs by transcriptional read-through into and subsequent epigenetic silencing of its downstream neighbor, *MSH2*, resulting in the LS phenotype (Ligtenberg et al., 2009).

The role of the MMR machinery is to maintain genomic integrity by correcting base-pair and small insertion-deletion mismatches that are generated during DNA replication. Two heterodimeric protein complexes, MutS-α and MutS-β, recognize the mismatch. MutS-α is a heterodimer of *MSH2* and *MSH6* proteins and MutS-β is an *MSH2/MSH3* heterodimer, see Figure 1 (Masuda et al., 2011). Either MutS-α and MutS-β heterodimers can recognize insertion/deletion loops with more than two bases, but MutS-α preferentially recognizes single base-pair mismatches or, one or two base pair insertion-deletion loops (Koessler et al., 2008). The repair components of the MMR machinery involve three other heterodimer pairs: MutL-α (*MLH1/PMS2*), MutL-β (*MLH1/PMS1*), and MutL-γ (*MLH1/MLH3*).

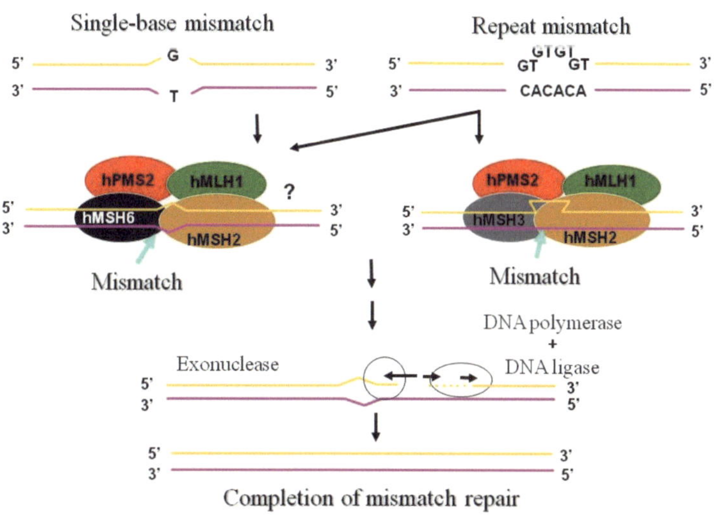

(Reproduced from Masuda et al., 2011).

Fig. 1. The DNA Mismatch Repair (MMR) machinery in humans.

In general, affected patients with LS carry a germline mutation in one allele of a MMR gene and acquire a second mutation within the tumor. Common mechanisms of the "second hit" include allele inactivation by mutation, loss of heterozygosity, or promoter hypermethylation leading to epigenetic silencing. Biallelic inactivation of MMR genes results in genomic instability due to failure in the repair of base pair mismatches that occur commonly during DNA replication (approximately 1 in 10^6 base pairs). DNA mismatches commonly occur in regions of tandem repeats of short DNA sequences called microsatellites that make up about 3% of human DNA (Baudhuin et al., 2005). Normally, the MMR machinery corrects errors in microsatellites, but mutations in the MMR genes in tumors cause expansion or contraction of these regions compared to normal tissue. These genetic alterations in microsatellite length are termed "microsatellite instability" (MSI) and are the molecular signature of LS-associated cancers (Lynch et al., 2009). Further, the increased mutation rate that results from MMR loss leads to alterations in nucleotide repeats in many other pathways; those that control cell growth, regulate cell death, and in the MMR genes themselves. Together, this accumulation of mutations drives the carcinogenetic process in LS.

3.1 MMR genes and the risk of endometrial cancer

The range of cancer risks in LS varies depending on the MMR gene involved. Approximately 70-80% of the clinical features of LS are accounted for by *MLH1* and *MSH2* mutations. Families with *MSH6* and *PMS2* mutations appear to have an attenuated cancer phenotype, presenting with a later age of diagnosis and a lower penetrance than *MLH1* and *MSH2*. *MSH6* may account for up to 15% and *PMS2* for up to 3-15% of all identified LS mutations (Hampel et al., 2005; Niessen et al., 2009). Recently, *EPCAM* has been thought to account for approximately 1-3% of LS mutations (Kuiper et al., 2011).

Endometrial cancer risk per MMR gene is as follows:

MLH1 and MSH2: Endometrial cancer in patients with *MLH1* and *MSH2* mutations often occur before the age of 50. The risk in *MLH1* and *MSH2* carriers is up to 20% by age 50 and up to 60% by age 70 according to some studies (Aarnio et al., 1999; Lynch et al., 2009). However, the diagnosis of EC after the age of 50 should still raise concern for LS if there is a positive family history.

MSH6**:** *MSH6* mutation carriers appear to have the highest risk for endometrial cancer (up to 71%) of the MMR genes, higher than that of colorectal cancer (CRC) (Hendricks et al., 2004). The average age of onset of EC in *MSH6* mutation-positive individuals is 54 years. One study identified a somewhat lower risk for endometrial cancer in *MSH6* mutation carriers, however the risk was significantly increased above the general population, and appeared to be higher than the risk for CRC in women with LS. They reported a risk for endometrial cancer to age 70 of 26% (95% CI: 18-36%) and risk to age 80 of 44% (95% CI: 30-58%) (Baglietto et al., 2009). These reports suggest that if a woman carries an *MLH1*, *MSH2* or *MSH6* mutation, her risk of EC may be even higher than her risk of CRC.

PMS2**:** One large series of *PMS2* carriers found the incidence of EC to be 7.5-fold higher than expected in the general population. This translates to a 15% risk to age 70 (Senter et al., 2008).

EPCAM**:** The clinical features of *EPCAM/TACSTD1* mutations as a cause of Lynch syndrome is still being defined. Recent studies evaluating *EPCAM* 3′-end mutation carriers for their clinical phenotype found the risk for EC was dependent upon the type and size of

EPCAM mutation (Kempers et al., 2011; Kupier et al., 2011). However, since deletions in *EPCAM* lead to disruption of the *MSH2* gene, following management guidelines for LS appears prudent at this point. Further research is needed to clarify the EC risks associated with *EPCAM* mutations and their association with LS.

3.2 Microsatellite instability

As discussed above, microsatellite instability (MSI) results from defects in the MMR machinery that correct the replication errors found in these regions of the human genome. MSI may occur via two mechanisms. MSI in the majority of EC is sporadic in nature, resulting from hypermethylation of the *MLH1* promoter leading to epigenetic silencing of the gene (Esteller et al., 1998). The second, and the one associated with LS, is a consequence of germline mutations in the DNA-MMR genes as discussed above. Thus, MSI is not pathognomonic of LS, and in fact, LS accounts for only a minority of MSI-high EC cases (Meyer et al., 2009).

MSI analysis may be performed on paraffin-embedded tissue sections. Amplification by PCR using five primers recommended by the National Cancer Institute-two mononucleotide (BAT25, BAT26) and three dinucleotide repeats (D2S123, D5S346, D173250)-are used to detect changes in the number of microsatellite repeats in tumor compared with normal tissue (Boland et al., 1998). Tumors are classified using the five marker panel as follows: MSI-high (MSI-H, highly unstable) if two or more of the five markers are positive, MSI-low (MSI-L, low instability) if one of the markers is positive, and MS-stable (MS-S, no instability) if none of the markers show MSI. MSI analysis has some limitations when used to detect LS-associated endometrial cancers. Many, but not all the ECs that are diagnosed in LS are MSI-H, while most, but not all MSI-H endometrial cancers are sporadic (Garg & Soslow, 2009). Thus, MSI analysis may fail to detect some LS-associated ECs, while it may turn out positive in a large percentage of sporadic ECs.

3.3 Immunohistochemistry

Mutations in the MMR genes typically result in truncated or absent protein products. Immunohistochemistry (IHC) staining using antibodies to the C-terminus of the MMR proteins can be used to identify LS-associated tumors for the absence of these gene products (Weissman et al., 2011). Like CRC, IHC in endometrial cancer has shown efficacy for identification of LS. However, results must be interpreted with caution since both absent MMR gene product and *MLH1* promoter hypermethylation are found in up to one-third of endometrioid adenocarcinomas (Modica et al., 2007).

Further, more than one gene product may be absent. This may be due to the heterodimerization of the MMR proteins. Thus, a loss in *MLH1* staining is almost always coupled with concurrent loss of *PMS2*, and loss of *MSH2* staining is accompanied by loss of *MSH6*. A deleterious mutation in either primary proteins *MLH1* and *MSH2* will most likely result in loss of the entire heterodimer (Wei et al., 2002). As an example, a lack of tumor staining for *MLH1* and *PMS2* is most likely the result of *MLH1* protein absence. In contrast, *PMS2* and *MSH6* are secondary proteins, and a deleterious mutation in either gene will result in loss of that isolated protein. In addition, large deletions in the upstream *EPCAM* gene can cause inactivation and absence of *MSH2* expression by IHC. As many as 20-25% of cases suspected of having a mutation in *MSH2*, are actually caused by germline deletions in *EPCAM* (Rumilla et al., 2011)

Assays to detect methylation of the *MLH1* promoter that can recognize epigenetic mechanisms that lead to MSI-H, should be considered along with IHC for MMR gene testing (Whelan et al., 2002). For example, studies have shown that methylation of the small proximal region in the *MLH1* promoter located -248 to -178 relative to the gene transcription start site invariably correlates with loss of *MLH1* expression (Kang et al., 2002). If methylation is present, the patient most likely has sporadic tumor rather than LS-associated carcinoma.

IHC has been shown to be a convenient and readily performed test for the detection of germline MMR gene mutations. There are, however, studies of mutations in the MMR genes that are not detected by IHC (Vasen et al., 2004). In fact, by most reports, there is an approximate 5-10 % false negative rate with both IHC and MSI. That is, up to 90-95% of CRCs and ECs seen in LS patients are MSI-H or lack at least one MMR protein product on IHC testing (Ferreira et al., 2009). Therefore, most experts recommend that IHC and MSI testing in combination, along with family and personal history, be used to maximize identification of patients at risk for LS so that germline genetic testing may confirm the diagnosis.

4. Identifying patients at risk for Lynch syndrome

In 1991, the International Collaborative Group on Hereditary Nonpolyposis Colorectal Cancer established research criteria, which became known as the Amsterdam Criteria (AC I), for the diagnosis of LS (Vasen et al., 1991). These criteria were broadened in 1999 as the Amsterdam Criteria II (AC II) to recognize a diagnostic role for extra-colonic tumors and suggested that LS-associated cancers should be suspected in relatives (Vasen et al., 1999) (see Table 1).

AC I
At least 3 relatives with histologically verified colorectal cancer (CRC):
One is a first-degree relative of the other 2;
At least 2 successive generations affected;
At least 1 of the with CRC diagnosed at <50 years of age;
Familial adenomatous polyposis (FAP) should be excluded.
AC II
At least 3 relatives must have a cancer associated with Lynch Syndrome (CRC, EC, stomach, ovary, ureter, renal pelvis, brain, small bowel, hepato-biliary, sebaceous tumors):
One is a first-degree relative of the other 2;
At least 2 successive generations affected
At least 1 of the LS-associated cancers diagnosed at <50 years of age;
FAP should be excluded in any CRC cases;
Tumors should be verified whenever possible.

(adapted from Vasen et al., 1991 & Vasen et al., 1999).

Table 1. Amsterdam Criteria I and II.

Individuals meeting the AC I were presumptively defined as having LS. However, once MSI analyses and genetic testing became available, it became clear that certain families who met AC II criteria did not have an identifiable MMR germline mutation (Lindor et al., 2005). In fact, approximately half of patients with LS will be missed by these criteria and approximately half will meet the criteria and not have LS ie., do not carry MSI or MMR variations; but a high familial risk of uncertain etiology. The term "familial colorectal cancer type X" has been suggested for these patients to distinguish them from those with LS (Lindor et al., 2005).

As a result of this major limitation of the AC, the Bethesda Guidelines were originally developed (1997) and revised (2004) to help identify patients with CRC or other LS-associated cancers who should be screened for MSI (Umar et al., 2004). If found to have microsatellite unstable cancers, these patients should undergo subsequent germline MMR genetic testing (see Table 2).

Tumors from individuals should be tested for MSI if:
CRC[1] diagnosed in a patient who is <50 years of age;
Presence of synchronous, or metachronous LS-associated tumors[2], regardless of age;
CRC with MSI-H histology[3] diagnosed in a patient who is <60 years of age;
CRC diagnosed in a patient with 1 or more first-degree relatives with an LS-associated cancer[2], with one of the cancers being diagnosed under 50 years of age;
CRC diagnosed in a patient with 2 or more first- or second-degree relatives with LS-associated cancers[2] regardless of age.

(adapted from Umar et al., 2004 and NCCN Guidelines Version 2.2011).

[1] Endometrial cancer <50 years of age is not included in the guidelines, however, current evidence suggests that these individuals should be evaluated for LS.

[2] LS-associated cancers include: CRC, EC, stomach, ovarian, ureter/renal pelvis, pancreas, hepatobiliary tract, brain (glioblastomas as seen in Turcot syndrome), small bowel, sebaceous adenomas and keratoacanthomas (seen in Muir-Torre syndrome).

[3] Presence of tumor infiltrating lymphocytes, Crohn's-like lymphocytic reaction, mucinous (signet-ring) differentiation, or medullary growth pattern.

Table 2. Revised Bethesda Guidelines.

Despite the revised Bethesda criteria, multiple studies show the guidelines have low specificity, with approximately 80% of individuals who meet the criteria will not have LS (Hampel et al., 2005, 2006). Concerns that both the AC and Bethesda guidelines may miss a substantial portion of patients with LS, most investigators agree that all CRC cases be screened for MSI and that any case identified as MSI-H and/or show absence of ≥1 MMR protein, undergo further genetic testing for LS (EGAPP recommendations, 2009). Further, even with normal MSI and IHC, it is important to consider both the patient and their family history when determining to proceed with germline testing for LS.

While it appears that these guidelines focus on CRC patients, it is important to know that they are at high risk of developing a synchronous or metachronous cancers, especially of the colon, rectum, endometrium and/or ovary (Lu et al., 2005; Lynch et al., 1977; Mecklin & Jarvinen, 1986; Watson et al., 2001). An early study found that among 33 families with "cancer family syndrome", the risk of a second LS-associated cancer was approximately 30% within 10 years of the initial cancer diagnosis and up to 50% within 15 years of the initial cancer diagnosis (Mecklin & Jarvinen, 1986). Another report found the annual metachronous

CRC rates to be 2.1% and 1.7% between *MLH1* and *MSH2* families, respectively, as compared to 0.33% for the general population (Lin et al., 1998). In a study by Lu et al., dual primary cancers (CRC and gynecologic-endometrial or ovarian) were reported in 16 women (14%) of 117 women with LS (Lu et al, 2005). An earlier study found synchronous and metachronous cancers: endometrial (21 patients), CRC (28 patients), and either gastric, small bowel, or urinary tract cancers (6 patients), in 80 women with LS-associated ovarian cancer (Watson et al., 2001).

The Society of Gynecologic Oncologists Education Committee published guidelines to identify women with a personal or family history of EC or ovarian cancer, and synchronous or metachronous CRC, whom may benefit from genetic risk assessment for LS (Lancaster et al., 2007) (see Table 3).

Genetic risk assessment RECOMMENDED: Patients with >20-25% chance of having LS	Genetic risk assessment may be HELFUL: Patients with >5-10% chance of having LS
EC or ovarian cancer with a synchronous or metachronous CRC with the first cancer diagnosed < age 50;	**EC or ovarian cancer with synchronous or metachronous CRC or other LS-associated cancers* with the first cancer diagnosed at any age;**
EC or CRC and meet AC II criteria;	**EC or CRC diagnosed < age 50;**
First or second-degree relative with a known germline mutation in a MMR gene.	**EC or CRC with 2 or more first or second-degree relatives with LS-associated cancers*;**
	First or second-degree relative that meets the above criteria.

(adapted from Lancaster et al., 2007).

*LS-associated cancers include: CRC, EC, stomach, ovarian, ureter/renal pelvis, pancreas, hepatobiliary tract, brain (glioblastomas as seen in Turcot syndrome), small bowel, sebaceous adenomas and keratoacanthomas (seen in Muir-Torre syndrome).

Table 3. Society of Gynecologic Oncologist: Guidelines for Lynch Syndrome Risk Assessment.

5. Managing Lynch syndrome cancer risks

Any discussion with individuals and family members at risk for hereditary cancer must occur in the context of a high risk cancer clinic with available medical interventions or referral made to address these risks. The benefits and limitations of surveillance and risk reducing surgery should be individualized, and when possible, evidence based. Over the past few years, a number of studies and recommendations have been published that document the available strategies to guide management of these at-risk individuals with LS (Lindor et al., 2006; NCCN Practice Guidelines 2011; Schmeler et al., 2006; Winawer et al., 2003).

5.1 Surveillance

Both EC and ovarian cancer are likely to develop before the menopause in women diagnosed with LS. Endometrial cancer screening in women with LS who are asymptomatic consists of annual endometrial sampling beginning at age 30 to 35 or five to ten years prior to the earliest age of the family member diagnosed with a LS-associated cancer (Lindor et al., 2006; NCCN Practice Guidelines 2011). A recent Finnish study evaluated the efficacy of screening with endometrial biopsy and transvaginal ultrasound (TVUS) among 175 mutation-positive women age 35 or older with LS (Renkonen-Sinisalo et al., 2007). They found that surveillance intrauterine biopsy detected 8 women with EC and 4 ECs were indicated by TVUS. Although no statistically significant differences were observed in cancer stage or survival when compared with 83 women with EC who did not undergo surveillance, this strategy detected earlier cancers and there were no deaths in the surveillance group.

Studies have shown that endometrial thickness measurement to detect EC has a high false-positive rate in women with LS, and in particular premenopausal women where endometrial thickness is highly variable (Dove-Edwin et al., 2002). Conversely, in postmenopausal women, atypical endometrial thickness is less variable. In this population, TVUS and endometrial sampling have similar sensitivities, and early detection is common because most women present with abnormal uterine bleeding (Dijkhuizen et al., 2000).

The primary role of TVUS appears to be in ovarian cancer screening in women with LS. LS is associated with an increased risk of ovarian cancer, estimated at 12% by age 70 compared with 1.5% in the general population (Barrow et al., 2009). Although there are no data regarding ovarian cancer screening in women with LS, most experts recommend an annual pelvic exam, TVUS, and CA125 serum tumor marker, every 6 to 12 months, starting at age 30 to 35 or five to ten years prior to the earliest age of the family member diagnosed with a LS-associated cancer (Lindor et al., 2006; NCCN Practice Guidelines 2011). Since ovarian cancer is much less common than EC in women with LS, it is unknown whether these screening strategies decrease morbidity and mortality.

Although not the emphasis of this chapter, CRC surveillance recommendations in individuals with LS include, colonscopy every one to two years, beginning at age 20 to 25 or two to five years prior to the earliest diagnosis if it is before age 25 (Lindor et al, 2006; NCCN Practice Guidelines 2011). For *MSH6* and *PMS2* mutation positive carriers, colonoscopy is recommended at age 30 to 35 or 10 years prior to the youngest age of diagnosis in the family, whichever comes first (NCCN Practice Guidelines 2011; Senter et al., 2008). In support of this strategy, one study showed that colonoscopy every 3 years reduced the CRC risk by 50% and decreased overall mortality by about 65% (Jarvinen et al., 2000). In a further study, the cumulative risk of CRC after a 10-year follow-up was 6% with a surveillance interval of 1-2 years compared to a 2-3 year surveillance (Vasen et al., 2010).

Lynch syndrome is associated with an increased risk for other cancers as well, including, gastric, small bowel, urothelial, pancreatic, and brain. It is imperative that the clinician caring for these individuals and their families with LS, refer to the National Comprehensive Cancer Network (NCCN) Guidelines for management options for these cancer risks.

5.2 Risk reducing surgery

Women with LS may consider prophylactic hysterectomy and bilateral salpino-oophorectomy (BSO) to substantially reduce the risk of endometrial and ovarian cancers (Guillem et al., 2006; NCCN Practice Guidelines 2011). In a large retrospective case-control study of 315 mutation-positive (*MLH1, MSH2,* or *MSH6*) women, risk-reducing hysterectomy with BSO proved to be an effective strategy for preventing endometrial and ovarian cancer (Schmeler et al., 2006). No women who had a hysterectomy developed EC compared with 69 of 210 (33%) of the controls (no hysterectomy). Further, no women who underwent a BSO developed ovarian cancer compared with 12 of 233 (5%) of the controls (no BSO). One ovarian cancer was diagnosed in a woman who underwent a hysterectomy. Risk-reducing surgery may take place at the time of CRC diagnosis or once child-bearing is completed. In addition, there are no recommendations for chemopreventive strategies in LS to decrease gynecologic cancer risks. Studies from Lu et al., suggest oral contraceptive pills or medroxyprogesterone acetate (Depo-Provera) may have the potential to prevent EC and/or ovarian cancer associated with LS (Lu et al., 2010).

Counseling regarding prophylactic surgery of this kind should include not only the risks inherent in surgery, but also premature menopause and its associated risks; menopausal vasomotor symptoms, estrogen therapy, osteoporosis, urogenital atrophy, and less clear, heart disease (Chen et al., 2007; Schmeler et al., 2006). Preoperative assessment should include colonoscopy, endometrial sampling, TVUS and a CA125 tumor marker. Preparation for a complete surgical staging should be available if occult carcinoma is found.

Cost-effectiveness decisions must be reviewed with the patient when embarking on a management strategy for surveillance or prevention of LS-associated cancers. One study compared different strategies in a hypothetical cohort of women with LS: 1) no prevention, 2) prophylactic hysterectomy and BSO at age 30, 3) prophylactic surgery at age 40, 4) annual screening with endometrial biopsy, TVUS and CA125 from age 30, and 5) annual screening from age 30 until prophylactic surgery at age 40 (combined strategy) (Kwon et al., 2008). The authors found that annual screening followed by prophylactic surgery at age 40 was the most effective gynecologic cancer prevention strategy, but the incremental benefit over risk-reducing surgery alone came with a substantial cost. Thus, a careful review of different strategies to improve the effectiveness and decrease the lifetime costs of these interventions is warranted in patients with LS.

6. Conclusion

Lynch Syndrome (hereditary nonpolyposis colorectal cancer) is an autosomal dominant disorder that is caused by germline mutations in one of several DNA-MMR genes (*MLH1, MSH2, MSH6, PMS2,* and *EPCAM*). The syndrome is characterized by an approximate lifetime risk of EC and CRC of 40% to 60% in affected individuals. Other LS-associated cancers (gastric, ovarian, urothelial, pancreas, hepatobiliary tract, brain, small bowel, skin) as well as, synchronous and metachronous cancers, may present in these patients and their families. Identification of these individuals meeting AC II and/or Bethesda guidelines should have their tumors tested for MSI and for MMR protein expression by IHC. Further genetic counseling and direct MMR gene testing of those at-risk individuals should be done in the context of an established high risk genetics/cancer clinic. Post-test genetic counseling regarding the risks and benefits of LS-associated cancer surveillance and prophylactic surgery strategies, should be performed with consideration of the informed consent, completed child-bearing, autonomy, cost-effectiveness and quality of life, for each individual patient.

7. References

Aarnio M, Sankila R, Pukkala E, Salovaara R, Aaltoner LA, de la Chapelle A, Peltomaki P, Meclin JP, Jarvinen HJ. Cancer Risk in Mutation Carriers of DNA-Mismatch Repair Genes. *International Journal of Cancer.* 1999;81:214-18.

American Cancer Society. (2011). *Cancer Facts & Figures 2011*. Atlanta: American Cancer Society.

Antoniou AC, Gayther SA, Stratton JF, Ponder BAJ, Easton DF. Risk Models for Familial Ovarian and Breast Cancer. *Genetic Epidemiology*. 2000;18:173-90.

Baglietto L, Lindor NM, Dowty JG, White DM, Wagner A, Gomez Garcia EB, Vriends AH. Risks of Lynch Syndrome Cancers for MSH6 Mutation Carriers. *Journal of the National Cancer Institute*. 2009;102(3):193-201.

Barrow E, Robinson L, Alduaij W, Shenton A, Clancy T, Lalloo F, Hill J, Evans DG. Cumulative Lifetime Incidence of Extracolonic Cancers in Lynch Syndrome: A Report of 121 Families with Proven Mutations. *Clinical Genetics*. 2009;75:141-9.

Baudhuin LM, Burgart LJ, Leontovich O, Thibodeau SN. Use of Microsatellite Instability and Immunohistochemistry for the Identification of Individuals at Risk for Lynch Syndrome. *Familial Cancer*. 2005;4:255-265.

Boks DES, Trujillo AP, Voogd AC, Morreau H, Kenter GG, Vasen HFA. Survival Analysis of Endometrial Carcinoma associated with Hereditary Nonpolyposis Colorectal Cancer. *International Journal of Cancer*. 2002;102;198-200.

Boland RC, Thibodeau SN, Hamilton SR, Sidransky D, Eshleman JR, Burt RW, Meltzer SJ, Rodriguez-Bigas MA, Fodde R, Ranzani NG, Srivastava S. A National Cancer Institute Workshop on Microsatellite Stability for Cancer Detection and Familial Predisposition: Development of International Criteria for the Determination of Microsatellite Stability in Colorectal Cancer. *Cancer Research*. 1998;58:5248- 5257.

Broaddus RR, Lynch HT, Chen LM, Daniels MS, Conrad P, Munsell MF, White KG, Luthra R, Lu KH. Pathologic Features of Endometrial Carcinoma Associated with HNPCC: a Comparison with Sporadic Endometrial Carcinoma. *Cancer*. 2006;106(1):87-94.

Carcangiu M, Radice P, Casalini P, Bertario L, Merola M, Sala P. Lynch Syndrome Related Endometrial Carcinomas Show a High Frequency of Nonendometrioid Types and of High FIGO grade Endometrioid Types. *International Journal of Surgical Pathology*. 2010;18(1):21-6.

Chen LM, Yang KY, Little SE, Cheung MK, Caughey AB. Gynecologic Cancer Prevention in Lynch Syndrome/Hereditary Nonpolyposis Colorectal Cancer Families. *Obstetrics & Gynecology*. 2007;110:18-25.

Dijkhuizen FP, Mol BW, Brolmann HA, Heintz AP. The Accuracy of Endometrial Sampling in the Diagnosis of Patients with Endometrial Carcinoma and Hyperplasia: A Meta-analysis. *Cancer*. 2000;89:1765- 72.

Dove-Edwin I, Boks D, Goff S, Kenter GG, Carpenter R, Vasen HF, Thomas HJ. The Outcome of Endometrial Carcinoma Surveillance by Ultrasound Scan in Women at Risk of Hereditary Nonpolyposis Colorectal Carcinoma and Familial Colorectal Carcinoma. *Cancer*. 2002;94:1708-12.

Esteller M, Levine R, Baylin SB, Ellenson LH, Herman JG. MLH1 Promoter Hypermethylation is associated with the Microsatellite Instability Phenotype in Sporadic Endometrial Carcinomas. *Oncogene*. 1998;17:2413-7.

Evaluation of Genomic Applications in Practice and Prevention (EGAPP) Working Group. Recommendations from the Working Group: Genetic Testing Strategies in Newly Diagnosed Individuals with Colorectal Cancer Aimed at Reducing Morbidity and Mortality from Lynch Syndrome in Relatives. *Genetics in Medicine*. 2009;11(1):35-41.

Felton KE, Gilchrist DM, Andrew SE. Constitutive deficiency in DNA mismatch repair: is it time Lynch III? *Clinical Genetics.* 2007;71:483-498.

Ferreira AM, Westers H, Wu Y, Niessen RC, Olderode-Berends M, van der Sluis T, van der Zee AG, Hollema H, Kleibeuker JH, Simons RH, Hofstra RM. Do Microsatellite Instability Profiles Really Differ between Colorectal and Endometrial Tumors? *Genes, Chromosomes & Cancer.* 2009;48:552-7.

Garg K and Soslow RA. Lynch Syndrome (Hereditary Non-polyposis Colorectal Cancer) and Endometrial Cancer. *Journal of Clinical Pathology.* 2009;62:679-684.

Guillem JG, Wood WC, Moley JF, Berchuck A, Karlan BY, Mutch DG, Gagel RF, Weitzel J, Morrow M, Weber BL, Giardiello F, Rodriguez-Bigas MA, Church J, Gruber S, Offit K. ASCO/SSO Review of Current Role of Risk-Reducing Surgery in Common Hereditary Cancer Syndromes. *Journal of Clinical Oncology.* 2006;24:4642-60.

Hampel H, Frankel WL, Martin E, Arnold M, Khanduja K, Kuebler P, Nakagawa H, Sotamaa K, Prior TW, Westman J, Panescu J, Fix D, Lockman J, Comeras I, de la Chapelle, A. Screening for Lynch Syndrome (Hereditary Nonpolyposis Colorectal Cancer). *NEJM.* 2005;352:1851-1860.

Hampel H, Frankel W, Panescu J, Lockman J, Sotamaa K, Fix D, Comeras I, Jeunesse JL, Nakagawa H Westman JA, Prior TW, Clendenning M, Penzone P, Lombardi J, Dunn P, Cohn DE, Coeland L, Eaton L, Fowler J, Lewandowski G, Vaccarello L, Bell J, Reid G, de la Chapelle A. Screening for Lynch Syndrome (Herediatary Nonpolyposis Colorectal Cancer) among Endometrial Cancer Patients. *Cancer Research.* 2006;66:7810.

Hendriks YM, Wagner A, Morreau H, Menko F, Stormorken A, Quehenberger F, Sandkuijl L, Moller P, Genuardi M, Houwelingen HV, Tops C, Puijenbroek MV, Verkuijlen P, Kenter G, Mil AV, Meijers- Heijboer H, Tan GB, Breuning MH, Fodde R, Winjen JT, Brocker-Vriends AHJT, Vasen H. Cancer Risk in Hereditary Nonpolyposis Colorectal Cancer due to MSH6 Mutations: Impact on Counseling and Surveillance. *Gastroenterology.* 2004;127:17-25.

Jarvinen HJ, Aarnio M, Mustonen H, Akatan-Collan K, Aaltonen LA, Peltomaki P, de la Chapelle A, Mecklin JP. Controlled 15-year Trial on Screening for Colorectal Cancer in Families with Hereditary Nonpolyposis Colorectal Cancer. *Gastroenterology.* 2000;118:829-34.

Kang GH, Lee S, Shim YH, Kim JC, Ro JY. Profile of Methylated CpG sites of hMLH1 Promoter in Primary Gastric Carcinoma with Microsatellite Instability. *Pathology International.* 2002;52(12):764-768.

Kempers M, Kuiper RP, Ockeloen CW, Chappuis PO, Hutter P, Rahner N, Schackert PHK, Steinke V, Holinski-Feder PE, Morak M, Kloor M, Buttner R, Verwiel ETP, Krieken JHV, Nagtegall ID, Goossens M, van der Post RS, Niessen RC, Sijmons RH, Kluijt I, Hogervorst FBL, Leter EM, Gille JJP, Aalfs CM, Redeker EJW, Hes FJ, Tops CMJ, van Nesselrooij BPM, van Gin ME, Gomez Garcia EB, Eccles DM, Bunyan DJ, Syngal S, Stoffel EM, Culver JO, Palomares MR, Graham T, Velsher L, Papp J, Olah E, Chan TL, Leung SY, van Kessel AG, Kiemeney LALM, Hoogerbrugge N, Ligtenberg MJL . Risk of Colorectal and Endometrial Cancer in EPCAM Deletion Positive Lynch Syndrome: a Cohort Study. *Lancet Oncology.* 2011;12:49-55.

Koessler T, Oestergaard MZ, Song H, Tyrer J, Perkins B, Dunning AM, Easton DF, Pharoah PDP. Common Variants in Mismatch Repair Genes and Risk of Colorectal Cancer. *Gut*. 2008;57:1097.

Koornstra JJ, Mourits MJE, Sijmons RH, Leliveld AM, Hollema H, Kleibeuker JH. Management of Extracolonic Tumors in Patients with Lynch Syndrome. *Lancet Oncology*. 2009;10:400-408.

Kupier RP, Vissers LELM, Venkatachalam R, Bodmer D, Hoenselaar E, Goossens M, Haufe A, Kamping E, Niessen RC, Hogevorst FBL, Gille JJP, Redeker B, Tops CMJ, van Gijn ME, van den Ouweland AMW, Rahner , Steinke V, Kahl P, Holinski-Feder E, Morak M, Kloor M, Stemmler S, Betz B, Hutter P, Bunyan DJ, Syngal S, Culver JO, Graham T, Chan TL, Nagtegaal ID, van Krieken JH, Schackert HK, Hoogerbrugge N, van Kessel AG, Ligtenberg MJL. Recurrence and Variability of Germline *EPCAM* Deletions in Lynch syndrome. *Human Mutation*. 2011;32:407-414.

Kwon JS, Sun CC, Peterson SK, White KG, Daniels MS, Boyd-Rogers SG, Lu KH. Cost-effective Analysis of Prevention Stratgies for Gynecologic Cancers in Lynch Syndrome. *Cancer*. 2008;113:326-335.

Lancaster JM, Powell CB, Kauff ND, Cass I, Chen LM, Lu KH, Mutch DG, Berchuck A, Karland BY, Herzog TJ. Society of Gynecologic Oncologists Education Committee Statement on Risk Assessment for Inherited Gynecologic Cancer Predispositions. *Gynecology Oncology*. 2007;107:159-62.

Ligtenberg MJ, Kuiper RP, Chan TL, Goossens M, Hebeda KM, Voorendt M, Lee TYH, Bodmer D, Hoenselaar E, Hendriks-Cornelissen SJB, Tsui WY, Kong CK, Brunner HG, van Kessel AG, Yuem ST, van Krieken JH, Leung SY, Hoogerbrugge N . Heritable Somatic Methylation and Inactivation of MSH2 in Families with Lynch Syndrome due to Deletion of the 3′ Exons of TACSTD1. *Nature Genetics*. 2009;41:112-7.

Lin KM, Shashidharan M, Ternent CA, Thorson AG, Blatchford GT, Christenson MA, Lanspa SJ, Lemon SJ, Watson P, Lynch H. Colorectal and Extracolonic Cancer Variations in MLH1/MSH2 Hereditary Nonpolyposis Colorectal Cancer Kindreds and the General Population. *Diseases of the Colon & Rectum*. 1998;41:428-33.

Lindor NM, Petersen GM, Hadley DW, Kinney AY, Miesfeldt S, Lu KH, Lynch P, Burke W, Press N. Recommendations for the Care of Individuals with an Inherited Predisposition to Lynch Syndrome: A Systematic Review. *JAMA*. 2006;296:1507-17.

Lindor NM, Rabe K, Petersen GM, Haile R, Casey G, Baron J, Gallinger S, Bapat B, Aronson M, Hopper J, Jass, J, LeMarchand L, Grove J, Potter J, Newcomb P, Terdiman JP, Conrad P, Moslein G, Goldberg R, Ziogas A, Anton-Culver H, de Andrade M, Siegmund K, Thibodeau SN, Boardman LA, Seminara D. Lower Cancer Incidence in Amsterdam-I Criteria Families without Mismatch Repair Deficiency: A Familial Colorectal Cancer Type X. *JAMA*. 2005;293:1979-1985.

Lu KH, et al. A Prospective, Multicenter Randomized Study of Oral Contraceptive versus Depo-Provera for the Prevention of Endometrial Cancer in Women with Lynch Syndrome. *SGO* 2010; Abstract 6.

Lu KH, Dinh M, Kohlmann W, Watson P, Green J, Syngal S, Bandipalliam P, Chen LM, Allen B, Conrad P, Terdiman J, Sun C, Daniels M, Burke T, Gershenson DM, Lynch H, Lynch P, Broaddus RR. Gynecologic Cancer as a "Sentinel Cancer" for Women with Hereditary Nonpolyposis Colorectal Cancer Syndrome. *Obstetrics & Gynecology*. 2005:105:569-74.

Lu KH, Schorge JO, Rodabaugh KJ, Daniels MS, Sun CC, Soliman PT, White KG, Luthra R, Gershenson DM, Broaddus RR . Prospective Determination of Prevalence of Lynch Syndrome in Young Women with Endometrial Cancer. *Journal of Clinical Oncology.* 2007;25(33):5158-5164.

Lynch HT & de la Chapelle A. Genomic Medicine: Hereditary Colorectal Cancer. *NEJM.* 2003;348:919- 32.

Lynch HT, Harris RE, Lynch PM, Guirgis HA, Lynch JF, Bardwil WA. Role of Heredity in Multiple Primary Cancer. *Cancer.* 1977;40:1849-54.

Lynch HT, Lynch PM, Lanspa SJ, Synder CL, Lynch JF, Boland CR. Review of the Lynch Syndrome: History, Molecular Genetics, Screening, Differential Diagnosis, and Medicolegal Ramifications. *Clinical Genet*ics. 2009;76:1-18.

Masuda K, Banno K, Yanokura M, Kobayashi Y, Kisu I, Ueki A, Ono A, Asahara N, Nomura H, Hirasawa A, Susumu N, Aoki D. Relationship between DNA Mismatch Repair Deficiency and Endometrial Cancer. *Molecular Biology International.* 2011;(ID256063):1-6.

Mecklin JP and Jarvinen HJ. Clinical Features of Colorectal Carcinoma in Cancer Family Syndrome. *Diseases of the Colon & Rectum.* 1986;29:160-4.

Meyer LA, Broaddus, RR, Lu KH. Endometrial Cancer and Lynch Syndrome: Clinical and Pathologic Considerations. *Cancer Control.* 2009;16:14-22.

Modica I, Soslow RA, Black D, Black D, Thornos C, Kauff N, Shia J. Utility of Immunohistochemistry in Predicting Microsatellite Instability in Endometrial Cancer. *American Journal of Surgical Pathology.* 2007;31:744-51.

NCCN Clinical Practice Guidelines in Oncology™ NCCN Guidelines Lynch Syndrome (Version 2.2011). National Comprehensive Cancer Network. Current version available at http://www.nccn.org.

NCCN Clinical Practice Guidelines in Oncology™ Colorectal Cancer Screening (Version 2.2011). National Comprehensive Cancer Network. Current version available at http://www.nccn.org.

Niessen RC, Kleibeuker JH, Westers H, Jager POJ, Rozeveld D, Bos KK, Boersmavan-EK W, Hollema H, Sijmons RH, Hofstra RMW. PMS2 Involvement in Patients Suspected of Lynch Syndrome. *Genes, Chromosomes & Cancer.* 2009;48:322-29.

Renkonen-Sinisalo L, Butzow R, Leminen A, Lehtovirta P, Mecklin JP, Jarvinen HJ. Surveillance for Endometrial Cancer in Hereditary Non-Polyposis Colorectal Cancer Syndrome. *International Journal of Cancer.* 2007;120:821-4.

Rumilla K, Schowalter KV, Lindor NM, Tomas BC, Mensink KA, Gallinger S, HolterS, Newcomb PA, Potter JD, Jenkins MA, Hopper JL, Long TI, Weisenberger DJ, Haile RW, Casey G, Laird PW, Merchand LL, Thibodeau SN. Frequency of Deletions of EPCAM (TACSTD1) in MSH2-associated Lynch Syndrome Cases. *Journal of Molecular Diagnostics.* 2011;13-93-99.

Senter L, Clendenning M, Sotamaa K, Hempel H, Green J, Potter JD, Lindblom A, Lagestedt K, Thibodeau SN, Lindor NM, Young J, Winship I, Dowty JG, White DM, Hopper JL, Baglietto L, Jenkins MA, de la Chapelle A. The Clinical Phenotype of Lynch Syndrome due to Germ-Line PMS2 Mutations. *Gastroenterology.* 2008;135(2):419-28.

Schmeler KM, Lynch HT, Chen LM, Munsell MF, Soliman PT, Clark MB, Daniels MS, White KG, Boyd- Rogers SG, Conrad PG, Yang KY, Rubin MM, Sun CC, Slomovitz BM, Gershenson DM, Lu KH. Prophylactic Surgery to Reduce the Risk of Gynecologic Cancers in the Lynch Syndrome. *NEJM*. 2006;354:261-69.

Stoffel E, Mukherjee B, Raymond VM, Tayob N, Kastrinos F, Sparr J, Wang F, Bandipalliam P, Syngal S, Gruber SB. Calculation of Risk of Colorectal and Endometrial Cancer among Patients with Lynch Syndrome. *Gastroenterology*. 2009;137:1621-7.

Umar A, Boland CR, Terdiman JP, Syngal S, de la Chapelle A, Ruschoff J, Fishel R, Lindor NM, Burgart LJ, Hamelin R, Hamilton SR, Hiatt RA, Jass J, Lindblom Annika, Lynch HT, Peltomaki P, Ramsey SD, Rodriguez-Bigas MA, Vasen HFA, Hawk ET, Barrett JC, Freedman AN, Srivastava S. Revised Bethesda Guidelines for Hereditary Nonpolyposis Colorectal Cancer (Lynch Syndrome) and Microsatellite Instability. *Journal of the National Cancer Institute.* 200496:261-68.

van den Bos M, van den Hoven M, Jongejan E, van der Leij F, Michels M, Schakenraad S, Aben K, Hoogerbrugge N, Ligtenberg M, van Krieken JH. More Differences Between HNPCC-related and Sporadic Carcinomas From the Endometrium as Compared to the Colon. *American Journal of Surgical Pathology.* 2004;28:706–11.

Vasen HFA, Hendriks Y, de Jong AE, van Puijenbroek M, Tops C, Brocker-Vriends AHJT, Wijnen JTh, Morreau H . Identification of HNPCC by Molecular Analysis of Colorectal and Endometrial Tumors. *Disease Markers.* 2004;20:207-13.

Vasen HF, Mecklin JP, Meera KP, Lynch HT. The International Collaborative Group on Hereditary Nonpolyposis Colorectal Cancer (ICG-HNPCC). *Diseases of the Colon & Rectum.* 1991;34:424-425.

Vasen HF, Watson P, Mecklin JP, Lynch HT. New Clinical Criteria for Hereditary Nonpolyposis Colorectal Cancer (HNPCC, Lynch Syndrome) Proposed by the International Collaborative Group on HNPCC. *Gastroenterology.* 1999;116:1453-6.

Vasen HF, Watson P, Mecklin JP, Jass JR, Green JS, Nomizu T, Muller H, Lynch HT. The Epidemiology of Endometrial Cancer in Hereditary Nonpolyposis Colorectal Cancer. *Anticancer Research.* 1994;14(4B):1675-1678.

Vasen HF, Adbirahman M, Brohet R, Langers AM, Kleibeuker JH, van Kouwen M, Koomstra JJ, Boot H, Cats A, Dekker E, Sanduleanu S, Poley JW, Hardwick JC, de Vos Tot Nederveen Cappel Wh, van der Meulen-de Jong AE, Tan TG, Jacobs MA, Mohamed FL, de Boer SY, van de Meeberg PC, Verhulst ML, Salemans JM, van Bentem N, Westerveld BD, Vecht J, Nagengast FM. One to 2-year Surveillance Intervals Reduce the Risk of Colorectal Cancer in Families with Lynch Syndrome. *Gastroenterology.* 2010;138:2300-06.

Watson P, Butzow R, Lynch HT, Lynch HT, Mecklin J-P, Jarvinen HJ, Vasen HFA, Madrensky L, Fidalgo P, Bernstein I, International Collaborative Group on HNPCC . The Clinical Features of Ovarian Cancer in Hereditary Nonpolyposis Colorectal Cancer. *Gynecology Oncology.* 2001;82:223-8.

Wei K, Kucherlapati R, Edelmann W. Mouse Models for Human DNA Mismatch-Repair Gene Defects. *Trends in Molecular Medicine.* 2002;8(7):346-353.

Weissman SM, Bellcross C, Bittner CC, Freivogel ME, Haidle JL, Kaurah P, Leininger A, Palaniappan S, Steenblock K, Vu TM, Daniels MS. Genetic Counseling Considerations in the Evaluation of Families for Lynch Syndrome-A Review. *Journal of Genetic Counseling.* 2011;20:5-19.

Westin SN, Lacour RA, Urbauer DL, Luthra R, Bodurka DC, Lu KH, Broaddus RR. Carcinoma of the Lower Uterine Segment: A Newly Described Association with Lynch Syndrome. *Journal of Clinical Oncology*. 2008;26:5965-71.

Whelan AJ, Babb S, Mutch DG, Rader J, Herzog TJ, Todd C, Ivanovich JL, Goodfellow PJ. MSI in Endometrial Cancer: Absence of MLH1 Promoter Methylation is Associated with Increased Familial Risk for Cancers. *International Journal of Cancer*. 2002;99:697-704.

Winawer S, Fletcher R, Rex D, Bond J, Burt R, Ferrucci J, Ganiats T, Levin T, Woolf S, Johnson D, Kirk L, Litin S, Simmang C. Colorectal Cancer Screening and Surveillance: Clinical Guidelines and Rationale-Update Based on New Evidence. *Gastroenterology*. 2003;124:544-60.

Part 2

Modern Imaging and Radiotherapy

4

Diagnostic Value of Dynamic Contrast-Enhanced MRI in Endometrial Cancer

Ting Zhang, Ai-Lian Liu, Mei-Yu Sun, Ping Pan,
Jin-Zi Xing and Qing-Wei Song
Radiology Department of the First Affiliated Hospital of Dalian Medical University
China

1. Introduction

Endometrial cancer is the second most common cancer of the female reproductive organs after cervical cancer in China. The depth of myometrial invasion is the most important factor for treatment selection and prognosis prediction [1]. Magnetic resonance imaging (MRI) provides high spatial resolution and excellent soft tissue contrast. The contrast of tumors to uterine cavity and myometrium can be further improved with the use of contrast agents and the enhancement features of tumors at different stages can be analyzed quantitatively and dynamically [5]. However, the relationship between the clinical stages and differentiation degrees of endometrial cancer and the time-intensity curve (TIC) types or the enhancement rates is still not clear on the dynamic contrast-enhanced MRI (DCE-MRI). This study aimed to explore the relationship between the quantitative data of DCE-MRI and the staging of endometrial cancer by investigating the DCE-MRI characteristics of endometrial cancer at different stages, and thus to evaluate the usefulness of the quantitative data and the TIC types of MRI in the diagnosis of endometrial cancer and identification of their degrees of differentiation.

2. Methods

2.1 Cases

A retrospective analysis of 24 patients with endometrial cancer from April 2007 to July 2009 was performed. The diagnosis was confirmed with diagnostic curettage in all patients. The 24 patients received MRI examination in our hospital and of them, 15 patients underwent MRI within 1 week after surgery. The mean age of the patients was 55.8 years, ranging from 28 to 77. Eight patients were pre-menopausal and 16 were post-menopausal. The clinical symptoms included postmenopausal vaginal bleeding in 19 cases, increased vaginal discharge in 2 cases, increased menstrual flow and extended menstrual period in 1 case, and contact bleeding in 2 cases. Informed written consent was obtained from all patients.

2.2 MRI techniques

MRI was performed using GE 1.5T Signa HD Echospeed Superconducting Scanner with body phased-array. Intrauterine device was removed from each patient who had it and all patients were asked to drink about 500 ml water to make the bladder moderate full 1 h before the scanning. Conventional MRI was first performed with the sequences of SE T1-weighted imaging (T1WI) and fat-suppressed FSE T2-weighted imaging (T2WI). DCE-MRI was then performed in 9 patients with horizontal surface fast spoiled gradient echo (FSPGR) sequence and in 15 patients with sagittal liver volume T1-weighted ultra-fast three-dimensional imaging (liver acquisition with volume acceleration, LAVA). MR scanning ranged from the upper edge of the iliac wing to the level of bilateral femoral neck with patients in the supine position. For DCE-MRI, Gd-DTPA contrast agent (0.1 mmol/kg) was given to each patient through antecubital vein using a high-pressure syringe with a flow rate of 2.5 ml/s. Scanning was taken at 16, 32, 48, 64, and 300 seconds (s), respectively, after injection. The scanning parameters were summarized in Table 1.

2.3 Image analysis

2.3.1 Analysis of the tumor characteristics

2.3.1.1 General types

Two types were classified: diffuse type and focal type. Diffuse type was defined as extensive thickening of the uterine endometrium (>3 mm for menopause and >10 mm for pre-menopausal patients). The focal type was defined as the formation of soft-tissue mass.

2.3.1.2 Invasion depth

Two groups were divided. One group referred to the tumors with no myometrial invasion (intact junctional zone and homogeneous low signal on T2WI) or with superficial myometrial invasion (depth of the myometrial invasion, ≤1/2). Another group referred to the tumors with deep myometrial invasion (myometrial invasion, >1/2).

sequence	position	TR（ms）	TE（ms）	thickness（mm）	spacing（mm）	FOV (cm x cm)	matrix	NEX
SE T1WI	axial	400	8	6.0	1.0	32 × 32	320×192	2
fat-	axial	4000	125	6.0	1.0	32 × 32	320×192	4
suppressed	sagittal	3500	110	5.0	0.5	40 × 40	288×256	4
FSE T2WI	coronal	3500	110	5.0	0.5	40 × 40	288×256	4
	axial	155	1.4	6.0	1.0	32 × 32	320×192	1
FSPGR	sagittal	155	1.4	5.0	0.5	40 × 40	288×256	1
	coronal	155	1.4	5.0	0.5	40 × 40	288×256	1
LAVA	sagittal	6.1	1.1	3.0	-3.0	40 × 40	288×256	1

Note: FSPGR: fast spoiled gradient echo sequence; LAVA: liver volume three-dimensional ultra-fast T1WI sequence.

Table 1. The sequence parameters of MRI.

2.3.1.3 Cervical invasion

All tumors were divided into two groups: without cervical invasion and with cervical invasion.

2.3.1.4 Infiltration width

Tumors were classified into two groups. One group was the lesions limited within the uterus, and another group was those with invasion into the parametrium or adjacent organs, or with metastasis.

2.3.2 Region Of Interest (ROI)

The ROI of the tumors or ROI1 was selected from the scanning section with the maximum tumor diameter and the contrast-enhanced area of the solid part (> 0.1 cm^2). The control or ROI2 was selected from the adjacent unaffected myometrial tissue, and its size and shape were kept same to those of ROI1. Necrosis, hemorrhage, and other areas with heterogeneous signal were avoided on the basis of the characteristics of conventional MRI.

2.3.3 Quantitative measurements

The DCE TIC was obtained directly from the GE functool 4.3 workstation. The signal intensity in the different DCE phases was measured in the ROI1 and ROI2, respectively. The enhanced rate in each phase was calculated as enhanced rate = (SIpost-SIpre)/SIpre×100%. SIpost was the enhanced signal intensity in the ROI and SIpre was the corresponding signal intensity before the enhancement. The enhanced rate at 16 s was recorded as the arterial phase relative signal increase (ARSI%) and the enhanced rate at the curve peak was recorded as the maximal relative signal increase (MRSI%). The signal enhancement ratio (SER%) was calculated as SER% = (SImax-SIprior)/(SIe-SIprior) × 100%. SImax was the maximum signal intensity from the DCE TIC, and SIe was the signal intensity during the delayed period.

2.3.4 TIC types

The time period of enhancement to 32 s after injection of contrast agent was set to the early phase; the time period from 32 s to 64 s was set to the middle phase; the time period from 64 s was set to the late phase; and the time period from 300 s was set to the delayed phase. Thus the TIC of endometrial cancer could be divided into four types [6]: type I: early and rapid enhancement to the peak in the early phase with the ARSI% ≥ 60%; type II: similar enhancement pattern in the early phase to type I, but with the ARSI% <60%; type III: significant enhancement in the early phase with the ARSI% ≥ 60%, but showing continued enhancement in the middle and late phases; and type IV: lack of rapid enhancement in the early phase with ARSI% < 60%, but showing continued enhancement.

2.3.5 Endometrial cancer staging based on pathology

The pathological information of 15 postoperative cases was collected by two physicians. The general type, differentiation degree, and invasion depth on MRI were compared with the corresponding findings in pathology which was used as the gold standard. The other 9 cases without operative treatment were staged comprehensively based on the clinical information, mainly the gynecological specialized examination, B-mode ultrasound, cystoscopy, and colonoscopy [7].

2.4 Statistical analysis

Statistical analysis was performed with the SPSS 11.5 statistical software package. Paired t-test was used to compare the signal intensity in different DCE phases between cancer lesions and adjacent myometrial tissues. Two independent samples t-test was used to compare the differences of ARSI%, MRSI%, and SER% among groups. $P < 0.05$ was considered to be significant.

3. Results

3.1 Pathological findings and MRI features

3.1.1 Pathological findings

Pathologically, 16 tumors were adenocarcinoma, 5 were adenosquamous cell carcinoma, 1 was serous adenocarcinoma, 1 was papillary adenocarcinoma, and 1 was clear cell carcinoma. In addition, 12 of the 24 tumors were well differentiated and the other 12 were poorly differentiated.

3.1.2 Features of MRI

3.1.2.1 General types

Nineteen tumors exhibited diffuse type with the endometrial thickness of 1.12 ~ 10.35 cm (4.68 ± 0.33 cm in average). Five tumors exhibited focal type with the maximum diameter of 0.94 ~ 6.17 cm (3.27 ± 0.42 cm in average).

3.1.2.2 Depth of invasion

Fifteen tumors showed no invasion or superficial myometrial invasion, and the other 9 tumors showed deep myometrial invasion.

3.1.2.3 Cervical involvement

Nine tumors had no involvement of the cervix and 15 tumors invaded the cervix.

3.1.2.4 Infiltration width

There were 20 tumors without peripheral invasion, 1 tumor with parametrial invasion, 1 tumor with right sacral metastasis, and 2 tumors with lymph node metastasis.

3.2 DCE TIC types

All 24 tumors were enhanced at 16 s after contrast agent injection. Of them, 17 tumors showed lower or similar enhancement and the other 7 tumors showed significantly higher enhancement compared with the adjacent normal myometrium tissues. On TIC, 23 tumors exhibited continued enhancement in the late phase, and only 1 tumor exhibited decreased enhancement (Figures 1-4). Based on the TIC types, we found type I in 12 tumors (12/24), type II in 6 tumors (6 / 24), type III in 3 tumors (3 / 24), and type IV in 3 tumors (3 / 24). Types I and II curves with an early peak were observed in 18 tumors (18/24). ARSI% ≥ 60% in types I and III curves was observed in 15 tumors (15/24) (Figures 5-8).

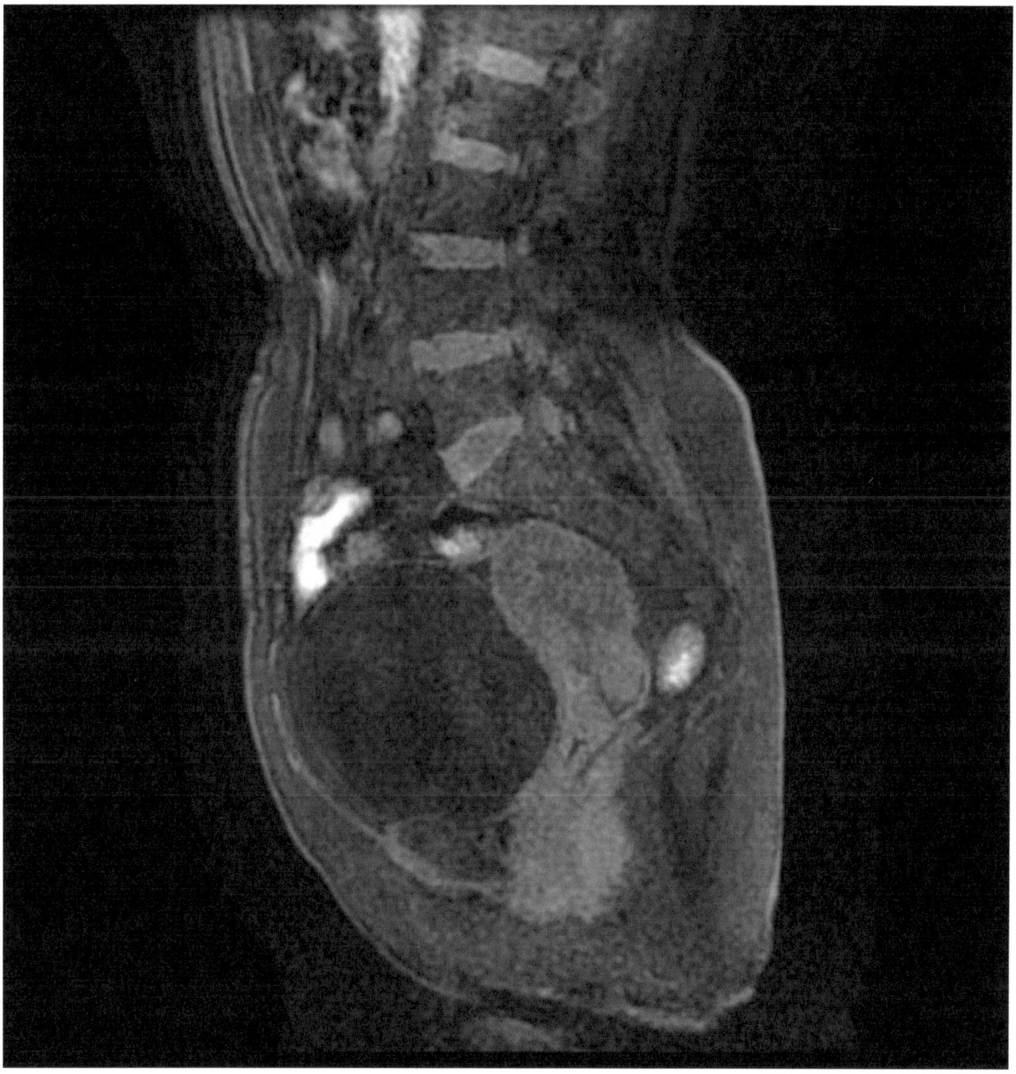

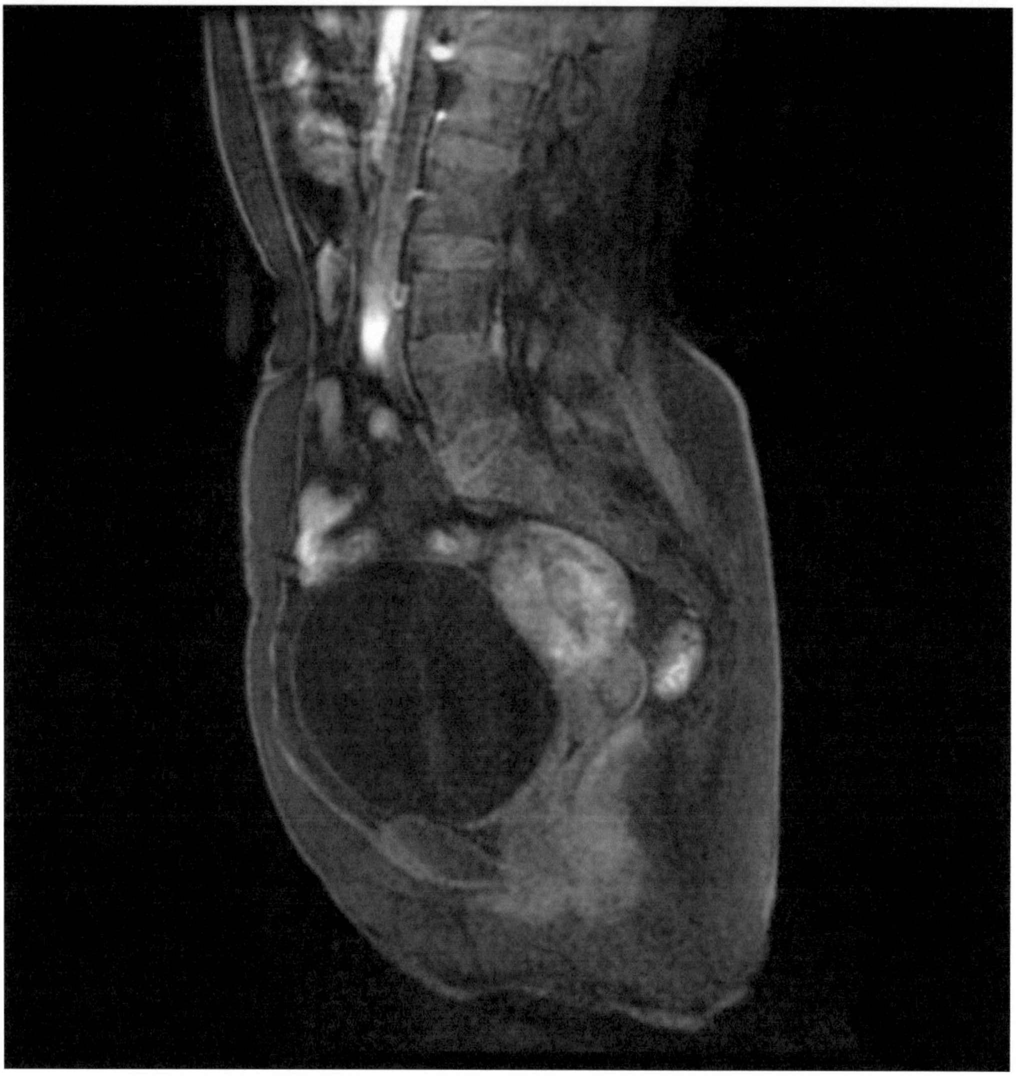

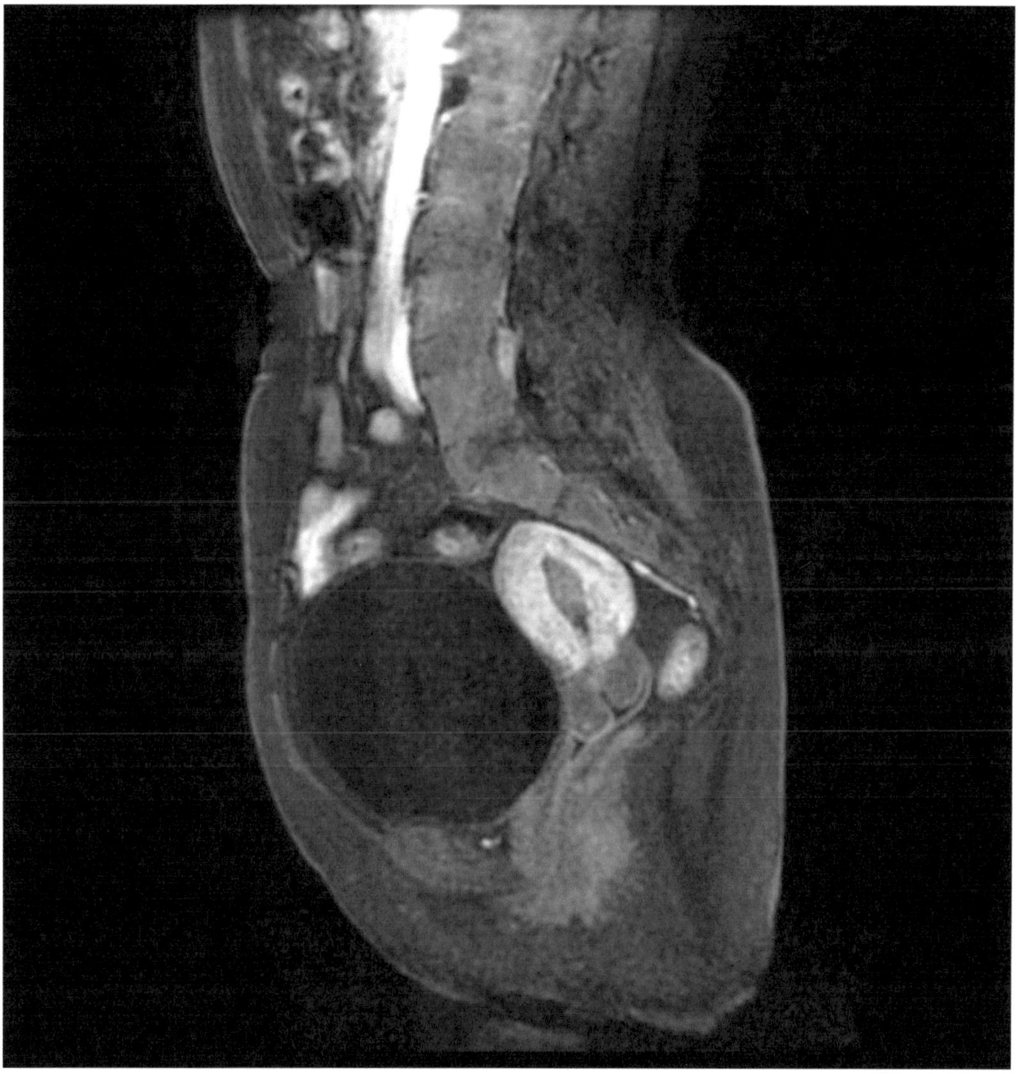

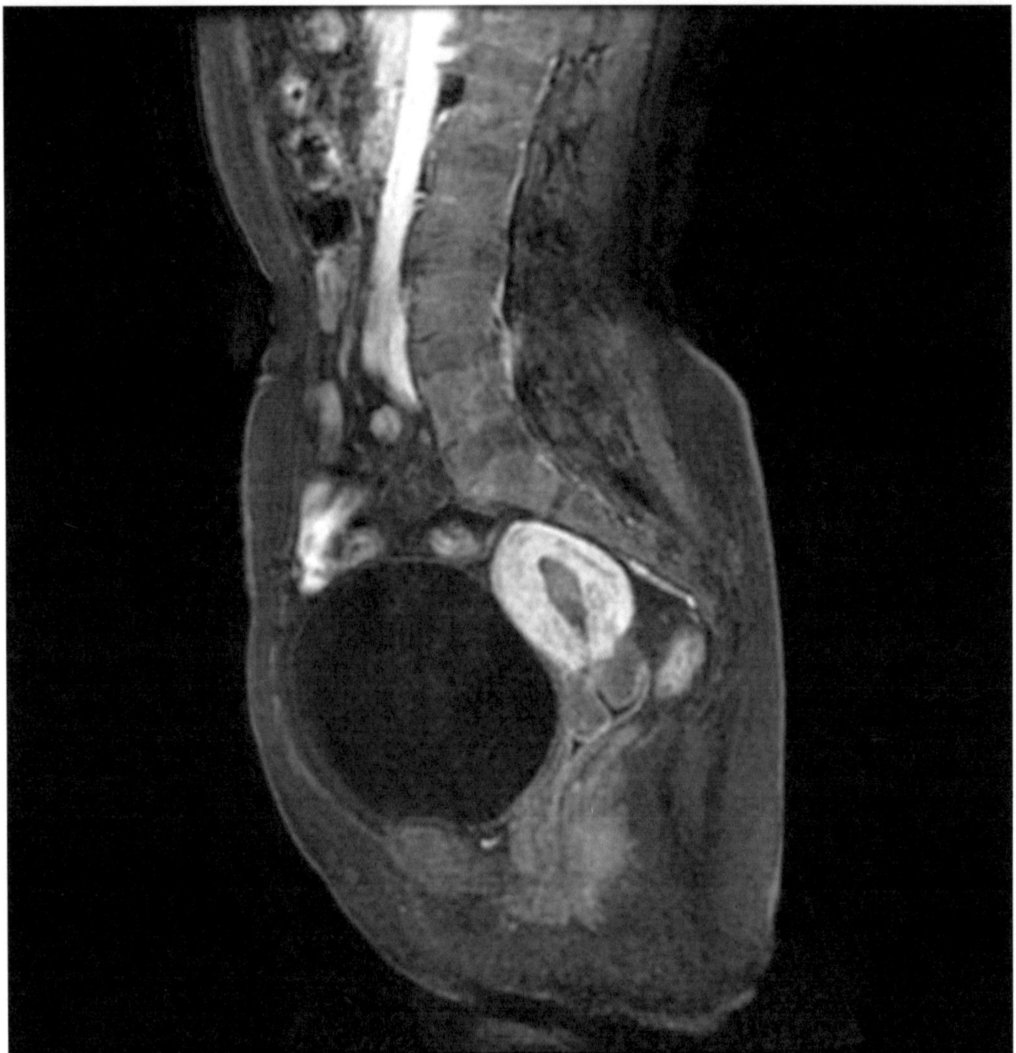

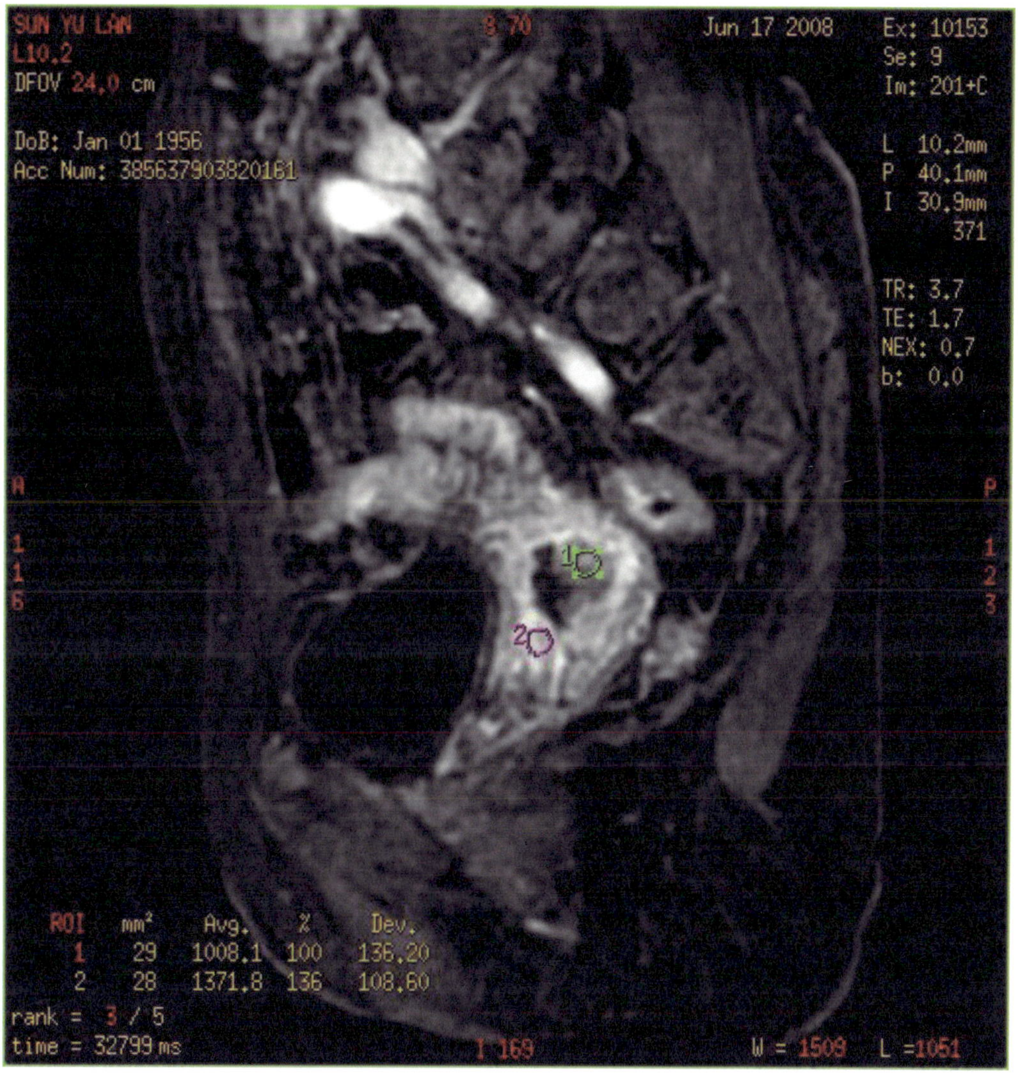
SUN YU LAN
L10.2
DFOV 24.0 cm
DoB: Jan 01 1956
Acc Num: 385637903820161
S 70
Jun 17 2008
Ex: 10153
Se: 9
Im: 201+C
L 10.2mm
P 40.1mm
I 30.9mm
371
TR: 3.7
TE: 1.7
NEX: 0.7
b: 0.0
A
P
1
2
ROI mm² Avg. % Dev.
1 29 1008.1 100 136.20
2 28 1371.8 136 108.60
rank = 3 / 5
time = 32799 ms
I 169
W = 1509 L =1051

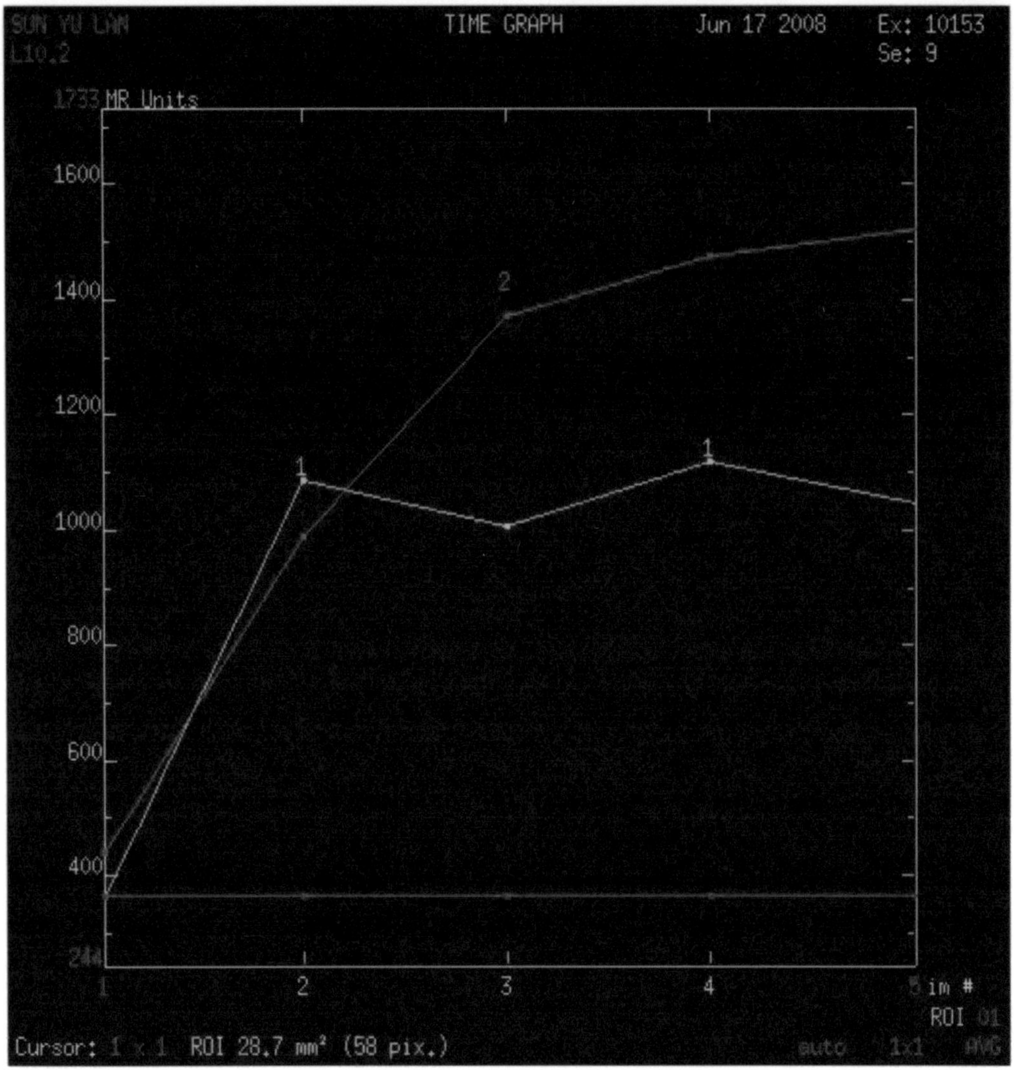
TIME GRAPH
Jun 17 2008
Ex: 10153
Se: 9
MR Units
1600
1400
1200
1000
800
600
400
2
3
4
im #
ROI
Cursor:
ROI 28.7 mm² (58 pix.)

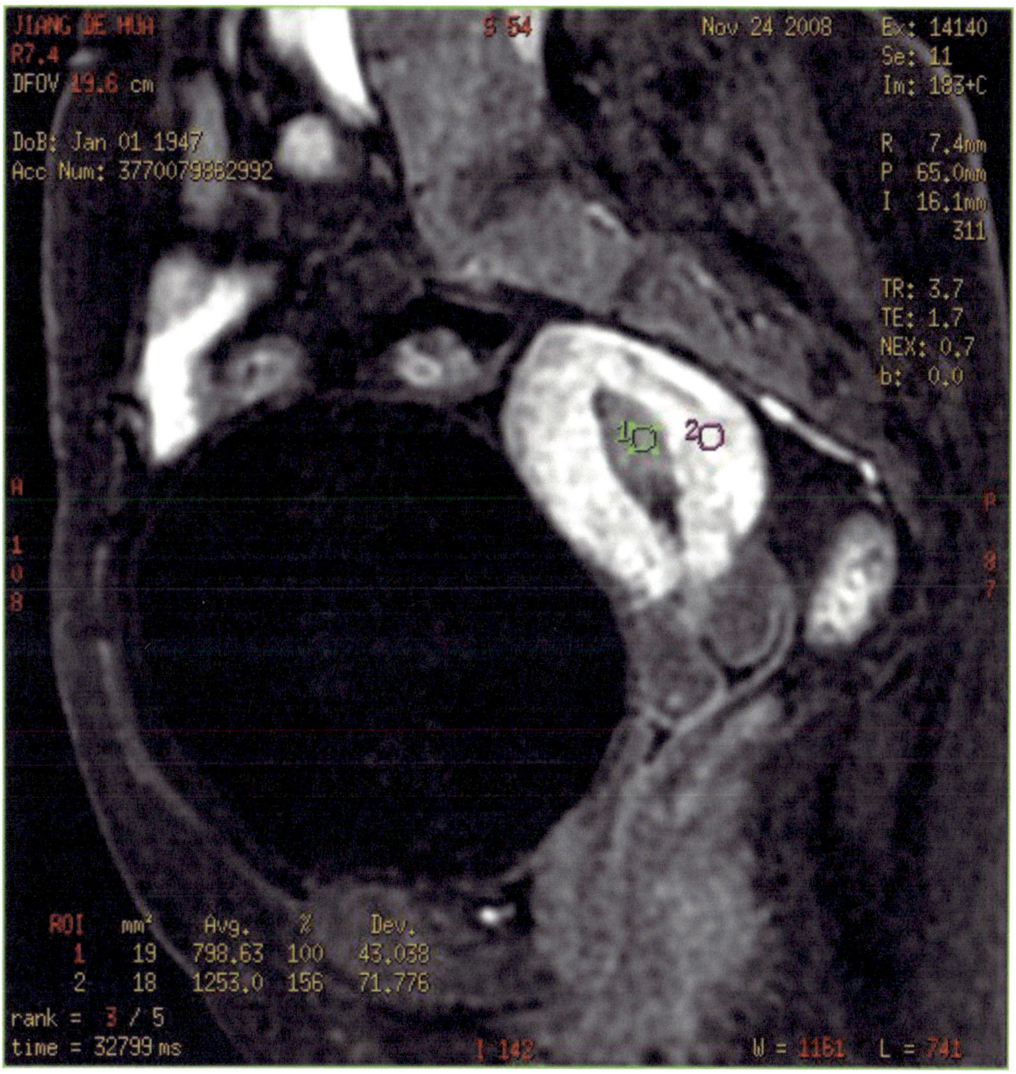
JIANG DE HUA
R7.4
DFOV 19.6 cm
DoB: Jan 01 1947
Acc Num: 3770079862992
S 54
Nov 24 2008
Ex: 14140
Se: 11
Im: 183+C
R 7.4mm
P 65.0mm
I 16.1mm
311
TR: 3.7
TE: 1.7
NEX: 0.7
b: 0.0
A
108
P
87
1
2
ROI mm² Avg. % Dev.
1 19 798.63 100 43.038
2 18 1253.0 156 71.776
rank = 3 / 5
time = 32799 ms
I 142
W = 1161 L = 741

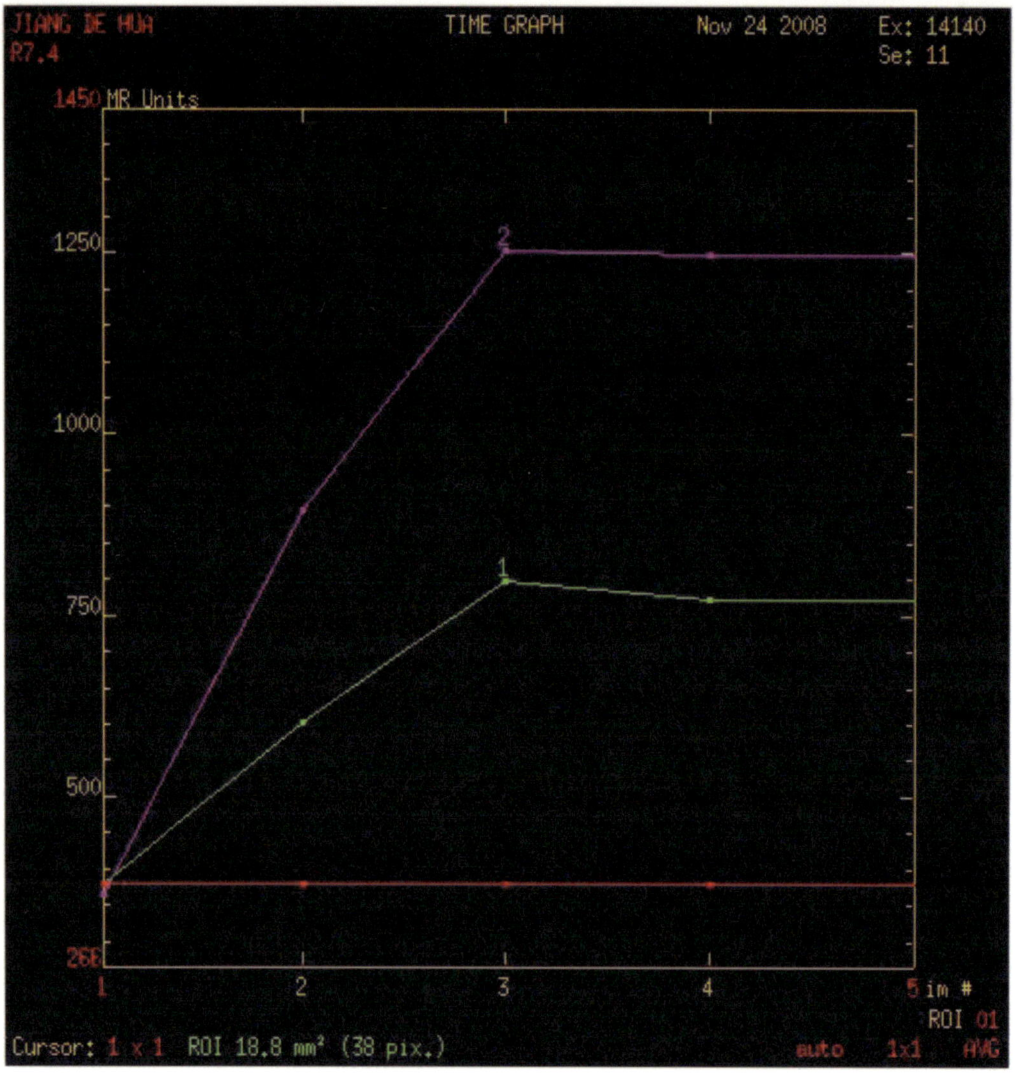
JIANG DE HUA
R7.4
TIME GRAPH
Nov 24 2008
Ex: 14140
Se: 11
1450 MR Units
1250
1000
750
500
266
1
2
3
4
5 im #
ROI 01
Cursor: 1 x 1 ROI 18.8 mm² (38 pix.)
auto 1x1 AVG

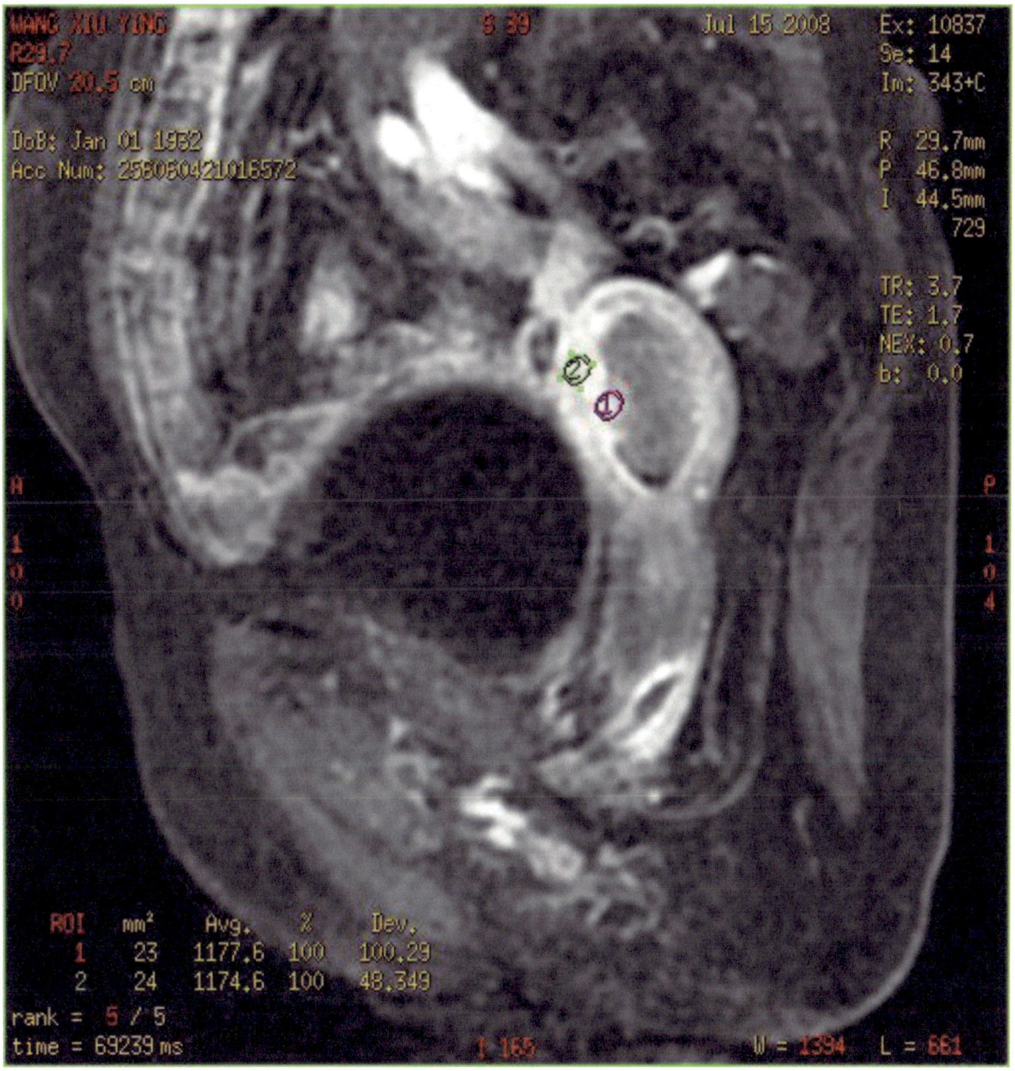
WANG XIU YING
R29.7
DFOV 20.5 cm
DoB: Jan 01 1932
Acc Num: 25606042101657Z
S 39
Jul 15 2008
Ex: 10837
Se: 14
Im: 343+C
R 29.7mm
P 46.8mm
I 44.5mm
729
TR: 3.7
TE: 1.7
NEX: 0.7
b: 0.0
A
P
1
0
0
1
0
4
ROI mm² Avg. % Dev.
1 23 1177.6 100 100.29
2 24 1174.6 100 48.349
rank = 5 / 5
time = 69239 ms
I 165
W = 1394
L = 661

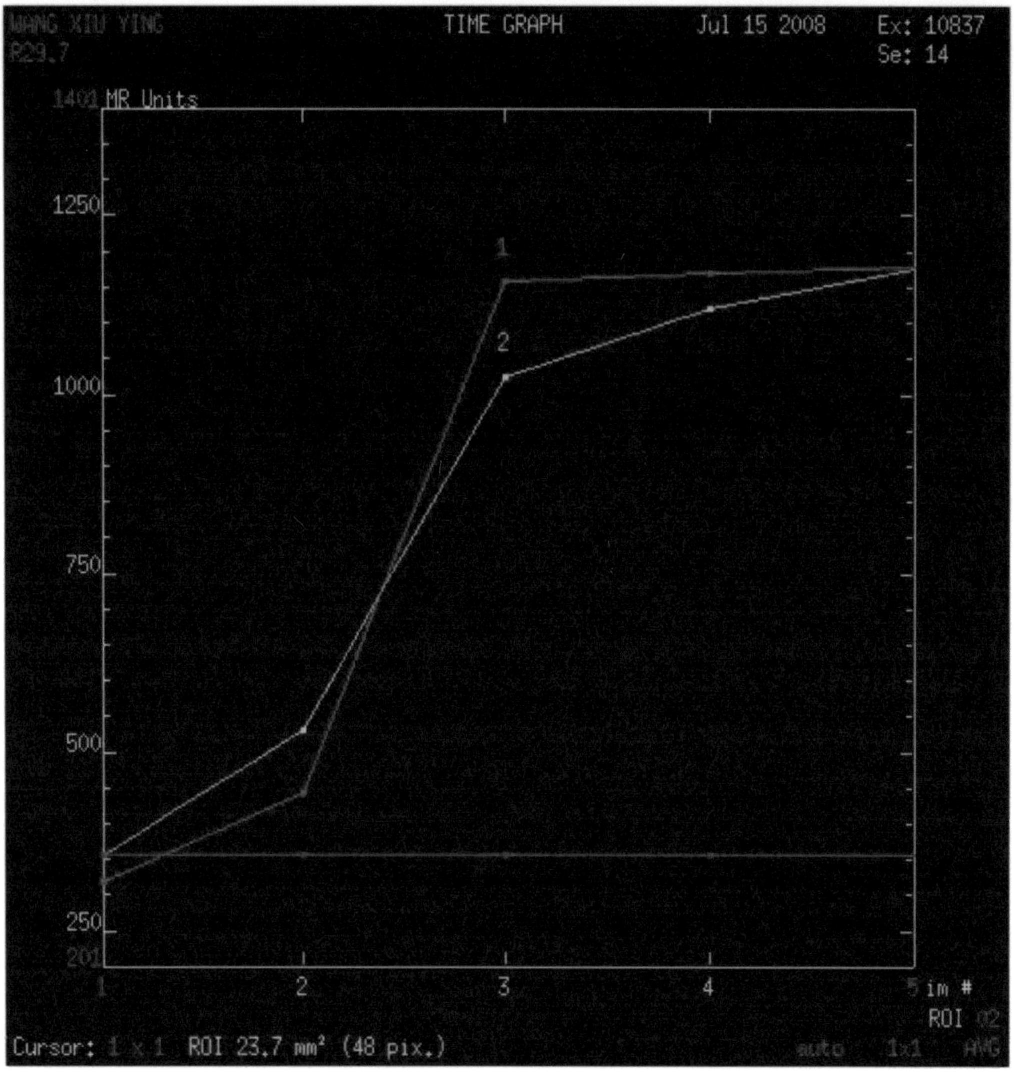
WANG XIU YING
R29.7
TIME GRAPH
Jul 15 2008
Ex: 10837
Se: 14
1401 MR Units
1250
1000
750
500
250
201
1
2
1
2
3
4
5 im #
ROI 02
Cursor: 1 x 1 ROI 23.7 mm² (48 pix.)
auto 1x1 AVG

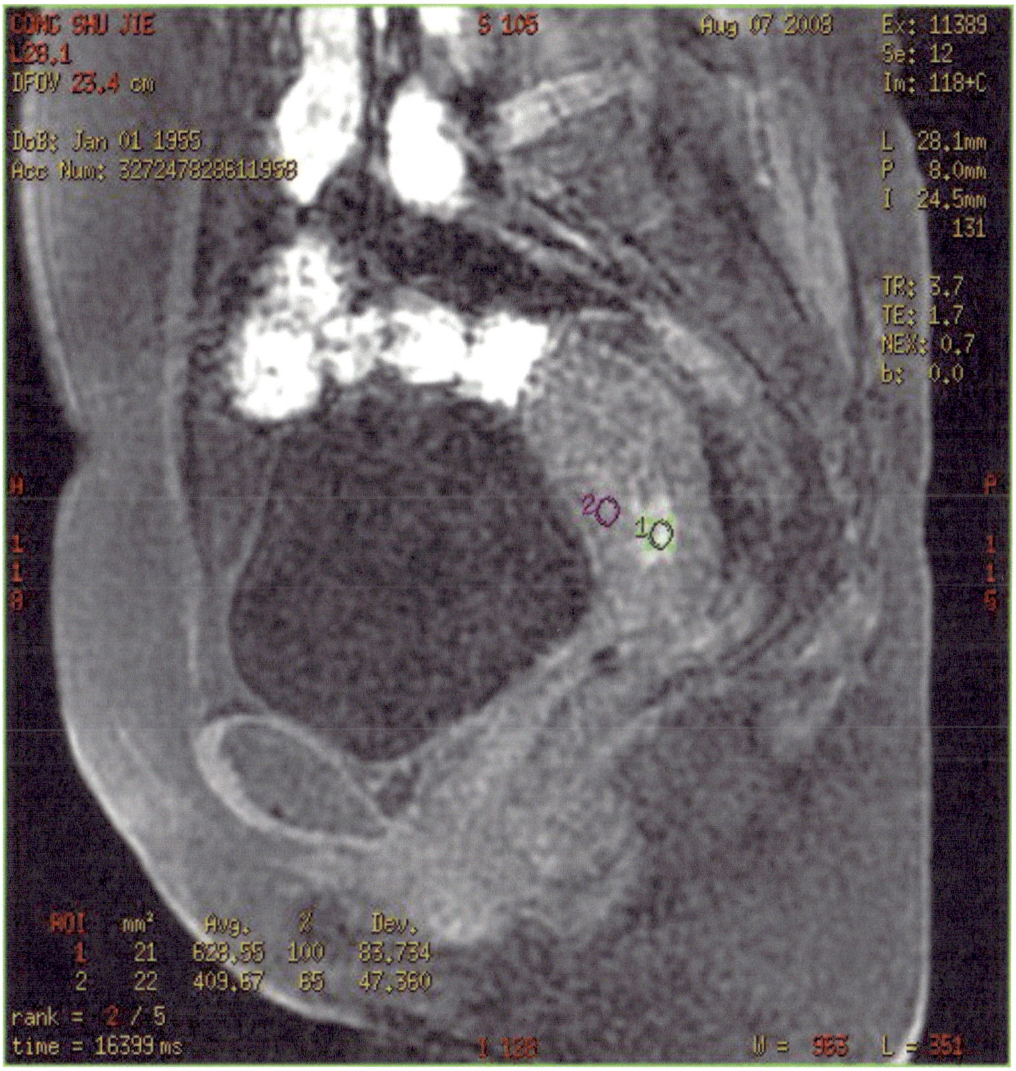
GONG SHU JIE
L28.1
DFOV 23.4 cm
DoB: Jan 01 1955
Acc Num: 327247828611958
S 105
Aug 07 2008
Ex: 11389
Se: 12
Im: 118+C
L 28.1mm
P 8.0mm
I 24.5mm
131
TR: 3.7
TE: 1.7
NEX: 0.7
b: 0.0
A
P
2O
1O
ROI mm² Avg. % Dev.
1 21 628.55 100 83.734
2 22 409.67 65 47.360
rank = 2 / 5
time = 16399 ms
W = 953 L = 351

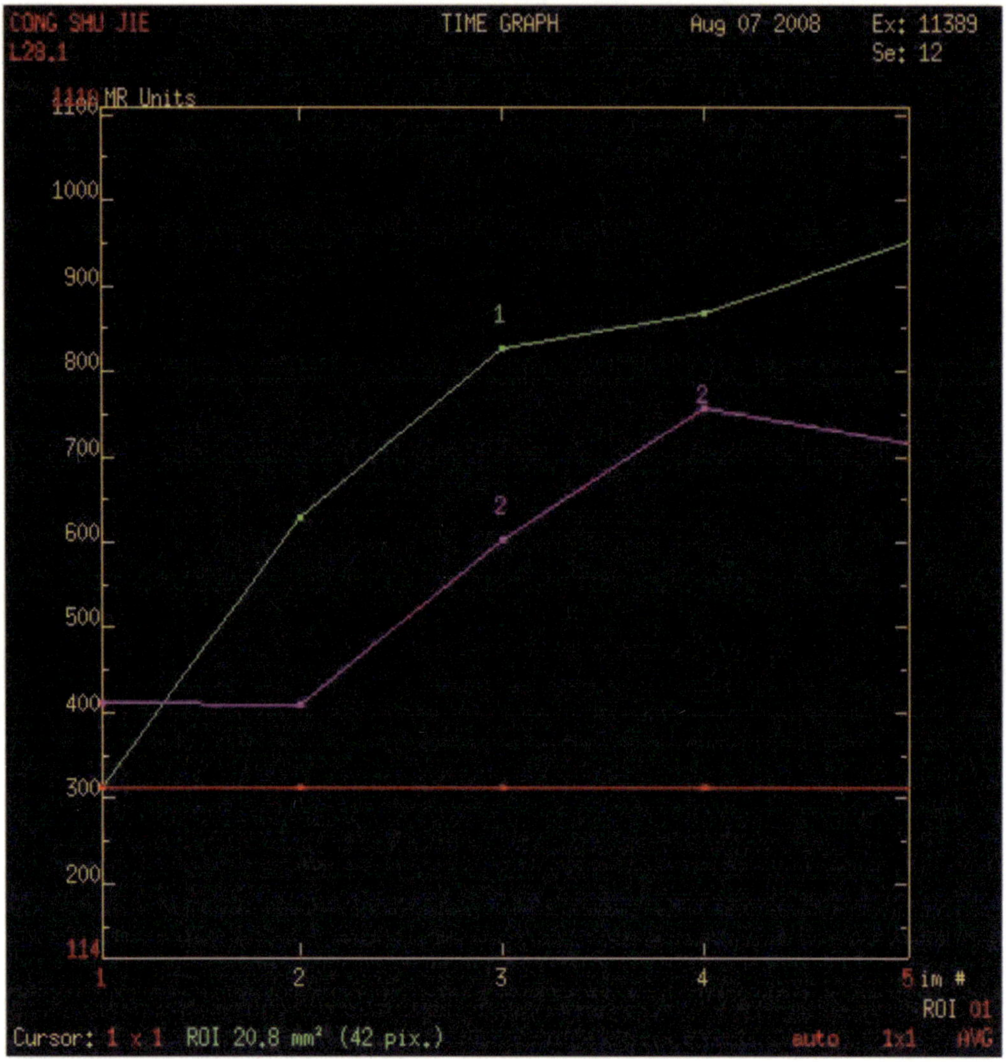

Fig. 1 to 4 female, 61 years old, endometrial adenocarcinoma. Figure 1 showed 0 s after the contrast agent injection, endometrial cancer lesions showed slightly lower signal, such as uterine tissue showed equal signal; Figure 2-4 16 s, 32 s and 64 s after the contrast agent injection, endometrial cancer lesions showed moderate enhancement, and normal uterine tissue was significantly enhanced, contrast between them was clear. Figure 5-12 Dynamic enhancement curves (TIC) type. Figure 5 endometrial cancer lesions (curve 1)was type I, ARSI% ≥ 60%, reached peak in early dynamic contrast-enhanced; normal tissue (curve 2) showed type III, ARSI% ≥ 60%, continuing to strengthen and enhance level higher than lesion; Figure 6 endometrial cancer lesions (curve 1) showed type II, ARSI% <60%, also reached its peak in the early dynamics; normal tissue (curve 2) showed type I, strengthening was higher than the lesion; Figure 7 endometrial cancer lesions (curve 1) showed type II curve, normal tissue (curve 2) showed type IV, ARSI% <60%, degree of enhancement was similar with lesions; Figure 8 endometrial cancer lesions (curve 1) showed type III, normal tissue (curve 2) showed type IV, the degree of enhancement below the lesion.

The signal intensities of the tumors in the early phase (16 s), delayed phase (300 s), or the curve peak were significantly lower than those of the adjacent normal tissue. The signal intensity in tumors was significantly higher in the delayed phase than in the early phase (Table 2). Also, the mean values were all significantly higher for SER% in the menopausal group than in the non-menopausal group, for ARSI% in the poorly differentiated group than in well differentiated group, and for ARSI% in the deep myometrial invasion group than in the superficial or no myometrial invasion group (all P < 0.05) (Table 3).

tissue	16 s	300 s	peak
endometrial carcinoma	716.48±215.10	802.71±289.34	879.33±280.96
normal	893.94±354.52	1110.83±288.83	1183.18±318.13
t	-2.911	-4.926	-4.7
P	P<0.01	P<0.01	P<0.01

Table 2. Comparison of the signal intensity in the early and delayed phases between normal tissues and endometrial carcinoma (%,±s).

enhanced rate	menopause		t	P	general types		t	P
	yes	no			diffuse	localized		
ARSI%	1.06±0.50	1.03±0.48	0.132	0.896	1.07±0.45	0.95±0.61	0.492	0.628
MRSI%	1.56±0.75	1.92±0.72	-1.139	0.267	1.69±0.78	1.68±0.67	0.016	0.988
SER%	1.27±0.23	1.07±0.19	2.095	0.048	1.22±0.24	1.12±0.22	0.87	0.394
enhanced ratc	differentiation degree		t	P	infiltration depth		t	P
	well	poorly			no / superficial	deep		
ARSI%	0.80±0.38	1.20±0.48	2.142	0.044	0.86±0.34	1.37±0.52	2.917	0.008
MRSI%	1.86±0.88	1.58±0.67	-0.862	0.398	1.66±0.75	1.73±0.78	0.231	0.819
SER%	1.13±0.22	1.25±0.24	1.17	0.254	1.17±0.23	1.25±0.24	0.762	0.454
enhanced rate	cervical involvement		t	P	Infiltration breadth		t	P
	yes	no			yes	no		
ARSI%	1.19±0.53	0.82±0.28	1.955	0.063	1.34±0.70	0.99±0.42	1.364	0.186
MRSI%	1.73±0.81	1.61±0.66	0.388	0.702	1.90±0.80	1.64±0.75	0.63	0.535
SER%	1.17±0.23	1.26±0.24	-0.848	0.406	1.27±0.31	1.19±0.22	0.643	0.527

Note: ARSI%: arterial phase relative signal increase; MRSI%: maximal relative signal increase; SER%: signal enhancement ratio.

Table 3. Comparison of the ARSI%, MRSI%, and SER% between designated groups (%,).

4. Discussion

4.1 Endometrial cancer characteristics of DCE-MRI

Currently, staging of uterine lesions is often determined based on the findings of multi-phase enhanced MRI in clinic, however, the selection of the enhanced phases is controversial [8]. DCE-MRI is a dynamic MR technology, focusing on the enhancement behaviors at different time points and reflecting the characteristics of tumor blood supply [9]. Therefore, the tumor blood vessels can be quantified to a certain extent, which makes it possible to study the microvascular characteristics non-invasively.

It has been reported [5] that a mild thin-like enhancement can be observed in the thin layer of tissue between endometrium and myometrium in the early phase of DCE-MRI, which is called subendometrial enhancement (SEE). Similarly, because of the difference in blood supply between tumor and myometrial tissue, the signal enhancement in tumors is significantly lower than that in normal tissue, which leads to increased contrast between tumor and myometrium. Until to the delayed phase, the tumor enhancement is increasing, but the intensity in tumor is still lower than that in myometrium. The maximum signal difference between tumor and myometrium can be observed at certain time, at which the tumor size and margin can be seen clearly and accurate estimation of the invasion depth to myometrium can be made. In the present study, all 24 endometrial tumors were enhanced on DCE-MRI. The enhancement degree in 17 tumors was lower than that in the normal tissue in the early phase, which was consistent with the literature. The remaining 7 tumors showed significantly stronger enhancement than the normal tissues, and of the tumors, 3 were poorly differentiated adenocarcinoma, 1 was clear cell carcinoma, and 1 was serous carcinoma. These results suggest that the enhancement degree may be associated with the degree of malignancy as more abundant blood supply in higher malignant tumors. Only 1 tumor showed decreased contrast enhancement in the delayed phase, which was inconsistent with the report in the literature. The maximum signal intensity in the delayed phase was lower in the tumors than in the adjacent normal tissue, but the signal intensity difference between tumors and normal tissues was higher in the delayed phase than in the early phase, consistent with the previous reports [10-11], indicating that the delayed phase (300 s) was more favorable to delineate the lesions on DCE-MRI.

4.2 Quantitative evaluation of enhancement and TIC curves

Enhanced patterns of tumors reflect the trend of enhancement, however there is no quantitative criterion for the enhancement evaluation. In recent years, many investigators measured the degree of the lesion enhancement with ARSI%, MRSI%, SER%, and other indicators, in addition to the detection sensitivity, noise, etc. These indicators reflect the degree of tumor angiogenesis and the status of blood supply. ARSI% reflects the relative degree of enhancement in the early phase, MRSI% reflects the maximum degree of enhancement, and SER% reflects the relative degree of enhancement in the delayed phase.

Our study showed that the mean value of ARSI% was significantly higher in poorly differentiated tumors than in well differentiated tumors, which was consistent with the findings by Yamashit et al. [12] who showed that the poorer the tumor differentiation was, the richer blood supply in the early phase there was. They also showed that ARSI% could be used to evaluate the prognosis to a certain extent. Bronow et al. found [1] that the metastasis probabilities in the pelvic and para-aortic lymph nodes were 2.5% and 1.2%, respectively, if the tumor limited in the endometrium, while those probabilities were 46.4% and 28.5%, respectively, if tumors had deep myometrial invasion. Therefore, precise evaluation of the depth of myometrial invasion is critical for the clinical treatment selection and prognosis prediction. In our study, the ARSI% in deep myometrial invasion group was higher than in the no/superficial myometrial invasion group. The mean value of SER% in post-menopausal group was higher than in non-menopausal group, which may be due to the reasons of uterine atrophy, increased fiber content, and a larger extracellular space in post-menopausal women. Patients diagnosed with cervical involvement should expand the scope of operation, or take surgery after the radiotherapy. Seki et al. [5] used DCE sequences in the detection of cervical involvement and they showed diagnostic accuracy of 95%, higher than 85% obtained on T2WI. Our study showed that the mean value of ARSI% in cervical involvement group was higher than in the unaffected group, but the difference was not significant. Further study is necessary in a large sample of tumors.

Regarding the TIC curves of the 24 endometrial cancers, 18 (18/24) were types I and II with an early peak and16 (16/24) were types I and III with ARSI% ≥ 60% and an early enhancement. All these endometrial cancers were those with rich blood supply.

In short, the signal enhancement of endometrial cancers in different phases of DCE-MRI can be quantitatively measured, which reflects the status of the tumor's blood supply, and indirectly provides information on their biology. The data in the early and delayed phases of DCE-MRI could provide more relevant information for prognosis prediction and tumor stage determination.

5. References

[1] Bronow RC.Surgical staging in endometrial cancer: clinical pathologic findingof preoperative study. David Manual of Gynecologic Oncology, 1999 , 87:99

[2] Janus CL, Wlczky HP, Laufer N. Magnetic resonance Imagine of the menstrual cycle.Magn Reson Imagine.1998;6;669-674

[3] Lee EJ, Byun JY, Kim BS, et al. Staging of early endometrial carcinoma: assessment with T2 weighted and Gadolinium2enhanced T1-weighted MR imaging. Radiographics, 1999, 19:937

[4] Hardesty LA, Sumkin JH, Nath ME, et al. Use of preoperative MR imaging in the management of endomertrial carcinoma: coat analysis. Radiology, 2000, 15(1): 45-49

[5] Seki H , Takano T, Sakai K.Value of Dynamic MR Imaging in Assessing Endometrial Carcinoma Involvement of the Cervix [J].AJR , 2000 , 175(1) :171 176.

[6] Jun Shan, jian-Min Xu, Jing-Shan Gong, etc. The value of differential diagnosis to Ovarian benign and malignant tumor on enhanced MRI. Chinese Journal of Radiology, 2003, 11:1001-1006

[7] Van Vierzen PB, Massuger LF, et a1. Fast dynamic contrast enhanced MR imaging of cervical carcinoma. Clin Radiol, 1998, 53:183-192

[8] Seki H, Azumi R, Kimura M, et al. Stromal invasion by carcinoma of the cervix:assessment with dynamic MR imaging.AJR, 1997, 168:1579-1585.

[9] Aberle DR, Chiles C, Gatsonis C, et al. Imaging and cancer:research strategy of the American College of Radiology Imaging Network.Radiology, 2005, 235:741- 751.

[10] Seki H, Kirnura M, Sakai K. Myometrial invasion of endometrial carcinorma; assessment with dynamic MR and contrast-enhanced T1-weighted imagines. Clin Radiol.1997, 52(18):18-23

[11] Chaudhry S, Reinhold C, Guermazi A , et al.Benign and Malignant Disease of the Endometrium[J]. Top Magn Reson Imaging, 2003, 14(4) :339-357
[12] Yamashita Y, Fan ZM, Yamamoto H, et al. Spin echo and dynamic gadolinium enhanced FLASH MR imaging of hepatocellular carcinoma: correlation with histopathologic findings[J]. JMagn Reson Imaging, 1994, 4 (1) :83 - 90.

5

Modern External Beam Radiotherapy Techniques for Endometrial Cancer

Ruijie Yang and Junjie Wang
Peking University Third Hospital
China

1. Introduction

Endometrial cancer is one of the most common gynecological cancers in the world. The standard treatment of endometrial cancer includes hysterectomy with bilateral salpingo-oophorectomy, pelvic and/or para-aortic lymph node dissection/sampling, and/or adjuvant radiotherapy [1]. Selection of adjuvant therapy is based on an approximation of the risk of recurrence with features such as stage, tumor histology, lymphovascular space invasion, and patient age. Randomized trials indicated that whole pelvic radiation therapy (WPRT) reduced the rate of pelvic disease recurrence in patients who undergone hysterectomy for endometrial cancer with high risk of recurrence. Radiotherapy is generally administered as external irradiation alone and/or vaginal brachytherapy. The delivery technique is a critical part of the success of radiotherapy for patients with endometrial cancer. Careful consideration of the related factors involved and critical assessment of the techniques available are fundamental to good and effective practice. The purpose of this chapter is to review the modern external beam radiotherapy techniques available for endometrial cancer, including 3D-CRT (Three-dimensional Conformal Radiation Therapy), IMRT (Intensity-modulated Radiation Therapy), HT (Helical Tomotherapy) and VMAT (Volumetric Modulated Arc Therapy), in terms of their physics and technical characteristics, dosimetric advantage, planning and delivery efficiency, taking into account recent advances in this field. A novel conformal arc radiotherapy technique for postoperative WPRT of endometrial cancer will be proposed. The effect of intravenous contrast agent on dose distribution in treatment planning for postoperative WPRT of gynecologic cancer will also be discussed. In addition, the significance of selecting beam energy for the radiotherapy of endometrial cancer will also be covered. Finally, the clinical choice of different techniques will be discussed.

2. 3D-CRT

Three dimensional conformal radiation therapy (3D-CRT) is a technique where multiple beams of radiation are shaped to match the tumor's size and shape, limiting exposure to nearby tissue and organs. Whereas, radiation beams matched the height and width of the tumor in the conventional radiation therapy era, meaning that much of the healthy tissue had to be exposed to the beams. Usually, three dimensional imaging modalities (typically computerized tomography, CT) are used to define the relevant patient anatomy including tumor target(s) and normal tissues in 3D-CRT. Three dimensional dose calculation algorithms and dose analysis tools, and also three dimensional conformal treatment planning and delivery tools (blocks, multileaf collimators, beams' eye view) are used to maximize dose to the defined target and minimize dose to defined normal tissues. 3D-CRT has been shown to be more effective in killing tumors, while minimizing damage to the healthy surrounding tissue since it was implemented clinically in end of 1980s.

WPRT with 3D-CRT improves the dose distribution for the targets and also the critical structures of the endometrial cancer patients dramatically compared with the conventional four box fields. However, conventional WPRT with 3D-CRT exposes most of the contents of the true pelvis to the prescribed dose, due to the cup-shaped tissue volume produced by the pelvic floor and iliac lymph nodes [2]. In addition, a mount of small bowel tends to fall into the vacated space in the true pelvis after hysterectomy, increasing the amount of bowel treated to high dose. This in turn increases the risk of acute and late small bowel complications, limiting the dose that can be delivered to paravaginal and nodal tissues that are at risk for recurrence. Even with modest doses of radiation therapy (45-50 Gy), the risk of severe injury from postoperative radiation therapy is between 5% and 15%. Although severe chronic toxicities (proctitis, obstruction, fistulas) are uncommon, many women treated with WPRT suffer from a variety of chronic problems including intermittent diarrhea, intolerance to certain foods, and malabsorption of vitamins, lactose and bile acids [3].

3. IMRT

IMRT is an advanced mode of high-precision radiotherapy that utilizes computer-controlled linear accelerators to deliver precise radiation doses to a malignant tumor. In contradistinction to 3D-CRT, where the radiation intensity is generally uniform within the radiation portal, IMRT allows for the radiation dose to conform more precisely to the three-dimensional shape of the tumor by modulating the intensity of the radiation beam. Because the ratio of normal tissue dose to tumor dose is reduced to a minimum with IMRT, higher and more effective radiation doses can safely be delivered to tumors with fewer side effects compared with conventional radiotherapy techniques. IMRT has been shown to be a promising approach to give higher than conventional conformal dose with better sparing of bladder, rectum, and small bowel for WPRT [4-7]. The improved conformity of IMRT has been shown to significantly reduce the acute and late toxicities of organs at risk (OARs) for patients with endometrial cancer [8-9].

4. HT

HT is a new method of IMRT that delivers highly conformal dose distributions in a helical pattern. HT was first proposed by Mackie and is now commercially available from TomoTherapy (TomoTherapy Inc, Madison, WI, USA) [10]. In HT, a fan beam of radiation rotates around the patient who is translated through the bore of the tomotherapy machine as in conventional CT. The beam trajectory follows a helical path during delivery and is modulated by a binary MLC. Treatments are optimized from 51 projections and can be conceptualized as IMRT beams delivered from 51 equally spaced angles. The benefit of HT in improving dose homogeneity and a reduced dose to critical structures have been reported in prostate cancer [11], nasopharyngeal cancer [12], other head and neck cancer [13], breast cancer [14], and intracranial tumors [15].

5. VMAT

VMAT is a newer way of IMRT planning and delivery technique, in which the dose rate, MLC leaf positions, as well as the gantry rotation speed vary continuously during the treatment. It falls into the more general category of intensity-modulated arc therapy (IMAT), which was first proposed by Yu [16]. The most important characteristic of VMAT compared with the conventional IMRT is the higher delivery efficiency, with similar or better dose distribution. Cozzi et al [17] evaluated VMAT for the whole pelvic radiotherapy for cervix uteri cancer. They found Systematic and highly statistically significant reduction of bladder and rectum involvement with uncompromised target coverage compared to conventional IMRT.

A systematic study on 3D-CRT, IMRT and HT for WPRT in postoperative endometrial cancer patients has been performed and published by the Peking University Third Hospital [18]. They compared the dosimetric characteristics of 3D-CRT, IMRT and HT, and also systematically investigated the integral dose (ID) and low dose bath to organs at risk (OARs) and normal tissue (NT). They found that compared with the 3D-CRT plans, IMRT can achieve more conformal PTV coverage, lower volume of OARs and NT receiving dose higher than 20 Gy, and lower ID to OARs and NT, a little higher volume of NT receiving dose lower than 10 Gy. IMRT and HT did not increase the integral dose to NT significantly, although a larger volume of NT is irradiated to a low dose in the range of 2-10 Gy. The results were similar in HT, except that the volume of bowel and pelvic bones receiving dose of 5 Gy and 10 Gy increased, and the ID to NT increased slightly. But, the difference in ID to NT between HT and 3D-CRT is less than <5%. The mean conformity index was 0.67, 0.87 and 0.87 for 3D-CRT, IMRT and HT plans. Compared directly with IMRT, HT showed more homogeneous PTV dose and better sparing of rectum and bladder, but higher volume of bowel, pelvic bones and NT receiving dose lower than 20 Gy, and slightly higher ID to pelvic bones and NT.

6. Conformal arc

Conventional WPRT with 3D-CRT exposes most of the contents of the true pelvis to the prescribed dose. IMRT provides more conformal dose distribution and better sparing of critical structures for WPRT. However, IMRT is more complicated in planning and delivery, requiring more expensive equipments and time-consuming quality assurance, with many small, irregular, and off-center fields. Not all the institutions have the facilities and personnel for IMRT, especially in the developing countries and regions. Yang et al [19] explored and evaluated a novel conformal arc radiotherapy technique for postoperative WPRT of endometrial cancer. This technique involves two-axis conformal arc therapy (2A-CAT) each with 180 degrees rotation around two isocenters in two separate dose shaping structures, which were formed by cutting off the central 2.5 cm of PTV in the sagittal plane of the body. In order to produce concave and conformal dose distributions to protect the organs at risk, these two dose shaping structures were considered as the target volume for the dynamic MLC instead of the PTV itself. They demonstrated that the mean conformity index was 0.83, 0.61, and 0.88 for the 2A-CAT, 3DCRT and IMRT plans, respectively. The mean homogeneity index was 1.15, 1.08 and 1.10. The mean dose to small bowel and colon, rectum, bladder and pelvic bones was 1.19 Gy, 3.39 Gy, 4.65 Gy and 1.64 Gy lower with 2A-CAT than with 3DCRT ($p<0.05$), although a little higher than with IMRT. The mean dose to normal tissue was 1.87 Gy higher with 2A-CAT than with IMRT ($p=0.00$). The difference in mean dose to normal tissue in 2A-CAT and 3DCRT was not significant statistically. 2A-CAT offers more conformal dose distribution and better sparing of bowel, rectum and urinary bladder compared with 3D-CRT, although the dose uniformity and conformity is still inferior to IMRT.

This new 2A-CAT technique was found advantageous in many aspects. First, it only requires a linear accelerator equipped with a MLC device, it is more available than IMRT, and can be implemented in most institutions, while it may not be feasible to implement IMRT techniques in much of the developing world, where many gynecologic malignancies, in particular cervical cancer, are quite common. This technique, if adopted, may significantly improve the delivery of radiation in gynecology patients in parts of the world where IMRT may not be possible to implement. Second, it needs less manpower for planning (forward planning for 2A-CAT and inverse planning for IMRT), verification, and quality assurance. Since, in endometrial cancer, the geometrical correlation of the target volume and organs at risk is consistent, it is relatively easy to prepare a treatment plan template. Third, 2A-CAT has the added advantage of shorter fractional delivery time and less MU. The mean number of MU is 240, 451 and 877 for 3D-CRT, 2A-CAT and IMRT plans in their study. Lastly, this new 2A-CAT could be considered as a treatment of selection for postoperative WPRT of endometrial cancer patients, and likely for a wide group of postoperative or even preoperative and definitive WPRT indications, including cervical cancer, prostate cancer and rectal cancer. They are further exploring this 2A-CAT technique for these tumor sites. Eventually, it is possible that this practical 2A-CAT technique would have utility as a short-cut method and would become an accepted alternative for IMRT in external beam radiotherapy (EBRT) of these indications, especially in the not well equipped institutions in facilities and personnel. It will enhance the feasibility and availability of the clinical practice of high precision conformal radiotherapy with its simplicity, extensive availability combined with further improvement and refinement.

7. Beam energy

Higher energy photons were usually used in the conventional conformal radiotherapy for the endometrial cancer due to the higher penetration ability and better dose distribution in terms of the target coverage and sparing of the critical structures [20].

The basic teaching in radiotherapy has been that higher energies (≥10 MV) are preferred for deep-seated pelvic/abdominal lesions, particularly for larger target volumes or larger size patients. Recent work in the field of IMRT has suggested that this energy dependence disappears once beam modulation is added, especially when more beams are used although some researchers suggest that there is still a value to higher energies for deep-seated targets as the volume of the target increase [21]. The value to higher energies for deep-seated targets in IMRT is still a controversial issue. Yang et al [18] found that, the use of 18 MV reduced the IDs to the OARs, NT and the whole body compared with 6 MV for conformal plans. This is consistent with the essentials of radiotherapy physics found in the classic textbooks: higher penetrative quality, more pronounced build-up, lower skin dose, steeper dose gradients at the PTV margin, better dose conformation to the PTV, and more effective dose sparing of normal tissue make high energies the superior beam quality in many clinical situations, especially for the abdominal and pelvic targets. For IMRT plans, the use of 18 MV also reduced the IDs to normal tissue and the whole body, although no significant difference was found in the PTV coverage and IDs to OARs compared with the 6 MV plans. The mean integral dose to normal tissue was 2.4% lower with 18 MV plans (P=0.00). As an ancillary finding, they determined that there is an increase in monitor units (MUs) when lower energy was used in both 3D-CRT and IMRT plans. The mean MUs are 300 and 237 for 6MV-3DCRT and 18 MV-3DCRT plans, 1115 and 926 for 6MV-IMRT and 18MV-IMRT plans. It should be noted that, however, a limitation of their study is that the neutron peripheral dose was neglected in the 18 MV plans. The peripheral dose to distant normal tissue outside the radiation therapy patient's treated volume could be increased in IMRT due to the increased x-ray leakage radiation to the patient, and also from neutron leakage radiation associated with high energy x-ray beams (>10 MV).

8. The effect of intravenous contrast agent

The intravenous contrast agent (CA) during the CT simulation is helpful in accurately delineating the tumor targets and OARs for the patients with endometrial cancer due to the complex anatomy of the pelvic region, whereas, accurate contouring of the target volumes and OARs is the prerequisite to get a high degree of dose conformity in IMRT. In the treatment planning system, Hounsfield units (HU) of CT numbers are used for the dose calculation and heterogeneity correction. Iodine containing CAs, used during CT scan, lead to an increase of HU in tissues with increased CA uptake, and the high HU acts like high density tissue for dose calculation. But, the CA is only present during the CT simulation process, not during treatment. Therefore, it causes errors of the dose to be irradiated in a patient. Yang et al [22] examined the effect of intravenous contrast agent on dose distribution for postoperative whole pelvic radiotherapy (WPRT) of gynecologic cancer. They demonstrated that the doses calculated from the enhanced CTs were lower than those from the non-enhanced CTs, but the differences of mean dose to PTV, OARs and normal tissue were less than 1.0 Gy, the differences of the maximum dose to OARs and normal tissue were less than 2.0 Gy. The differences were not statistically significant between the non-enhanced and enhanced CTs. So, when the plans created from the enhanced CT are applied to a patient, the PTVs will receive more dose than planned. However, the degree of overdose seemed to be negligible clinically, because the concentration of CA was low and the volumes of the enhanced structures were small.

9. Summary

Technical innovations in the treatment planning and delivery of radiotherapy over the last three decades have changed dramatically the practice of radiation therapy. 3D-CRT is now firmly in place as the standard of practice in clinics around the world. IMRT represents a major advance in the delivery of radiotherapy which delivers higher than conventional conformal dose with better sparing of adjacent critical structures. The benefit of improved dose homogeneity and better sparing of critical structures in helical tomotherapy (HT) compared with conventional linac-based IMRT has also been reported. IMAT becomes more and more attractive due to its significant efficiency improvements with uncompromised target coverage, and the sparing of organs at risk and healthy tissue compared with conventional IMRT.

3D-CRT, IMRT, HT and IMAT are all advanced external beam radiation therapy techniques, each having their own relative merits. They differ in terms of the trade-offs between treatment planning time, treatment delivery time, and overall plan quality. IMRT plans can be created in a much shorter period of time as compared to either VMAT or tomotherapy, and VMAT (either single or dual arcs) has the lowest estimated treatment delivery time compared to both IMRT and tomotherapy. With respect to plan quality, it appears that tomotherapy can meet most of the dose-volume objectives, and can provide the most uniform dose to the PTV. For VMAT itself, the choice of 1 or 2 arcs represents a trade-off between plan quality and treatment time whereby single arc plans are expected to be deliverable in a shorter period of time. Adding an additional arc may improve the plan quality with an increase in the treatment time. However, a single arc that is delivered in less than 2 minutes may unduly compromise the plan quality for very complex cases.

VMAT reduces significantly the treatment time (beam on time) compared with both IMRT and tomotherapy. This in turn increases patient comfort, reduces patient motion and internal organ's displacement (e.g. bladder or rectum filling changes over time) during treatment. In addition to the shorter delivery time, VMAT is advantageous in its availability and versatility compared with helical tomotherapy. It can be implemented on the standard C-arm linacs, with wider utilization as, e.g., low and high energy photon beams, non-coplanar arcs in addition to dose rate, gantry speed and possibly collimator variations during delivery to better personalize treatments and increase conformal avoidance of radiotherapy.

The clinical interest of external beam radiotherapy for the gynecological cancer include the treatment of the primary site, and also the pelvic lymph nodes at various levels depending on stage, with proximity with highly sensitive OARs. As a result, gastrointestinal and genitourinary tracts are often highly involved and could lead to acute and late toxicities. The dose-volume objectives represent a significant challenge to the radiotherapy techniques, especially for the demanding cases. The dosimetric and clinical benefits of IMRT for postoperative WPRT have been demonstrated in endometrial cancer patients [8-9]. HT can deliver a more conformal dose to the target volume with greater degree of freedom of intensity modulation due to the helical pattern of dose delivery and unique binary MLC. The improved sparing of rectum and bladder of HT is expected to further reduce the acute and late toxicities, especially for the patients requiring local boost and concurrent/ sequential chemotherapy. However, these benefits of IMRT and HT are achieved generally at the cost of a greater volume of normal tissue in the irradiated volume receiving a low dose. Greater volume of pelvic bones exposed to a dose of 2-20 Gy could increase the risk of hematologic suppression [23] and bone fracture [24]. There has also been concern about the increase of normal tissue integral dose (ID) with multiple beams radiation therapy as a potential risk factor for the development of secondary malignancies in IMRT [25]. Given the life expectancy of the older patients with endometrial cancer, the risk of secondary cancers in the larger volume of NT irradiated to low dose may be small.

The study published by D'Souza and Rosen [26] suggested that the total energy deposited in a patient is relatively independent of treatment planning parameters (such as beam orientation or relative weighting when many beams are used) for deep-seated targets, the ID to NT increases with increasing size of the anatomic region for similar tumor sizes, decreases with increasing size of targets for similar anatomic region size. HT slightly increased the ID to NT and pelvic bones in reference [18] compared with IMRT. This might be attributable to the larger and longer target volumes exposed to more radiation beams in the helical pattern of radiation delivery. This finding also suggests that one technique cannot be considered the "end-all" for everything, the advantage that HT has over IMRT is that while HT reduces the dose received by critical structures at the expense of a greater volume of normal tissue exposed to a low dose. Each approach should be evaluated in terms of the specific objectives when selecting the best option for a given patient. If the objective is to always minimize ID to normal tissue, protons are emerging as an important option [27-28].

10. Acknowledgements

This work was supported by the National Natural Science Foundation of China (No. 81071237).

11. References

[1] Greven K, Winter K, Underhill K, et al. Preliminary analysis of RTOG 9708: Adjuvant postoperative radiotherapy combined with cisplatin/paclitaxel chemotherapy after surgery for patients with high-risk endometrial cancer. *Int J Radiat Oncol Biol Phys* 2004;59:168-173.

[2] Ahamad A, D'Souza W, Salehpour M, *et al*. Intensity-modulated radiation therapy after hysterectomy: comparison with conventional treatment and sensitivity of the normal-tissuesparing effect to margin size. *Int J Radiat Oncol Biol Phys* 2005;62:1117-24.

[3] Roeske JC, Lujan A, Rotmensch J, *et al*. Intensity-modulated whole pelvis radiation therapy in patients with gynecologic malignancies. *Int J Radiat Oncol Biol Phys* 2000;48:1613-1621.

[4] Lujan AE, Mundt AJ, Yamada SD, et al. Intensity-modulated radiotherapy as a means of reducing dose to bone marrow in gynecologic patients receiving whole pelvic radiotherapy. *Int J Radiat Oncol Biol Phys*, 2003, 57:516-521.

[5] Roeske JC, Lujan A, Rotmensch J, et al. Intensity-modulated whole pelvis radiation therapy in patients with gynecologic malignancies. *Int J Radiat Oncol Biol Phys*, 2000, 48:1613-1621.

[6] Mundt AJ, Lujan AE, Rotmensch J, et al. Intensity-modulated whole pelvic radiotherapy in women with gynecologic malignancies. *Int J Radiat Oncol Biol Phys*, 2002, 52:1330-7.

[7] Lorraine Portelance, K. S. Clifford Chao, Perry W. Grigsby et al. Intensity-modulated radiation therapy (IMRT) reduces small bowel, rectum, and bladder doses in patients with cervical cancer receiving pelvic and para-aortic irradiation. *Int J Radiat Oncol Biol Phys*, 2001, 51:261-266.

[8] Randall ME, Ibbott GS. Intensity-modulated radiation therapy for gynecologic cancers: Pitfalls, hazards, and cautions to be considered. *Semin Radiat Oncol*, 2006, 16:138-143.

[9] Brixey CJ, Roeske JC, Lujan AE, et al: Impact of intensity-modulated radiation therapy on acute hematologic toxicity in women with gynecologic malignancies. *Int J Radiat Oncol Biol Phys*, 2002, 54:1388-1396.

[10] Mackie TR, Holmes T, Swerdloff S, *et al*. Tomotherapy: a new concept for the delivery of conformal radiotherapy [J]. *Med Phys,* 1993, 20:1709-19.

[11] Aoyama. H.; Westerly, D.C.; Mackie, T.R.; *et al*. Integral radiation dose to normal structures with conformal external beam radiation. *Int. J. Radiat. Oncol. Biol. Phys.* 64:962-967; 2006.

[12] Lee, T.F.; Fang, F.M.; Chao, P.J.; *et al*. Dosimetric comparisons of helical tomotherapy and step-and-shoot intensity-modulated radiotherapy in nasopharyngeal carcinoma. *Radiother. Oncol.* 89:89-96; 2008.

[13] Sheng, K.; Molloy, J.A.; Read, P.W.; Intensity-modulated radiation therapy (IMRT) dosimetry of the head and neck: a comparison of treatment plans using linear

accelerator-based IMRT and helical tomotherapy. *Int. J. Radiat. Oncol. Biol. Phys.* 65:917-923; 2006.

[14] Caudrelier, J.M.; Morgan, S.C.; Montgomery, L.; *et al.* Helical tomotherapy for locoregional irradiation including the internal mammary chain in left-sided breast cancer: Dosimetric evaluation. *Radiother. Oncol.* 90:99-105; 2009.

[15] Han, C.; Liu, A.; Schultheiss, T.E.; *et al.* Dosimetric comparisons of helical tomotherapy treatment plans and step-and-shoot intensity-modulated radiosurgery treatment plans in intracranial stereotactic radiosurgery. *Int. J. Radiat. Oncol. Biol. Phys.* 65:608-616; 2006.

[16] C.X. Yu, M.J. Symons, M.N. Du, *et al.* A method for implementing dynamic photon beam intensity modulation using independent jaws and multileaf collimator [J]. *Phys Med Biol*, 1995, 40:769-787.

[17] Cozzi L, Dinshaw K A, Shrivastava SK, *et al.* A treatment planning study comparing volumetric arc modulation with RapidArc and fixed field IMRT for cervix uteri radiotherapy [J]. *Radiother Oncol*, 2008, 89:180-191.

[18] Ruijie Yang, Shouping Xu, Junjie Wang, Weijuan Jiang, Chuanbin Xie. Integral dose in three-dimensional conformal radiotherapy, intensity-modulated radiotherapy, and helical tomotherapy. *Clinical Oncology*. 2009, 21(9):706-712.

[19] Yang R, Jiang W, Wang J. A novel conformal arc technique for postoperative whole pelvic radiotherapy for endometrial cancer. *Int J Gynecol Cancer*. 2009, 19(9):1574-9.

[20] Laughlin JS, Mohan R, Kutcher GJ. Choice of optimum megavoltage for accelerators for photon beam treatment. *Int J Radiat Oncol Biol Phys*, 1986, 12(5):1551–7.

[21] Soderstrom S, Eklof A, Brahme A. Aspects on the optimal photon beam energy for radiation therapy. *Acta Oncologica*, 1999, 38(1):179-187.

[22] Ruijie Yang, Wenbao Wang, Yue Zhang, Yuan Lei, Weijuan Jiang, Yuliang Jiang, Lihong Zhu, Jina Li, Na Meng, Ang Qu, Hao Wang, Junjie Wang. Effect of intravenous contrast agent on dose distribution in treatment planning for postoperative whole pelvic radiotherapy of gynecological cancer. *Journal of Practical Oncology* (Chinese) 2010, 25(3): 311-314.

[23] Mell, L.K.; Tiryaki, H.; Ahn, K.H.; *et al.* Dosimetric comparison of bone marrow-sparing intensity-modulated radiotherapy versus conventional techniques for treatment of cervical cancer. *Int. J. Radiat. Oncol. Biol. Phys.* 71:1504-1510; 2008.

[24] Baxter N, Habermann EB, Tepper JE, *et al.* Risk of pelvic fractures in older women following pelvic irradiation [J]. *JAMA*, 2005, 294:2587-2593.

[25] Hall, E.J.; Wuu, C.S. Radiation-induced second cancers: The impact of 3D-CRT and IMRT. *Int. J. Radiat. Oncol. Biol. Phys.* 56:83-88; 2003.

[26] D'Souza, W.D.; Rosen, I.I. Nontumor integral dose variation in conventional radiotherapy treatment planning. *Med. Phys.* 30:2065-2071; 2003.

[27] Chang, J.Y.; Zhang, X.; Wang, X.; *et al.* Significant reduction of normal tissue dose by proton radiotherapy compared with three-dimensional conformal or intensity-modulated radiation therapy in Stage I or Stage III non-small-cell lung cancer. *Int. J. Radiat. Oncol. Biol. Phys.* 65:1087-1096; 2006.

[28] Fogliata, A, Yartsev, S, Nicolini, G, *et al.* On the performances of Intensity Modulated Protons, RapidArc and Helical Tomotherapy for selected paediatric cases. *Radiat Oncol.* 4:2; 2009.

Part 3

Surgery and Staging

6

Controversies in the Surgery of Endometrial Cancer

F. Odicino, G.C. Tisi, R. Miscioscia and B. Pasinetti
Division of Obstetrics and Gynecology
Department of Gynecologic Oncology,
Spedali Civili di Brescia,
University of Brescia, Brescia
Italy

1. Introduction

Endometrial cancer represents over 96% of uterine cancer and is the most common gynecologic cancer in the developed countries with an estimated prevalence of 142,200 women diagnosed in 2011 worldwide[1].

This cancer affects mainly postmenopausal women, 95% of cases occurring in patients over 40 years of age; nonetheless up to 14% of patients are premenopausal, and 5% of cases occurs under the age of 40 years.

The 26th Annual Report of the International Federation of Gynecology and Obstetrics (FIGO) states that 83% of endometrial cancer patients are diagnosed and treated at early stage (FIGO I and II) with 5 year actuarial survival rates ranging from 85% to 91%[2].

Different treatments plans can be proposed for cancer of uterine corpus, but the standard treatment for this disease has been and remains hysterectomy.

The FIGO (Fédération Internationale de Gynécologie Obstétrique) staging system for this pathology has been recently reviewed and approved at the TNM UICC Core Group meeting in Geneva at the beginning of May 2008[3] and subsequently adopted by the American Joint Committee on Cancer (AJCC).

The proposed changes to the staging for endometrial cancer are linked to the data provided by the FIGO Annual Report and confirmed by other publications (Table 1).

The surgical treatment for most patients affected by endometrial cancer includes the thorough a surgical exploration of the abdominal cavity with collection of free peritoneal fluid/ peritoneal washing for cytologic evaluation, total extrafascial hysterectomy with bilateral salpingoophorectomy. The traditional abdominal access is laparotomic with vertical midline incision. The removal of pelvic/paraortic lymph nodes is also required to perform an adequate staging according to FIGO guidelines.

Usually this cancer belongs to perimenopausal age, a small percentage of cases affecting younger women.

Most premenopausal patients have a favorable disease-free survival rate (93%) compared to older patients (86%), with a higher rate of low-grade and low-stage disease.

The overall good prognosis in young women affected by early stage endometrial cancer makes fertility-sparing management an attractive option to this group of patients.

Stage I*	Tumor confined to the corpus uteri
IA	No or less than half myometrial invasion
IB	Invasion to or more than half of the myometrium
Stage II*	Tumor invades cervical stroma, but does not extend beyond the uterus**
Stage III*	Local and/or regional spread of the tumor
IIIA	Tumor invades the serosa and/or adnexae***
IIIB	Vaginal and/or parametrial involvement
IIIC	Metastases to the pelvic and/or para-aortic lymph nodes
IIIC1	Positive pelvic nodes
IIIC2	Positive para-aortic lymph nodes with or without positive pelvic lymph nodes
Stage IV*	Tumor invades bladder and/or bowel mucosa, and/or distant metastases
IVA	Tumor invasion of bladder and/or bowel mucosa
IVB	Distant metastases, including intraabdominal metastases and/or inguinal lymph nodes

* Either G1, G2, or G3
** Endocervical glandular involvement only should be considered as Stage I and no longer as Stage II
*** Positive cytology has to be reported separately without changing the stage.

Table 1. Endometrial Cancer: New FIGO Staging.

The progressive increasing incidence of endometrial cancer in the last few decades combined with the increase of absolute number of under forty's with childbearing desire have forced clinicians to consider fertility-sparing options in treatment of this pathology. These strategies include endocrine treatment and surgical ovarian preservation.

Fertility-sparing endocrine treatment is founded on the use progestational agents. The clinical staging system proposed by the FIGO in 1971 is still applicable for patients who attempt for a medical fertility sparing option (table 2).

Stage characteristics	
I	Carcinoma is confined to the corpus
IA	Length of the uterine cavity is 8 cm or less
IB	Length of the uterine cavity is more than 8 cm
Histologic subtypes of adenocarcinoma	
G1	Highly differentiated adenomatous carcinoma
G2	Differentiated adenomatous carcinoma with partly solid areas
G3	Predominantly solid or entirely undifferentiated carcinoma
II	Carcinoma involves the corpus and cervix
III	Carcinoma extends outside the uterus but not outside the true pelvis
IV	Carcinoma extends outside the true pelvis or involves the bladder or rectum

Table 2. Corpus Cancer Clinical Staging, FIGO 1971.

The use of progestational agents is still a subject of investigation in young patients with early stage disease [4,5,6] and it has been shown to have reasonable success particularly in women with low-grade disease [7]. A recent multicenter phase II study of treatment with medroxyprogesterone acetate for endometrial carcinoma and for atypical hyperplasia in young women by Ushijima and colleagues found a complete response in 55% and 82% of cases respectively, with a 47% recurrence rate observed during the 2-year follow up period.

Progestational uterine-preserving treatment is a reasonable option in women affected by early stage, low-grade endometrial cancer, but these patients should be widely counseled about the high recurrence risk observed in cases responding to progestins (about 50% of cases), and thus recommended to close follow-up because of the substantial rate of recurrence.[4]

MRI, with its high soft tissue contrast resolution and multiplanar capability, has been evaluated in several series. Most of them reported data on the prediction of deep myometrial invasion. In these series the sensitivity of the radiological procedure ranges between 71% to 83%, the specificity between 74% to 96% with Negative and Positive Predictice Values between 86%-97% and 80%-91% respectively.[8 9 10]

If the requirement for conservative treatment is no myometrial invasion, then MRI is a poor screening test with an NPV of only 46%[11].

Ovarian preservation in young patients, preferably in early stage, low grade cases, may be considered taking into account the potential risk of missing occult ovarian metastases or coexisting synchronous ovarian primary tumors [12,5] and the potential risk of endocrine stimulation of residual microscopic endometrial cancer foci [13,14,15,16]

Twenty-three coexisting synchronous epithelial ovarian tumors and 3 metastatic disease were reported in a cohort of 102 women younger than 45 years with endometrial cancer, thus ovarian cancer accounting for 25% of the study cohort. In this report, 4 patients (15%) had normal preoperative imaging of the adnexa, and 4 (15%) had benign appearing ovaries at the time of intraoperative assessment. Recent results of a Surveillance, Epidemiology, and End Results Database (SEER) analysis on ovarian preservation applied to 402 out of 3269 evaluable premenopausal women with stage I endometrial cancer (12%) showed that ovarian preservation may be safe and had no effect on either cancer-specific survival or overall survival. However, it must be considered that young patients could harbor a genetic predisposition to multiple site primary cancer [17].

The Lynch syndrome is an autosomal-dominant cancer susceptibility syndrome associated with early-onset colon, rectal, ovary, small bowel, ureter/renal pelvis, and endometrial cancer. This syndrome occurs in nearly 10% of endometrial cancer patients less than 50 years of age, compared to the 2% to 5% of all endometrial cancer cases, and the risk of ovarian cancer in patients affected by HNPCC is 10% to 12%.

The omission of a bilateral salpingo-oophorectomy should be carefully counseled in these young high-risk patients, and all the known devices should be used to best define their effective risk of ovarian cancer, such as genetic evaluation of mismatch repair defects or BRCA1 and BRCA2 germ line gene mutations.

However in the preoperative counseling the clinician has to make the patient clearly understanding that a negative genetic evaluation does not eliminate the risk of synchronous or metachronous ovarian cancers.

Usually, overall surgical cure rates for endometrial cancer are high but, unfortunately, up to 25% of affected patients have a poor prognosis when the disease is widely spread at diagnosis or characterized by poor clinical-pathological risk factors such as high grade of histological differentiation, deep myometrial invasion or unfavorable histology (clear cells / serous papillary pattern). Treatment planning must be tailored depending on tumor grade, depth of myometrial invasion, and extension to cervical stroma: these factors are directly related to the risk of regional lymph node and distant metastasis, influencing overall prognosis.

Laparotomic surgery has been considered the standard surgical approach in patients affected by endometrial cancer. This surgery must include an initial exploration of the abdominal and pelvic cavities, peritoneal free fluid or washing collection for cytology, biopsy of any suspicious extra uterine lesion, total extrafascial hysterectomy with bilateral salpingo-oophorectomy. In order to complete the surgical staging, the dissection of pelvic and para-aortic lymph nodes are recommended by FIGO.

Vaginal hysterectomy has often been defined as the simplest and least morbid approach and different studies found similar treatment outcomes in stage I endometrial cancer patients treated with vaginal or laparotomic hysterectomy [18,19,20]. Still, limitations to vaginal approach are the lack of exploration and of cytological evaluation of the abdominal cavity, difficulty in performing salpingo-oophorectomy and the inability to perform a thorough evaluation of lymph nodes [19]. This surgical approach should be considered a valid alternative for high-risk patients with co-morbidities that can contraindicate abdominal procedures.[21,22]

In the latest years, hysterectomy and bilateral salpingo-oophorectomy performed by a laparoscopic-assisted-vaginal (LAVH) or total laparoscopic (TLH) approach have increasingly been integrated in the standard practice of endometrial cancer patients. These techniques are able to overcome some of the limitations of the vaginal approach.

Initial case reports and small single-institution retrospective series described laparoscopic technique and demonstrated its feasibility during the early '90s [23,24,25]; subsequently larger series, randomized small size trial, and finally a multi-institutional randomized controlled trial, evaluated the feasibility and survival outcomes of laparoscopy in endometrial cancer patients [26,27,28,29]. A small prospective trial [26] randomized 70 patients with FIGO stage I-III endometrial carcinoma to radical vaginal or laparoscopy-assisted simple hysterectomy or simple or radical abdominal hysterectomy with or without lymph node resection. The laparoscopic group showed significantly lower blood loss and transfusion rates, while the number of pelvic and para-aortic lymph nodes, duration of surgery, and incidence of postoperative complications were similar for both groups. A significantly shorter hospital stay was found in the laparoscopic group, in accordance with other Authors [35,36]. No significant differences were observed between the laparoscopic and laparotomy groups in terms of disease recurrence rate and long-term survival (97.3% vs. 93.3% and 83.9% vs. 90.9%, respectively).

The conclusion of this study was that laparoscopic staging combined with laparoscopically assisted vaginal hysterectomy can be recommended for the treatment of women with endometrial cancer, offering a less invasive approach that is associated with less intraoperative and postoperative morbidity.

Results of a large randomized trial (LAP II trial) from the Gynecologic Oncology Group (GOG) comparing laparoscopic hysterectomy with comprehensive surgical staging to the traditional laparotomy technique were recently published [29,30].

The study enrolled 2616 patients with clinical stage I to IIA uterine cancer and randomized 920 patients to the open arm, and 1,696 to laparoscopy. The conversion rate from laparoscopy to open procedure was 26%; it increased with increasing patient obesity. Median number of removed pelvic nodes was similar between each technique, while a statistically significant higher para-aortic node dissection rate was observed in the laparotomy group (97% versus 94%). Most importantly, the frequencies of patients found to have positive lymph nodes were the same in both groups (9%). The rate of postoperative complications, median blood loss, and median length of hospital stay were significantly lower in the laparoscopy group, despite the relatively high conversion rate.

The authors concluded that laparoscopic surgical staging is an acceptable and possibly a better option, particularly when the surgery can be successfully completed laparoscopically, even if the results specific to long-term oncologic outcomes are not known.
Age and obesity have been suggested as relative contraindications to laparoscopic surgery. Similar conclusions where reached by Scribner et al. [31]
The authors concluded that, with the growth of an aging patient population, the laparoscopic management of endometrial cancer is a viable option.
Obese patients have also been suggested to be poor laparoscopic candidates due to difficulties in establishing pneumoperitoneum, poorer visualization, inability to tolerate steep Trendelenburg positioning needed to facilitate the surgery, and difficulties with ventilation. It is important to mention that complete surgical staging is more difficult in obese patients regardless of the surgical approach.
In a study of Eltabbakh et al. comparing LAVH and abdominal approach in women with BMI between 28 and 60 [32] laparoscopic conversion was required only in 8% of patients: laparoscopic surgery was associated with a longer operative time (195
minutes vs. 138 minutes), more pelvic nodes (mean 11 vs. 5), less pain medicine requirement, and shorter hospital stay (2.5 vs. 5.6 days) were recorded.
Total laparoscopic hysterectomy has also been shown to be feasible in heavier patients [33]. In the prospective GOG series, there was ≥80% success rate with patients with a BMI of 27 or less, but even at a BMI of 35, 65% could have successful laparoscopic surgery. [34]
In conclusion, the surgical approach and the technique used to remove the uterus with the ovaries does not represent a source of controversy since the comprehensive surgical pathological evaluation should be accomplished with different approaches. [25]
Minimal access surgery is being applied increasingly in gynecological oncology and is now a commonplace in the surgical treatment of endometrial cancer.
The widespread adoption of laparoscopy has been slow due to the prolonged learning curve needed to become proficient in such a technique. The development of robotic surgery has facilitated the use of laparoscopy due to the faster and easier learning curve.
In robotic surgery, the main surgeon sits at the surgeon console located away from the patient, places his index fingers and thumbs in the master rings and along with foot pedals is able to control all the robotic instruments held by the patient-side cart through a computer-based technology. Endometrial cancer is particularly suited for robotic surgery for several reasons. The majority of women with endometrial cancers are obese and at greater risk for postoperative wound complications, and would benefit from a minimally invasive procedure with smaller incisions, resulting in less risk for wound problems. However, at the same time obesity increases the degree of difficulty of management via laparoscopy: the level of difficulty of operating in an obese patient via robotic surgery is minimal. In a retrospective comparison of obese women and morbidly obese women undergoing traditional laparoscopic approach vs. robotic-assisted approach, better surgical outcomes were observed in the group undergoing robotic-assisted laparoscopy. [35]
Actually there are no published data of survival in endometrial cancer patients treated with robotic system that has been introduced in clinical practice short time ago. However, early case series thus far reported suggests that robotic surgery for endometrial cancer is feasible and safe. The use of robotic-assisted laparoscopy for the management of endometrial cancer is expected to be rapid, paralleling the growth that has been observed with radical prostatectomy.
Another important issue in the management of endometrial cancer is the tailoring of "radicality" according to the "clinical stage" of the disease.

Radical hysterectomy is the standard of care of early stage cervical cancer (IA2–IB1), but its role in endometrial cancer remains unclear [36]. A radical surgical approach to endometrial cancer requires the uterus to be removed with parametria, paracolpos, and an adequate vaginal cuff, and ensures wider tumor-free resection margins than those obtained with total abdominal hysterectomy. The main goals of the radical surgical approach for stage I endometrial cancer are a better local control of the disease and a reduction in the use of adjuvant radiation with its possible related complications.

A multicenter randomized Italian trial [37] aimed to determine whether a modified radical (Piver– Rutledge class II) hysterectomy can improve survival and loco regional control compared to the standard extrafascial (Piver–Rutledge class I) hysterectomy. The Authors randomized 520 early stage endometrial cancer patients and evaluated the difference between Class I vs. Class II group in terms of loco regional control, disease-free and overall survival, and treatment-related morbidity.

Intraoperative and postoperative complications rates were similar in the two arms, but there were slight imbalances with respect to urinary complications. Although class II hysterectomy turned out to be feasible in most patients enrolled onto our study (only 19 of the 279 assigned to class II underwent class I hysterectomy), it was far longer (20 min) and was associated with greater blood loss (50 ml) than class I.

The univariate and multivariate estimates of the HRs of recurrence confirm that class II hysterectomy offers no benefit.

The identification of spread to draining lymph node basins is considered of outmost importance since it can change the prognosis and modify the use of postoperative therapies. However no consensus exists regarding the role and the extension of lymphadenectomy in the primary surgical setting and more controversial is the therapeutical role of this procedure.

In women submitted to systematic lymphadenectomy without clinical suspect of nodal metastasis, pelvic lymph node involvement may be assessed in 8 to 28% of patients. [38, 39].

The risk of pelvic and/or paraortic nodal metastases [2] depends on hystotype, myometrial invasion and hystological grade of differentiation, ranging from 0% up to 20% in M0G1 and M3G3 patients (see Table 3).

Myometrial invasion	P-A-(%)	P+A-(%)	P-A+(%)	P+A+(%)
Unknown	97.42	1.81	0.17	0.60
M0	94.20	3.40	0.60	1.80
M≤50%	93.88	4.56	0.62	0.94
M>50%	73.90	18.41	1.56	6.14

P-, P+: negative, positive pelvic nodes;
A-, A+: negative, positive aortic nodes;
M0: no myometrial invasion
M≤50%: myometrial invasion ≤50%
M>50%: myometrial invasion >50 %.

Table 3. Carcinoma of the corpus uteri. Patients treated in 1999-2001. Lymhnodal status (a).

Even if there is no evidence that risk/benefit balance is in favor of lymphadenectomy however this procedure can cause potentially significant morbidity in approximately 11% of cases [40].

The relevance of lymph node status is of outmost importance for the prognosis of this disease. For this reason this procedure represents a fundamental step in staging the disease [3]. The main risks attributable to nodal dissections include increased operative time, potential for blood loss associated with vascular injuries eventually requiring blood transfusion, genitofemoral nerve injury with resulting numbness and paresthesias over medial thighs, lymphocysts formation, and lymphedema.

Many believe that nodal dissection should be reserved for those with sufficient risk of nodal disease. Most important factors related to incidence of nodal metastases are tumor grade and depth of myometrial invasion as we can see analyzing data of GOG 33 study [38]. Patients with grade 1 lesion with inner part of myometrium involved showed a 3% risk of nodal metastasis defined by the Authors "negligible". Patients with grade 3 lesions with deep myometrial invasion showed a 34% risk of nodal localizations.

Clear cell tumors and serous papillary tumors are more often affected by nodal metastasis (30-50% of risk independently by prognostic factors on surgical specimen) [41].

Usually the risks related to nodal resection are acceptable, if this procedure is managed by skilled and well trained physicians, and this procedure deeply influences the use of postoperative treatment: less indications for radiation therapy or use of vaginal cuff brachytherapy instead of whole pelvic external irradiation [42 43]. Without nodal information, physicians must rely on uterine factors to estimate the probability for nodal disease and pelvic failure to determine the need for postoperative radiation. This estimation can result in a substantial increase in the use of radiation.

The advantages of systematic lymphadenectomy are evidenced in some retrospective studies. Other observational studies, however, have not shown any such benefit. Until 2011 no class I evidence paper had been published.

MRC ASTEC trial [44] enrolled 1408 women with proven endometrial carcinoma from 85 centers in four countries.

This randomized trial did not showed any evidence of benefit with systematic lymphadenectomy for endometrial cancer in terms of overall, disease-specific, and recurrence-free survival. Overall morbidity was low, but there was a substantial increase in the incidence of lymphedema in the lymphadenectomy group compared with standard surgery. The Authors concluded that the balance of risks and benefits for systematic iliac and obturator lymphadenectomy does not favor this intervention, with no clear evidence of benefit in terms of overall or recurrence-free survival and increased risk of lymphedema. These results suggest that lymphadenectomy in patients affected by endometrial cancer, whose neoplasm is preoperatively diagnosed as confined to the corpus, has no therapeutic effect and is therefore not justified as a therapeutic procedure. Nevertheless this surgical procedure is required for surgical staging in order to identify those patients who will have benefit from adjuvant treatment.

It must be noted that this trial received a number of criticisms concerning the inclusion of a large number of women at low risk of nodal metastases and variable extent of nodal dissection between recruiting centers.

An Italian randomized prospective study [45] recruited 514 patients with preoperative FIGO stage I endometrial carcinoma (Stage IB with grade 1 lesions were excluded from randomization), randomly assigned to undergo pelvic systematic lymphadenectomy or no lymphadenectomy whose anatomical and numerical extent was clearly defined in the study design. No lack of consistency between the centers and uniformly high nodal counts were detected.

According to the Authors, pelvic systematic lymphadenectomy did not change the natural history of the disease since the pattern of disease recurrence, was similar between the two groups. However, pelvic lymphadenectomy did allow for a more accurate prognosis on the basis of the pathological lymph node assessment and, in this trial, provided for approximately 10% of the upstaging to surgical stage IIIC ($P < .001$).

The role of para-aortic lymphadenectomy is another field of debate: the anatomic extent and level of dissection remain ill defined for patients undergoing para-aortic node sampling or systematic dissection. [46,47,48,49]

Reports that address the routes of lymphatic dissemination in endometrial cancer have suggested that the principal connections are between the uterine corpus and the external iliac and obturator basins [50,51,52]. A direct route may exist from the corpus to the paraaortic node-bearing basins by the lymphatic channels adjacent to the gonadal vessels within the infundibulopelvic ligament [51,52]. Other reports have also suggested a potential direct lymphatic communication between the external iliac and obturator basins and the paraaortic node-bearing tissue [48,53]. Therefore, an a priori assertion exists that the paraaortic node-bearing tissue in the region of the origin and insertion of the gonadal arteries and veins, respectively, would be favored sites for nodal involvement.

In absence of metastatic pelvic nodes, isolated positive para-aortic nodes are identified in a small number of patients. The historical data from GOG 33 showed that isolated para-aortic nodal metastases occurred in 2% of patients. These data also suggest that when positive, outcomes are improved in patients who have complete surgical resection of para-aortic nodes. This effect may be simply be a consequence of better staging rather than a true therapeutic effect. Another explanation may be that extensive lymphadenectomy reflects overall better care. The use of Radiation therapy responding to positivity of para-aortic nodes may be another explanation of better survival in patients submitted to this procedure [54].

The risks of paraortic nodal involvement are essentially the same that predicts the pelvic nodal spread (depth of myometrial invasion, nuclear grading, and the presence of lymph-vascular space involvement) [46,55]. Mariani et al. showed that patients at high risk for para-aortic nodal disease (based on invasion >50%, palpable positive pelvic nodes, positive adnexa) who did not have para-aortic dissection or who had biopsy only and who were managed as though para-aortic nodes were positive had 5-year survival of 71% compared to 85% for those patients with positive para-aortic nodes who did undergo complete resection [56].

At the present time, the superior extent of para-aortic dissection should be at least to the level of the inferior mesenteric artery (IMA). The Mayo Clinic group retrospectively in their series observed that the routinely performed lymphadenectomies only up to the IMA potentially miss 38% to 46% of patients with positive para-aortic nodes because of the high rate of isolated involvement above the IMA. Furthermore, 63% of patients in Mayo's series with positive lymph nodes below the IMA also had positive nodes above the IMA that would have escaped detection if the dissection had been limited to the lower node basins. Thus, the node-bearing tissue between the IMA and the renal vessels appears in their experience of outmost importance for the assessment of the extent of disease and thus for determination of overall treatment dispositions. [56] This extended para-aortic dissection is feasible laparoscopically as well laparotomically [57]. Prospective data describing the frequency of high para-aortic/renal nodes are awaited.

More recently a large prospective trial compared the outcomes after complete pelvic lymphadenectomy or combined pelvic and para-aortic lymphadenectomy. The trial was non-randomized and was conducted at two sites, one in which pelvic lymphadenectomy was standard and a second where combined pelvic and para-aortic dissection was standard. More than 600 women were included. The authors report significantly increased overall survival in women undergoing para-aortic dissection and argue that women at intermediate or high risk of disease recurrence should have both pelvic and para-aortic lymphadenectomy [58]. No benefit was seen in low risk patients. Although the groups were comparable in most respects with a similar proportion of non-endometrioid carcinomas, 77% of women in the pelvic/para-aortic group received systemic chemotherapy compared with only 45% of women in the pelvic node group. These results do not argue convincingly for para-aortic lymphadenectomy in women at higher risk of disease recurrence or distant metastasis but do suggest that this is an area that should be addressed by a properly constructed clinical trial.

A recent Cochrane Review [59] assessed that published data do not support the routine use of pelvic lymphadenectomy in the treatment of endometrial cancer thought to be confined to the uterus at presentation. There was no statistically significant difference in survival between the groups. Meta-analysis indicated no significant difference in overall and recurrence-free survival between women who received lymphadenectomy and those who received no lymphadenectomy (pooled HR = 1.07, 95% CI: 0.81 to 1.43 and HR = 1.23, 95% CI: 0.96 to 1.58 for overall and recurrence-free survival respectively) and, in terms of harmful effects of treatment, women who did not receive lymphadenectomy showed a clear benefit. No good quality data were found which assessed the role of para-aortic lymphadenectomy, or removal of grossly enlarged lymph nodes. Further research is needed to allow more individualized treatment strategies, ensuring that women with more aggressive cancers receive appropriate treatment, whilst not exposing women with a better prognosis to potentially serious side effects. In addition, it is imperative to assess the impact of any intervention on quality of life in any future study, particularly for a cancer with good survival rates.

Although lymphadenectomy continues to be controversial for some, over the last 30 years our knowledge of the lymph node involvement in endometrial cancer has increased and how that information can be used to benefit our patients. Lymphadenectomy in endometrial cancer is certainly diagnostic and it may be also therapeutic if systematic pelvic and para-aortic procedures are performed. At the present time low risk patients can avoid this surgical assessment but there is no general agreement in the definition of the "low risk category". Recent data, and a new molecular staging system could improve our knowledge and would probably lead to a consensus in the near future.

2. Debulking

Endometrial cancer is often diagnosed at a stage I disease (71%) [60]. A low percentage of cases present at an advanced stage, defined by FIGO stage III and IV. Nonetheless, rare histopathologic types of endometrial cancer, such as papillary-serous (4% of cases) and clear cell carcinomas (2% of cases) frequently present at an advanced stage, both accounting for 14% of advanced stage (FIGO III and IV) compared with 4% of early stage (FIGO I and II) endometrial cancer patients [61,62].

The management of endometrial cancer is reviewed in several papers; still, limited evidence is available how to manage patients with advanced stage disease. The treatment of this relatively rare group of patients is frequently individualised and it depends on the surgical ability to resect disease.

In patients with macroscopic intraperitoneal disease it is debated if optimal surgical cytoreduction is indicated, and in these cases options include the resection of the easily removable disease such as uterus, adnexa, and omentum, versus performing a wider cytoreductive effort. Different retrospective studies evaluated the impact of surgical cytoreduction on the outcome of advanced endometrial cancer patients, suggesting that survival correlates with the volume of residual disease.

Goff et al [63] analysed 47 cases of stage IV endometrial cancer, observing a statistically significant improvement of median survival in the cases of no bulky disease at the end of surgery compared to patients not completely cytoreducted (18 vs. 8 months respectively).
Chi et al [64] also found a significatively longer median survival in the subgroup of patients treated with optimal cytoreduction (residual tumor < 2 cm) among 55 cases of stage IV endometrial cancer, compared to patients with residual tumor > 2 cm (31 months vs. 12 months).
Bristow et al [65] defines optimal cytoreduction as largest residual tumor < 1 cm and showed that median survival was 34 months after optimal cytoreduction compared to 11 months when suboptimal cytoreduction was performed, with a residual tumor > 1 cm, and again the difference were statistically significative.
In conclusion, it can be assessed that in all cases with no firm contraindication for surgery, primary treatment should include surgery, with an exception for patients with distant metastases: for these cases there may be a limited role of surgery such as to provide control of vaginal bleeding.
Still, the warranty for an optimal cytoreduction in cases with disease outside the uterus is only based on some retrospective studies made on relative small number of patients, different stage of disease are often included and different definitions of surgical cytoreduction are employed. Thus, these studies are difficult to compare, and no randomized trial has been carried out to confirm the advantage of optimal cytoreduction on survival.
Nonetheless, available data suggest that an optimal cytoreduction in advanced stage endometrial cancer is associated with improved survival of these patients.

3. Refferences

[1] Global cancer statistics. Jemal A, Bray F, Center MM, Ferlay J, Ward E, Forman D.CA Cancer J Clin. 2011 Mar-Apr;61(2):69-90. Epub 2011 Feb 4.

[2] Carcinoma of the corpus uteri. FIGO 26th Annual Report on the Results of Treatment in Gynecological Cancer.Creasman WT, Odicino F, Maisonneuve P, Quinn MA, Beller U, Benedet JL, Heintz AP, Ngan HY, Pecorelli S. Int J Gynaecol Obstet. 2006 Nov;95 Suppl 1:S105-43.

[3] Revised FIGO staging for carcinoma of the vulva, cervix, and endometrium. Pecorelli S. Int J Gynaecol Obstet. 2009 May;105(2):103-4.

[4] J Clin Oncol. 2007 Jul 1;25(19):2798-803. Multicenter phase II study of fertility-sparing treatment with medroxyprogesterone acetate for endometrial carcinoma and atypical hyperplasia in young women. Ushijima K, Yahata H, Yoshikawa H, Konishi I, Yasugi T, Saito T, Nakanishi T, Sasaki H, Saji F, Iwasaka T, Hatae M, Kodama S, Saito T, Terakawa N, Yaegashi N, Hiura M, Sakamoto A, Tsuda H, Fukunaga M, Kamura T.

[5] Outcome of fertility-sparing treatment with progestins in young patients with endometrial cancer. Gotlieb WH, Beiner ME, Shalmon B, Korach Y, Segal Y, Zmira N, Koupolovic J, Ben-Baruch G. Obstet Gynecol. 2003 Oct;102(4):718-25. Review.

[6] Progestin alone as primary treatment of endometrial carcinoma in premenopausal women. Report of seven cases and review of the literature. Kim YB, Holschneider CH, Ghosh K, Nieberg RK, Montz FJ. Cancer. 1997 Jan 15;79(2):320-7.

[7] Hormonal therapy for the management of grade 1 endometrial adenocarcinoma: a literature review. Ramirez PT, Frumovitz M, Bodurka DC, Sun CC, Levenback C. Gynecol Oncol. 2004 Oct;95(1):133-8.
[8] Intraoperative evaluation of depth of myometrial invasion in stage I endometrial adenocarcinoma. Doering DL, Barnhill D, Weiser EB, Burke TW, Woodward JE, Park RC. Obstet Gynecol 1989
[9] Clinical value of intraoperative gross examination in endometrial cancer. Franchi M, Ghezzi F, Melpignano M, Cherchi PL, Scarabelli C, Apolloni C, et al. Gynecol Oncol 2000;76:357
[10] Accuracy of intraoperative frozen-section diagnosis in stage I endometrial adenocarcinoma. .Kucera E, Kainz C, Reinthaller A, Sliutz G, Leodolter S, Kucera H, et al. Gynecol Obstet Invest 2000;49:62
[11] Predictive Value of Magnetic Resonance Imaging in Assessing Myometrial Invasion in Endometrial Cancer. Is Radiological Staging Sufficient for Planning Conservative Treatment? Cade TJ, MBBS, Quinn MA, McNally OM, Neesham D, Pyman J, Dobrotwir A. Int J Gynecol Cancer 2010;20: 1166
[12] Feasibility of ovarian preservation in patients with early stage endometrial carcinoma. Lee TS, Jung JY, Kim JW, Park NH, Song YS, Kang SB, Lee HP. Gynecol Oncol. 2007 Jan;104(1):52-7.
[13] Responses to estradiol in a human endometrial adenocarcinoma cell line (Ishikawa). Holinka CF, Hata H, Kuramoto H, Gurpide E. J Steroid Biochem. 1986 Jan;24(1):85-9.
[14] Association of exogenous estrogen and endometrial carcinoma. Smith DC, Prentice R, Thompson DJ, Herrmann WL. N Engl J Med. 1975 Dec 4;293(23):1164-7.
[15] Increased risk of endometrial carcinoma among users of conjugated estrogens. Ziel HK, Finkle WD. N Engl J Med. 1975 Dec 4;293(23):1167-70.
[16] Coexisting ovarian malignancy in young women with endometrial cancer. Walsh C, Holschneider C, Hoang Y, Tieu K, Karlan B, Cass I. Obstet Gynecol. 2005 Oct;106(4):693-9.
[17] Hereditary colorectal cancer syndromes: molecular genetics, genetic counseling, diagnosis and management. Lynch HT, Lynch JF, Lynch PM, Attard T. Fam Cancer. 2008;7(1):27-39
[18] Evaluation of different surgical approaches in the treatment of endometrial cancer at FIGO stage I. Candiani GB, Belloni C, Maggi R, Colombo G, Frigoli A, Carinelli SG. Gynecol Oncol. 1990 Apr;37(1):6-8.
[19] Vaginal hysterectomy versus abdominal hysterectomy for the treatment of stage I endometrial adenocarcinoma. Massi G, Savino L, Susini T. Am J Obstet Gynecol. 1996 Apr;174(4):1320-6.
[20] Role of vaginal surgery in the 1st stage endometrial cancer. Experience of the Florence School. Scarselli G, Savino L, Ceccherini R, Barciulli F, Massi GB. Eur J Gynaecol Oncol. 1992;13(1 Suppl):15-9.
[21] Use of vaginal hysterectomy for the management of stage I endometrial cancer in the medically compromised patient. Bloss JD, Berman ML, Bloss LP, Buller RE. Gynecol Oncol. 1991 Jan;40(1):74-7.
[22] Lymph node yield from laparoscopic lymphadenectomy in cervical cancer: a comparative study. Fowler JM, Carter JR, Carlson JW, Maslonkowski R, Byers LJ, Carson LF, Twiggs LB. Gynecol Oncol. 1993 Nov;51(2):187-92.

[23] Combined laparoscopic and vaginal surgery for the management of two cases of stage I endometrial cancer. Childers JM, Surwit EA. Gynecol Oncol. 1992 Apr;45(1):46-51.

[24] Laparoscopic lymphadenectomy and vaginal or laparoscopic hysterectomy with bilateral salpingo-oophorectomy for endometrial cancer: morbidity and survival. Magrina JF, Mutone NF, Weaver AL, Magtibay PM, Fowler RS, Cornella JL. Am J Obstet Gynecol. 1999 Aug;181(2):376-81.

[25] Laparoscopic-assisted vaginal hysterectomy for endometrial cancer: clinical outcomes and hospital charges. Gemignani ML, Curtin JP, Zelmanovich J, Patel DA, Venkatraman E, Barakat RR. Gynecol Oncol. 1999 Apr;73(1):5-11.

[26] Feasibility of laparoscopic management of presumed stage I endometrial carcinoma and assessment of accuracy of myoinvasion estimates by frozen section: a gynecologic oncology group study. Homesley HD, Boike G, Spiegel GW. Int J Gynecol Cancer. 2004 Mar-Apr;14(2):341-7.

[27] Laparoscopic-assisted vaginal versus abdominal surgery in patients with endometrial cancer--a prospective randomized trial. Malur S, Possover M, Michels W, Schneider A. Gynecol Oncol. 2001 Feb;80(2):239-44.

[28] Analysis of survival after laparoscopy in women with endometrial carcinoma. Eltabbakh GH. Cancer. 2002 Nov 1;95(9):1894-901.

[29] Laparoscopy compared with laparotomy for comprehensive surgical staging of uterine cancer: Gynecologic Oncology Group Study LAP2. Walker JL, Piedmonte MR, Spirtos NM, Eisenkop SM, Schlaerth JB, Mannel RS, Spiegel G, Barakat R, Pearl ML, Sharma SK. J Clin Oncol. 2009 Nov 10;27(32):5331-6.

[30] Quality of life of patients with endometrial cancer undergoing laparoscopic International Federation of Gynecology and Obstetrics staging compared with laparotomy: a Gynecologic Oncology Group study. Kornblith AB, Huang HQ, Walker JL, Spirtos NM, Rotmensch J, Cella D. J Clin Oncol 2009;27:5337–42.

[31] Surgical manangement of early stage endometrial cancer in the elderly: is laparoscopy feasible? Scribner D, Walker J, Johnson G, et al. Gynecol Oncol 2001;83:563–568.

[32] Hysterectomy for obese women with endometrial cancer: laparoscopy or laparotomy. Eltabbakh G, Shamonki M, Moody J Gynecol Oncol 2000;78:329–335

[33] Total laparoscopic hysterectomy for uterine pathology: impact of body mass index on outcomes. O'Hanlan K, Dibble S, Fisher D. Gynecol Oncol 2006;103:938–941

[34] Phase III trial of laparoscopy versus laparotomy for surgical resection and comprehensive surgical staging of uterine cancer: a Gynecologic Oncology Group study. Walker J, Mannel R, Piedmonte M, et al. Gynecol Oncol 2006;101(S1):11–12; abstr 22.

[35] What is the optimal minimally invasive surgical procedure for endometrial cancer staging in the obese and morbidly obese woman? Gehrig PA, Cantrell LA, Shafer A, Abaid LN, Mendivil A, Boggess JF. Gynecol Oncol. 2008 Oct;111(1):41-5.

[36] Randomised study of radical surgery versus radiotherapy for stage Ib-IIa cervical cancer. Landoni F, Maneo A, Colombo A, Placa F, Milani R, Perego P, Favini G, Ferri L, Mangioni C. Lancet. 1997 Aug 23;350(9077):535-40.

[37] Modified radical hysterectomy versus extrafascial hysterectomy in the treatment of stage I endometrial cancer: results from the ILIADE randomized study. Signorelli M, Lissoni AA, Cormio G, Katsaros D, Pellegrino A, Selvaggi L, Ghezzi F, Scambia

G, Zola P, Grassi R, Milani R, Giannice R, Caspani G, Mangioni C, Floriani I, Rulli E, Fossati R. Ann Surg Oncol. 2009 Dec;16(12):3431-41.

[38] Surgical pathologic spread patterns of endometrial cancer. A Gynecologic Oncology Group Study. Creasman WT, Morrow CP, Bundy BN, Homesley HD, Graham JE, Heller PB. Cancer. 1987 Oct 15;60(8 Suppl):2035-41.

[39] The incidence of pelvic lymph node metastasis by FIGO staging for patients with adequately surgically staged endometrial adenocarcinoma of endometrioid histology. Chi DS, Barakat RR, Palayekar MJ, Levine DA, Sonoda Y, Alektiar K, Brown CL, Abu-Rustum NR. Int J Gynecol Cancer. 2008 Mar-Apr;18(2):269-73.

[40] The morbidity of surgery and adjuvant radiotherapy in the management of endometrial carcinoma. Nunns D, Williamson K, Swaney L, Davy M. Int J Gynecol Cancer. 2000 May;10(3):233-238.

[41] Uterine papillary serous carcinoma: patterns of metastatic spread. Goff BA, Kato D, Schmidt RA, Ek M, Ferry JA, Muntz HG, Cain JM, Tamimi HK, Figge DC, Greer BE. Gynecol Oncol. 1994 Sep;54(3):264-8.

[42] Twelve-year experience in the management of endometrial cancer: a change in surgical and postoperative radiation approaches. Barakat RR, Lev G, Hummer AJ, Sonoda Y, Chi DS, Alektiar KM, Abu-Rustum NR. Gynecol Oncol. 2007 Apr;105(1):150-6.

[43] The impact of complete surgical staging on adjuvant treatment decisions in endometrial cancer. Goudge C, Bernhard S, Cloven NG, Morris P. Gynecol Oncol. 2004 May;93(2):536-9.

[44] Efficacy of systematic pelvic lymphadenectomy in endometrial cancer (MRC ASTEC trial): a randomised study. ASTEC study group, Kitchener H, Swart AM, Qian Q, Amos C, Parmar MK. Lancet. 2009 Jan 10;373(9658):125-36.

[45] Systematic pelvic lymphadenectomy vs. no lymphadenectomy in early-stage endometrial carcinoma: randomized clinical trial. Benedetti Panici P, Basile S, Maneschi F, Alberto Lissoni A, Signorelli M, Scambia G, Angioli R, Tateo S, Mangili G, Katsaros D, Garozzo G, Campagnutta E, Donadello N, Greggi S, Melpignano M, Raspagliesi F, Ragni N, Cormio G, Grassi R, Franchi M, Giannarelli D, Fossati R, Torri V, Amoroso M, Crocè C, Mangioni C. J Natl Cancer Inst. 2008 Dec 3;100(23):1707-16.

[46] Analysis of clinicopathologic factors predicting para-aortic lymph node metastasis in endometrial cancer. Nomura H, Aoki D, Suzuki N, Susumu N, Suzuki A, Tamada Y, Kataoka F, Higashiguchi A, Ezawa S, Nozawa S. Int J Gynecol Cancer. 2006 Mar-Apr;16(2):799-804.

[47] Retrospective analysis of selective lymphadenectomy in apparent early-stage endometrial cancer. Cragun JM, Havrilesky LJ, Calingaert B, Synan I, Secord AA, Soper JT, Clarke-Pearson DL, Berchuck A. J Clin Oncol. 2005 Jun 1;23(16):3668-75.

[48] Analysis of FIGO Stage IIIc endometrial cancer patients. McMeekin DS, Lashbrook D, Gold M, Johnson G, Walker JL, Mannel R. Gynecol Oncol. 2001 May;81(2):273-8.

[49] Advanced endometrial cancer: is lymphadenectomy necessary or sufficient? Scott Miller D. Gynecol Oncol. 2006 May;101(2):191-3.

[50] A clinical and pathologic study on para-aortic lymph node metastasis in endometrial carcinoma. Hirahatake K, Hareyama H, Sakuragi N, Nishiya M, Makinoda S, Fujimoto S. J Surg Oncol 1997;65:82–7.

[51] Indispensability of pelvic and paraaortic lymphadenectomy in endometrial cancers. Gynecol Oncol 1997;64:411–7. Yokoyama Y, Maruyama H, Sato S, Saito Y
[52] Lymphatic drainage of the uterus: preliminary results of an experimental study [French]. Lécuru F, Neji K, Robin F, Darles C, de Bièvre P, Taurelle R. J Gynecol Obstet Biol Reprod (Paris) 1997;26:418–23.
[53] Route of lymphatic spread: a study of 112 consecutive patients with endometrial cancer. Mariani A, Webb MJ, Keeney GL, Podratz KC. Gynecol Oncol 2001;81:100–4.
[54] The outcomes of 27,063 women with unstaged endometrioid uterine cancer. Chan JK, Wu H, Cheung MK, Shin JY, Osann K, Kapp DS. Gynecol Oncol. 2007 Aug;106(2):282-8.
[55] The role of pelvic and/or para-aortic lymphadenectomy in surgical management of apparently early carcinosarcoma of uterus. Park JY, Kim DY, Kim JH, Kim YM, Kim YT, Nam JH. Ann Surg Oncol. 2010 Mar;17(3):861-8.
[56] Prospective assessment of lymphatic dissemination in endometrial cancer: a paradigm shift in surgical staging. Mariani A, Dowdy SC, Cliby WA, Gostout BS, Jones MB, Wilson TO, Podratz KC. Gynecol Oncol. 2008 Apr;109(1):11-8.
[57] Laparoscopic paraaortic left-sided transperitoneal infrarenal lymphadenectomy in patients with gynecologic malignancies: technique and results. Köhler C, Tozzi R, Klemm P, Schneider A. Gynecol Oncol. 2003 Oct;91(1):139-48.
[58] Survival effect of para-aortic lymphadenectomy in endometrial cancer (SEPAL study): a retrospective cohort analysis. Todo Y, Kato H, Kaneuchi M, Watari H, Takeda M, Sakuragi N. Lancet. 2010 Apr 3;375(9721):1165-72.
[59] Lymphadenectomy for the management of endometrial cancer (Review) May K, Bryant A, Dickinson HO, Kehoe S, Morrison J The Cochrane Library 2010, Issue 1
[60] F.H. van Wijk, M.E.L. van der Burg, Curt W. Burgeret al. Management of Surgical Stage III and IV Endometrioid Endometrial Carcinoma. An Overview. Int J Gynecol Cancer 2009;19: 431-446
[61] Creasman W, Odicino F, Maisonneuve P, et al. Carcinoma of the corpus uteri. Int J Gynaecol Obstet. 2006;95:S105-S143.
[62] Boruta DM 2nd, Gehrig PA, Groben PA, et al. Uterine serous and grade 3 endometrioid carcinomas: is there a survival difference? Cancer. 2004;101:2214-2221
[63] Goff BA, Goodman A, Muntz HG, et al. Surgical stage IV endometrial carcinoma: a study of 47 cases. Gynecol Oncol. 1994;52: 237-240.
[64] Chi DS, Welshinger M, Venkatraman ES, et al. The role of surgical cytoreduction in Stage IV endometrial carcinoma. Gynecol Oncol. 1997;67:56-60.
[65] Bristow RE, Zerbe MJ, Rosenshein NB, et al. Stage IVB endometrial carcinoma: the role of cytoreductive surgery and determinants of survival. Gynecol Oncol. 2000;78:85-91.

7

Controversies Regarding the Utility of Lymphadenectomy in Endometrial Cancer

Frederik Peeters and Lucy Gilbert
McGill University
Canada

1. Introduction

The value of lymphadenectomy (LND) in the management of endometrial cancer remains controversial. Although it is required for the surgical staging of the disease (FIGO 2009) and its prognostic value is indisputable, its therapeutic benefit remains a matter of debate. Furthermore, systematic pelvic (PLND) and para-aortic lymphadenectomy (PaLND) cause morbidity, even when performed using minimally invasive surgical techniques. A reliable means of sentinel lymph node (SLN) mapping may be the way forward. In this chapter we review the literature surrounding this topic, identify areas for research and suggest a pragmatic approach to managing this dilemma.

2. Overview

The lifetime risk of a woman in the United States to develop uterine cancer is 2.5%. It is the fourth most common cancer in women and accounts for 6% of all female cancers and 3% of cancer-related deaths (Jemal et al., 2010). Two different clinico-pathological subtypes of endometrial cancer are recognized: Type I, which is endometrioid and estrogen-related, and Type II, which is non-endometrioid and non-estrogen-related.

When the disease is confined to the uterus, a hysterectomy and bilateral salpingo oophorectomy would constitute adequate treatment. If the disease has spread outside the uterus, adjuvant treatment is required to maximize the potential for cure. At the time of diagnosis approximately 85% of endometrioid cancers are confined to the uterine corpus and are therefore associated with a favorable five-year survival rate of 83% (Creasman et al., 2006). In the Western world at least 85% of newly diagnosed endometrial cancers are endometrioid in type (Amant et al., 2005; Creasman et al., 2006). As the propensity for lymph node metastasis in these patients can vary from clinically negligible to 20%, depending on the grade and stage of presentation, management of this subtype is fraught with ambiguity. In non-endometrioid cancers, 35% have already spread beyond the uterine corpus at presentation. Among the non-endometrioid uterine cancers, clear cell and papillary serous cancers are the worst offenders, with extra-uterine metastasis occurring in 33% and 41% of cases, respectively, which is reflected in correspondingly low five-year survival rates of 63% and 53%, respectively (Creasman et al., 2006).

Following primary surgical treatment, adjuvant treatment is tailored according to the risk of lymph node metastasis and recurrent disease. The current method of risk stratification uses patient-related factors as well as the definitive pathological findings identified to be associated with increased risk of lymph node metastasis and recurrence to group patients into low-, intermediate- and high-risk categories. Other determinate factors are age, tumor grade, non-endometrioid subtype and extension of the disease, including depth of myometrial invasion and lymphovascular space invasion (LVSI) (Creasman et al., 1987; Kadar et al., 1992; Keys et al., 2004; Morrow et al., 1991).

Risk group			Risk of metastatic LN (%)	Risk of recurrence at 5 years (%)
Low		Ia, Grade I & II	<3	<5
Intermediate Risk factors (RF): age, grade III, LVSI present, deep myometrial invasion (>50%)	Low	others	3-5	10-15
	High	≥70 years + 1 RF ≥50 years + 2 RF any age with 3 RF	10-30	20-25
High		Stage II-IV, non-endometrioid uterine cancers	>30	>25

Table 1. Classification of endometrial cancers adjusted to FIGO 2009.

The disadvantage of this system is that lymph node metastasis is presumed rather than known for certain, and a proportion of patients will be over-treated with adjuvant treatment. Furthermore, if removal of the affected nodes has a therapeutic value, and evidence suggests it has (please refer to section 6), patients would miss out on the survival advantage conferred by a systematic lymphadenectomy. Having access to information about lymph node status pre-operatively would allow surgery to be tailored accordingly. Below, we discuss the currently available methods for pre-operative assessment of the spread of disease.

3. Pre-operative assessment of the spread of disease

3.1 CA 125

Four studies have evaluated the role of CA 125 in evaluation of patients with endometrial cancer. All four conclude that a high CA 125 cut-off, ranging from 20 to 40U/ml., is an independent risk factor for extra-uterine disease or lymph node metastasis. Nevertheless, its sensitivity and specificity are only around 80% (Chung et al., 2006; Han et al., 2010; Hsieh et al., 2002; Sood et al., 1997). This means that 1 in 5 patients will be over-treated and 1 in 5 undertreated.

3.2 Imaging

3.2.1 Ultrasound

Most patients with endometrial cancer will have a transvaginal ultrasound (TVS) as it is the imaging procedure of choice to assess post-menopausal bleeding, the most common presenting symptom. TVS is a non-invasive, readily available and inexpensive test that has a very high sensitivity of 96% for raising suspicion about the presence of endometrial cancer when using a cut-off of ≥5mm endometrial thickness. Its specificity varies between 61% and 81% for all endometrial diseases (Fleischer, 1997; Smith-Bindman et al., 1998). False-negative rates have been reported at around 1% and are due to adenomyosis or distortion of the endometrial lining by fibroids (Smith-Bindman et al., 1998). If morphologic features such as endometrial heterogeneity were added to endometrial thickness, then specificity and the false-negative rate might be improved (Dubinsky, 2004).

After the diagnosis of endometrial cancer is made, TVS could provide information about the depth of myometrial invasion. Loubeyre et al. (2011) reviewed the correlation between the depth of myometrial invasion on TVS and the final pathology in eight studies with a total of 605 patients with endometrial cancer. They found the sensitivity to be 80% (range 58% to 95%) and so too the specificity (range 71% to 92%). Evaluation of cervical involvement by TVS is less informative, with sensitivities varying between 54% and 88% and specificity between 87% and 100% (Celik et al., 2010; Lee et al., 2011; Loubeyre et al., 2011).

The weaknesses of TVS are that it is operator-dependent and lymph nodes cannot be properly evaluated.

3.2.2 CT

CT scan is considered inferior to TVS in determining the depth of myometrial invasion (accuracy around 60%). The ability of CT scan to identify cervical involvement has not been properly investigated. The value of multidetector CT in the staging of endometrial cancer has yet to be explored (Lee et al., 2011; Loubeyre et al., 2011). Using a 1cm cut-off to evaluate pelvic and para-aortic lymph nodes, the sensitivity of CT is only 50% (range 44% to 66%)—no better than flipping a coin; its specificity is 95% (range 73% to 98%) (Lee et al., 2011). This poor correlation is due to the fact that only 39% of metastatic lymph nodes are enlarged and 37% are smaller than 2mm (Creasman et al., 1987; Mariani et al., 2000). For the same reason, MRI and PET-CT have similar results in detecting metastatic lymph nodes.

3.2.3 MRI

The imaging procedure of choice to assess patients with endometrial cancer is MRI, but it is an expensive test and, as mentioned before, is ineffective in detecting metastatic lymph nodes. However, MRI is superior to TVS and CT in evaluating the depth of myometrial invasion as well as cervical involvement (Loubreyre et al., 2011; Lee et al., 2011, on behalf of the American College of Radiology). Loubeyre et al. (2011) reviewed the correlation between depth of myometrial invasion on MRI and final pathology in nine studies with a total of 1,115 patients with endometrial cancer. Sensitivity ranged from 56% to 88% and specificity from 74% to 100%. This group also reviewed the correlation between cervical involvement on MRI and final pathology in five studies with a total of 623 patients with endometrial cancer. Sensitivity ranged from 47% to 72% and specificity from 83% to 100%. In its pre-treatment evaluation of endometrial cancer, the American College of Radiology indicates that the accuracy of MRI in predicting myometrial involvement ranges from 85% to 92%, cervical involvement from 86% to 95% and overall staging from 85% to 93% (Lee et al., 2011).

3.2.4 PET

The role of PET in endometrial cancer is more in the detection of disease recurrence than in the pre-operative evaluation of extra-uterine disease (Lee et al., 2011).

4. Pre-operative assessment of grade and histological subtype of the disease

4.1 Pathology

In addition to a TVS, a patient with post-menopausal bleeding needs a tissue diagnosis. This can be done by pipelle biopsy (office endometrial biopsy) or dilatation and curettage (D&C). The sensitivity of pipelle biopsy in detecting endometrial cancer is 99.6%. The sensitivity of D&C is similar; it serves as the diagnostic procedure when pipelle biopsy is not feasible or is inadequate (Dijkhuizen et al., 2000). After the diagnosis of endometrial cancer is made, pre-operative assessment of the aggressiveness of the disease is very important to tailor the surgery. Patients with a high-grade endometrial cancer have a 15% to 20% risk of having metastatic lymph nodes (Creasman et al., 1987). Therefore, the ability to grade the tumor accurately on the diagnostic sample, be it a pipelle biopsy or a D&C, is crucial.

A D&C reflects the final FIGO grade more accurately than a pipelle biopsy. Leitao et al., (2009) reported a higher grade at the time of hysterectomy in 8.7% of patients when the diagnosis was made with a D&C, compared to 17.4% with a pipelle biopsy. Obermaier et al. (1999) found that 20% of Grade 1 endometrial cancers on D&C were upgraded to Grade 2 (or Grade 3 in 2% to 3% of cases) while 4% were downgraded at final pathology. In summary, pre-operative FIGO Grade 1 endometrioid endometrial cancer correlates in 80% to 85% of cases with the grade on the final hysterectomy specimen. The difference between pipelle biopsy and D&C does not warrant extra anesthesia. Changing from the three-grade FIGO system to a binary system does not improve accuracy sufficiently to warrant replacing the FIGO system, which is currently in use worldwide. However, molecular tests may have greater potential to support the binary system in the future (Clarke & Gilks, 2010). In a review of Stage III cases treated at our institution, we found that less than half were suspected preoperatively (Denschlag et al., 2007). A recent French multicentre study on sentinel lymph node mapping, found that 29% of tumors thought to be grade 1 preoperatively or intraoperatively, were upgraded to grade 2 or 3 or at final histology and 7% of patients thought to have type I tumors had type 2 endometrial cancer at definitive histology (Ballester et all 2010).

4.2 Conclusion

Identifying metastatic lymph nodes by currently available imaging techniques is only as sensitive as flipping a coin (50%). Assessing risk factors for metastatic lymph nodes, such as depth of myometrial invasion and cervical involvement, is most accurate with MRI, reaching at least 85% (in study circumstances) for both risk factors. Pre-operative assessment of Grade 1 tumors correlates with the final grade in 80% to 85% of cases.

This means that approximately one patient in five is underestimated pre-operatively for risk factors that include depth of myometrial invasion and/or cervical involvement and/or tumor grade. Consequently, tailoring surgery based on pre-operative assessment alone is not adequate.

5. Intra-operative assessment

5.1 Palpation of lymph nodes

Intra-operative palpation of pelvic or para-aortic lymph nodes will reveal only 39% of the metastatic lymph nodes (Mariani et al., 2000). Creasman et al. (1987) have already shown that 37% of metastatic lymph nodes are smaller than 2mm. So neither pre-operative imaging nor intra-operative palpation is accurate enough to dispense with surgical excision.

5.2 Gross inspection

Assessment of the depth of myometrial invasion of an endometrial cancer by gross visual examination has been studied in three prospective studies (ranging from 148 to 403 patients). Compared to definite hystopathological findings, sensitivity varies from 71% to 79% and specificity from 93% to 96%. Evaluation of cervical involvement by gross inspection has never been studied (Loubreyre et al., 2011).

5.3 Frozen section

Given our inability to predict lymph node metastasis pre-operatively with accuracy, can intra-operative frozen section analysis help determine which patients should have a systematic PLND and PaLND? The literature on this is conflicting.

Correlations of 58% to 96% for grade with intra-operative frozen section analysis and final pathologic results have been reported. A similar variation is reported in the accuracy of intra-operative section analysis of depth of myometrial invasion (72% to 95%) as well as of cervical involvement (66% to 97%) (Frumovitz et al., 2004; Loubeyre et al., 2011).

Several retrospective studies, which used a combination of risk factors (grade and depth of myometrial invasion, histological subtype) to compare intra-operative frozen section analysis and final pathologic results, found that the correlation was not sufficient to dispense with surgical staging (Frumovitz et al., 2004; Denschlag et al., 2007; Papadia et al., 2009). According to Papadia et al., 78% of patients undergo appropriate surgery, while 16% are under-staged and 6% over-staged.

5.4 Adding tumor size

In an attempt to increase the accuracy of frozen section analysis, several investigators have studied the benefit of factoring in tumor size as determined intraoperatively. In 1987 Schink et al. described that patients with clinical Stage 1 endometrial cancer had only a 4% risk of lymph node metastasis if their endometrial cancer was ≤2cm. The Mayo Clinic in Rochester, Minnesota, uses a thorough intra-operative frozen section to identify a sub-group of patients with endometrioid adenocarcinoma in whom the risk of lymph node metastasis is negligible and who therefore do not warrant lymphadenectomy. The characteristics are: Type I, Grades 1 and 2; myometrial invasion less than 50%; primary tumor diameter less than 2cm, (Mariani et al. 2008).

The concept of adding tumor size to improve the ability of frozen section to correctly identify low-risk patients was evaluated by Yanazume et al. (2011) in a retrospective study of 228 patients. They used tumor size of ≤3cm as their cut off. This study found that a Grade 1 or 2 endometrial cancer, with a tumor diameter of ≤3cm and ≤50% myometrial invasion, accurately predicts the absence of lymph node metastasis.

5.5 Conclusion

The palpation of lymph nodes during a laparotomy should not be used to determine the need for a systematic PLND and PaLND. Frozen section analysis is useful to distinguish a benign from a malignant lesion, but it has limitations with regard to time involvement, inadequate sampling (only part of the tumor) and the technique of rapid freezing itself. However, despite these constraints, a detailed and thorough intra-operative frozen section that assesses subtype, grade, myometrial invasion and tumor size is preferable to the alternatives, namely, that of an unnecessary lymphadenectomy with its attendant complications in low risk patients, or not carrying out a systematic lymphadenectomy in patients at high risk of lymph node metastasis.

6. Surgical staging

As discussed in the previous section, it is clear that surgical staging and knowledge of lymph node status plays a very important role in the management of patients with endometrial cancer. What is not clear is what constitutes an adequate LND. The practice varies from selective sampling of accessible nodes to systematic LND. Is the latter necessary? Is a PLND adequate or is a PaLND required in addition to a PLND? If a PaLND is required, what are the limits of dissection? What are the additional risks of a LND? When are these additional risks justified? Does LND have a therapeutic effect? Below, we discuss the studies that have tried to address these questions.

6.1 Definitions

For a systematic PLND, all lymph nodes and fatty tissue between the external and internal iliac arteries, from the bifurcation of the common iliac artery up to the circumflex vein and above the obturator nerve, should be removed. A systematic PaLND includes resection of all lymph nodes and fatty tissue overlying the common iliac artery, vena cava and aorta anteriorly up to the renal vessels and extending laterally to the edge of the psoas major muscle.

6.2 The randomized controlled trials on lymphadenectomy

To date, two randomized controlled trials (Benedetti Panici et al. in 2008 and the MRC ASTEC trial 2009) have investigated whether the addition of PLND to standard hysterectomy with bilateral salpingo-oophorectomy improved overall survival and disease-free survival in patients with preoperative Stage I endometrial cancer.

6.2.1 Benedetti Panici et al., 2008

In this Italian RCT, the role of systemic PLND or no PLND in early-stage endometrioid or adenosquamous endometrial cancer (FIGO 1988) was examined. Patients with Stages IA and IB Grade I, were excluded; 514 patients were randomized to undergo PLND (n=264) or not (n=250). A minimum of 22 PLNs were removed; median was 30. PaLND and adjuvant radiotherapy were left to the discretion of the treating physician; 26% in the PLND group had PaLND compared to 2% in the no-PLND group; the median number of PaLN's removed in the LND group was four. The proportion of patients who received adjuvant radiotherapy was similar in both groups: ±31-35%. At a median follow-up time of 49 months, no difference in the disease-free or overall survival rates was seen between the two groups. The estimated blood loss and the number of intra-operative complications were similar in both arms, but operating time and hospital stay were longer in the PLND group. Furthermore, more post-operative complications were noted in the PLND group, predominantly due to the formation of lymphocysts and lymphedema (35 versus 4). The PLND group was diagnosed with 13% metastatic LN versus only 3% in the no-PLND group. The authors concluded that although disease-free or overall survival is not improved, a systemic PLND significantly improved surgical staging.

6.2.2 ASTEC Trial, 2009

Eighty-five centers in four countries participated in the ASTEC Trial, randomizing 1,408 women with histologically proven endometrial cancer that was pre-operatively (clinically) thought to be confined to the uterus (despite PLN enlargement on CT or MRI), to standard surgery with or without systemic PLND. At a median follow-up time of 37 months there was no difference in disease-free or overall survival in both groups. According to the authors, PLND cannot be recommended as a routine procedure for therapeutic purposes outside of clinical trials.

However, the ASTEC Trial had several serious shortcomings:

- 20% of patients in the systemic PLND group had ≤4 nodes removed; only 40% of the patients in the systemic PLND group had >14 PLN harvested.
- Furthermore, about half the cases were well-differentiated Stage IA or IB, where the risk of nodal metastasis is 3% to 5%.
- In a large prospective RCT, risk factors tend to be equalized in the two arms. Nevertheless, the PLND group had 3% more poor histotypes, 3% more Grade 3 lesions, 3% more LVSI and 10% more deep myometrial invasion. Although these are minor variances, in large groups this could influence small differences.
- Patients were randomized to receive adjuvant therapy regardless of node status.

6.3 Observational studies on the effect of lymphadenectomy on survival

6.3.1 Cragun et al., 2005

In a retrospective analysis of 509 patients, Cragun et al. (2005) noted that patients with poorly differentiated cancers having more than 11 pelvic nodes removed had improved overall survival (hazard ratio [HR] 0.25; $P < .0001$) and progression-free survival (HR 0.26; $P < .0001$) compared with patients having poorly differentiated cancers with 11 or fewer nodes removed. Among patients with cancers of Grades 1 to 2, the number of nodes removed was not predictive of survival. In multivariate analysis, a more extensive node resection remained a significant prognostic factor for improved survival in intermediate-/high-risk patients after adjusting for other factors including age, year of diagnosis, stage, grade, adjuvant radiotherapy and the presence of positive nodes ($P < .001$). Performance of *selective* PaLND was not associated with survival.

6.3.2 Chan et al., 2006

Further evidence for the prognostic and therapeutic benefits for a thorough LND came from Chan et al., who used the United States National Cancer Institute's Surveillance, Epidemiology and End Results Program dataset of 39,396 women with endometrioid uterine cancer. They compared 12,333 patients who underwent surgical-staging procedures, including LND, with 27,063 patients who did not receive a LND to determine the potential therapeutic role of LND in women with endometrioid corpus cancer. They found that the five-year disease-specific survival was significantly improved by lymphadenectomy, and that with increasingly high-risk disease, the survival advantage conferred by LND was progressively greater. The five-year disease-specific survival for Stages I, II, III and IV patients who underwent LND was 95.5%, 90.4%, 73.8% and 53.3%, respectively, compared with 96.6%, 82.2%, 63.1% and 26.9% for those who did not ($P > 0.05$ for Stage I, $P < 0.001$ for Stages II to IV). In the subset of patients with Stage I, Grade 3 disease, those who underwent LND, had a better disease-specific survival than those who did not (90% versus 85%; P 1⁄4 0.0001). However, no benefit for LND was identified for patients with Stage I, Grade 1 (P 1⁄4 0.26) and Grade 2 (P 1⁄4 0.14) disease.

The group also used the data from the 12,333 patients who underwent LND to determine whether the node count or extent of the LND had a therapeutic benefit, and they found that it did in women with intermediate-/high-risk endometrioid cancer but not those with low-risk endometrial cancer. In the intermediate-/high-risk patients (Stage IB, Grade 3; Stages IC and II to IV, all grades), a more extensive lymph node resection (1, 2-5, 6-10, 11-20, and >20) was associated with improved five-year disease-specific survivals across all five groups at 75.3%, 81.5%, 84.1%, 85.3% and 86.8%, respectively (P < .001). For Stage IIIC to IV patients with nodal disease, the extent of node resection significantly improved survival from 51.0%, 53.0%, 53.0% and 60.0%, to 72.0%, (P <.001). However, no significant benefit of lymph node resection in low-risk patients could be demonstrated (Stage IA, all grades; Stage IB, Grade 1 and 2 disease; P ¼ 0.23). In multivariate analysis, a more extensive node resection remained a significant prognostic factor for improved survival in intermediate-/high-risk patients after adjusting for other factors, including age, year of diagnosis, stage, grade, adjuvant radiotherapy and the presence of positive nodes (P <.001). In a follow-through study on 11,443 patients, Chan et al. (2007) investigated the association between the number of lymph nodes examined and the probability of detecting at least a single lymph node involved by metastatic disease in patients with endometrioid corpus cancer to define what constitutes an adequate LND. Their results suggest that the ideal node count is 21 to 25 lymph nodes. Although these are retrospective analyses, the strength of the data lies in the size of the sample and the fact that the study population reflects real-life practices across a range of units from community hospitals to tertiary-care academic centers. The limitations include the lack of detail regarding the location and size of the lymph nodes resected, specifically on what the contribution of PaLND is to the sample.

6.3.3 Para-aortic lymphadenectomy

There is evidence that patients with high-intermediate and high-risk endometrial cancer have 10% to 25% risk of metastatic PaLN (Kadar et al., 1992; Keys et al., 2004; Morrow et al., 1991). About 50% of patients with metastatic PLN have metastasis in the PaLN (Mariani et al., 2008; Watari et al., 2005). Sixteen percent of patients with high-risk endometrial cancer have metastasis only to the PaLN and not to the PLN (Mariani et al., 2008) and 77% of patients with para-aortic metastases harbor disease above the inferior mesenteric artery. It would appear that PaLND, when indicated, should be systematic and extend to the renal vessels. Although Abu-Rustum et al. (2009) reported that in their patients only 1% had isolated para-arotic metastasis (with negative pelvic nodes), they used a count of eight pelvic nodes as indicating a satisfactory pelvic lymphadenectomy and the retrieval of one para-arotic lymph node below the inferior mesenteric artery as evidence of a PaLND. Most gynecologic oncologists consider these LN counts inadequate to make firm conclusions.

6.3.4 SEPAL study 2010

Given the discordance between the findings of the large observational studies (Cragun 2005, Chan 2006, 2007a, 2007b) indicating a significant advantage in survival conferred by an extensive lymphadenectomy, and the RCTs indicating otherwise, Yukiharu Todo and colleagues investigated whether it was the addition of PaLND that improved survival in endometrial cancer (SEPAL). They studied cohorts from two tertiary-care gynecologic oncology units in the city of Sapporo, Japan. Although their study is retrospective, bias was kept to a minimum as the centers differed in the use of PaLND, which was practiced as a routine standard of care in one center and not in the other. The cohorts from both centers had systematic PLND; median pelvic lymph node count 34 (21 to 42) in the PLND group (325 patients) versus 59 (46 to 73) in the PLND and PaLND group (n=346). The number of PaLN counts in the two groups were 0 versus 23 (16 to 30). Patients at intermediate or high risk of recurrence were offered adjuvant radiotherapy or chemotherapy. Overall survival was significantly longer in the PLND and PaLND group than in the PLND group (HR 0.53, 95% CI 0.38 to 0.76; p=0.0005). This association was noted in 407 patients at intermediate or high risk (p=0.0009), but not in low-risk patients. Multivariate analysis of prognostic factors showed that in patients with intermediate or high risk of recurrence, PLND and PaLND reduced the risk of death compared with PLND (0.44, 0.30 to 0.64; p<0.0001). Analysis of 328 patients with intermediate or high risk who were treated with adjuvant radiotherapy or chemotherapy showed that patient survival improved with PLND and PaLND (0.48, 0.29 to 0.83; p=0.0049) and with adjuvant chemotherapy (0.59, 0.37 to 1.00; p=0.0465) independently of one another. The authors concluded that combined PLND and PaLND is recommended as treatment for patients with endometrial carcinoma of intermediate or high risk of recurrence.

6.4 Caveat with lymph node counts

Although there is much debate on constitutes the optimum pathological sampling of pelvic lymph nodes in endometrial cancer, the importance of counting the number of lymph nodes detectable in the pathologic specimens is incontrovertible (Berney et al., 2010). Weingärtner et al. (1996) reported on the average number of PLNs found at the time of autopsy. In 30 human cadavers (19 males and 11 females, mean age of death 64 years), it was found that there were 22.7+10.2 lymph nodes (ranging from 8 to 56) in the pelvis. It has been clearly established that lymph nodes undergo fatty involution that increases with age (>72 years), BMI (>27.8), diabetes, hypothyroidism and previous chemotherapy. A recent study confirmed this phenomenon for superficial lymph nodes in the cervical, axillary and inguinal regions. The fatty degeneration of lymph nodes makes their identification unreliable with either imaging or palpation at the time of surgery or during gross pathologic examination (Arango et al., 2000; Giovagnorio et al., 2005). Consequently, the value of lymph node counts in the elderly and in obese women with endometrial cancer is highly dependent on the thoroughness of the pathology technician.

6.5 Conclusion

In summary, it is clear that patients who have low-grade endometrioid adenocarcinoma with minimal myometrial invasion have very low risk of lymph node metastasis and do not benefit from a LND. Patients at risk of lymph node metastasis require a systematic PLND as well as PaLND. The latter should extend up to the renal vessels.

7. Morbidity of lymphadenectomy and benefits of minimally invasive approach

One of the factors that precludes LND in patients with endometrial cancer is the morbidity associated with an LND. Given that the risk factors for endometrial cancer are old age, diabetes, hypertension and obesity, it follows that a substantial number of women diagnosed with endometrial cancer have these co-morbidities, thus making them high risk for prolonged and technically complicated surgery. Several studies have tried to assess the additional risks posed by a systematic LND and the benefits of performing the surgery by laparoscopy or robotic surgery.

In a large retrospective study, Cragun et al. (2005) summarized the morbidities of LND by laparotomy. Two to three percent of patients had small bowel obstruction or ileus, deep vein thrombosis and lymphocysts requiring drainage. Patients undergoing PLND and PaLND required longer anesthesia time and hospital stay and had greater blood loss compared to those who had PLND alone. Up to 8% of patients had a wound infection. Chronic lymphedema of the lower limbs was observed in 2.5% (Abu-Rustum et al., 2006).

Querleu et al. (2006) audited 1,000 patients who had a *laparoscopic LND*. Only 1.3% were converted to laparotomy. Intra- and early post-operative complication and lymphocyst formation rates were 2.0%(bowel complication 0.7%; urinary tract complications 0.5%; nerve injuries 0.5%), 2.9% and 7.1%, respectively.

7.1 RCTs comparing laparotomy to minimally invasive surgery for endometrial cancer

In the LAP-2 study, an RCT carried out by the Gynecologic Oncology Group (GOG), 2,616 patients with endometrial carcinoma confined to the uterus were randomly assigned to laparoscopy or laparotomy (Walker, 2009). All patients had complete surgical staging including PLND and PaLND. Laparoscopic-assisted vaginal hysterectomy, total laparoscopic hysterectomy or robotic-assisted total laparoscopic hysterectomy was allowed. They found that laparoscopy resulted in similar intra-operative complications, fewer post-operative moderate or severe adverse events (14% versus 21% by laparotomy, $p<0.0001$), shorter hospital stay, less use of pain medication and quicker resumption of daily activities but required longer operating time. Twenty five percent of patients randomized to laparoscopy were converted to laparotomy. Patients at higher risk for a conversion to laparotomy were elderly (>63 years) and those with metastatic disease and a high BMI (17% in patients with a BMI of 25kg/m^2, 26% with a BMI of 35kg/m^2, 57% with a BMI >40kg/m^2).

In an Australian RCT (n=361), which also compared total laparoscopic hysterectomy with abdominal hysterectomy in early endometrial carcinoma, 52% of the patients had a pelvic or para-aortic lymphadenectomy. Only 2.4% of patients assigned to laparoscopy were converted to laparotomy. Patients who had laparoscopic surgery reported significantly greater improvement in QoL from baseline compared with those who had laparotomy, this difference persisted for up to 6 months after surgery. Operating time was significantly longer in the laparoscopy group (138 minutes [SD 43]) versus 109 minutes [SD 34]; $p=0.001$). Intra-operative adverse events were similar between groups (laparotomy 5.6% versus laparoscopy 7.4%]; $p=0.53$), but postoperatively, twice as many patients in the laparotomy group experienced adverse events of Grade 3 or higher (23.2% versus 11.6%; $p=0.004$). The authors concluded that QoL improvements from baseline during early and later phases of recovery, and the adverse event profile, favor laparoscopy over laparotomy for the treatment of Stage I endometrial cancer.

Other studies that investigated the feasibility of minimally invasive surgery (laparoscopy and robot-assisted surgery) in elderly and obese patients concluded that neither age nor BMI is a contraindication to minimally invasive procedures, as it is these patients who benefit the most (Boggess et al., 2008; Gehrig et al., 2008; Janda et al., 2010; Obermair et al., 2005; Scribner et al., 2001).

8. Radiotherapy (RT)

Can adjuvant radiotherapy increase disease-free and/or overall survival after standard surgery? In other words, can radiotherapy make up for incomplete staging if the characteristics of the cancer at final pathology appear to be worse? Several studies have addressed this question.

8.1 Studies

The Postoperative Radiation Therapy in Endometrial Cancer (PORTEC) Trial randomized 715 patients with Stage IB (Grades 2 and 3) and with IC (Grades 1 and 2) endometrial cancer after standard surgery without PLND to observation or pelvic RT with 46 Gy. Although the five-year actuarial locoregional recurrence rates were 4% in the radiotherapy group and 14% in the control group (p=0.001, the overall survival rates were similar in the two groups: 81% (radiotherapy) and 85% (controls), p=0.31. Endometrial-cancer-related death rates were 9% in the radiotherapy group and 6% in the control group (p=0.37). Treatment-related complications occurred in 25% of radiotherapy patients and in 6% of the controls (p=0.0001). One third of the complications were Grade 2 or higher. Seven out of eight Grade 3 to 4 complications were in the radiotherapy group (2%). The observation that the higher incidence of locoregional recurrences in the control group is not reflected in the overall survival was explained by the post-relapse survival. Twenty-three out of 51 patients with a locoregional relapse died, of whom only seven died due to their locoregional recurrence. By contrast, 21 of 30 patients with distant metastases as first failure died, of whom 19 died from the metastases. Salvage treatment of vaginal relapse was often successful. After vaginal recurrence, the two year survival rate was 79% in contrast to 21% after pelvic or distant relapse. At three years, the survival was 69% and 13%, respectively (p=0.001). As for the survival after first relapse by treatment arm, the survival rate was better for patients in the control group than for patients in the radiotherapy group (p=0.02). The authors concluded that post-operative radiotherapy in Stage 1 endometrial carcinoma reduces locoregional recurrence but has no impact on overall survival and that radiotherapy increases treatment-related morbidity. Therefore, a trade-off between the risk of locoregional recurrence and the survival rate after salvage treatment on the one hand, and the morbidity and cost of adjuvant pelvic radiotherapy on the other, has to be made for each subgroup of Stage 1 endometrial carcinoma. These findings further support the need for a systematic LND whenever possible for patients with intermediate or high risk of endometrial cancer.

8.2 Conclusion

Adjuvant radiotherapy cannot be substituted for a systematic LND in intermediate- and high-risk endometrial cancer patients.

9. Areas for future research

9.1 Sentinel Lymph Node (SLN)

From the evidence presented above, it is clear that for patients with endometrial cancer who are at risk of lymph node metastasis, the site of metastasis can be in the pelvic LNs or the para-aortic LN chain up to the renal vessels. Removal of metastatic lymph nodes has prognostic and therapeutic value. On the other hand, the addition of a systematic PLND and PaLND to a standard hysterectomy and bilateral salpingo-oophorectomy, increases the technical difficulty of the surgery, requires more operating time and increases the risk of intra-operative and postoperative complications. These problems apply even when a minimally invasive surgical approach is adopted. Therefore, the challenge is to identify a surgical technique that provides accurate staging information about nodal status, while avoiding unnecessary morbidity.

Sentinel lymph node detection might resolve this dilemma. This technique is based upon the observation that in several types of cancer, tumor cells migrate from the primary tumor to one or a few lymph nodes before metastasizing to other lymph nodes (melanoma, breast, cervix, vulva) (Altgassen et al., 2008; Hauspy et al., 2007a&b). Lymphatic mapping by sentinel lymph node (SLN) detection offers a means of assessing the lymph node status of primary tumors with respect to metastases, without having to resort to formal LND.

In a meta-analysis of various techniques to assess lymph node status in endometrial cancer, Selmanet al. (2008) showed that SLN biopsy was more accurate than MRI and CT scan. In endometrial cancer, several approaches have been attempted: serosal injection during surgery, cervical injection or peri-tumoral injection using hysteroscopic assistance. With cervical injection, detection rates of sentinel lymph nodes in low-risk endometrial cancer reach 85% (Abu-Rustum et al., 2009). A recent study in early invasive cancer suggested that SLN biopsy is a more sensitive procedure to detect pelvic lymph node metastasis compared to the classic PLND due to more extensive sectioning by the pathologist of this LN, its occasionally unusual location (common iliac or para-aortic) and the surgeon's thorough search for this blue or "hot" node (Gortzak-Uzan et al., 2010). Similarly, in early-stage endometrial cancer, SLN mapping appears to be a more sensitive procedure for detecting PLN metastasis compared to the classic PLND for the same reasons: the surgeon's thorough search for this sentinel node and extensive sectioning by the pathologist of the sentinel lymph node (Khoury-Collado et al., 2011).

A French multicentre study (SENTI-ENDO) prospectively evaluated the ability of cervical dual injection of technetium and patent blue to identify SLN in patients with endometrial cancer (Ballester et al 2011). One hundred thirty-three patients were enrolled at nine centers in France. At least one SLN was detected in 111 of the 125 eligible patients; 17% had pelvic lymph node metastases and 5% had an associated SLN in the para-aortic area. Three patients had false-negative results (two had metastatic nodes in the contralateral pelvic area and one in the para-aortic area), giving an NPV of 97% (95% CI 91 to 99) and sensitivity of 84% (62 to 95). All three of the patients in whom the SLN was negative in the presence of metastatic nodes had Type 2 endometrial cancer. Ultrastaging detected metastases, which were missed by conventional histology in nine of 111 (8%) patients with detected SLNs, representing nine of the 19 patients (47%) with metastases. SLN biopsy upstaged 10% of patients with low-risk and 15% of those with intermediate-risk endometrial cancer.

This study highlights the danger of omitting lymphadenectomy in patients with early-stage endometrial cancer, as suggested by the ASTEC study, as 11% of patients at low risk for lymph node metastasis (Grade 1, endometrioid cancer with no myometrial invasion), had positive lymph node metastasis. The authors conclude that SLN biopsy with cervical dual labeling could be a trade-off between systematic LND and no dissection at all in patients with low or intermediate risk endometrial cancer.

The limitations with this study are that the investigators used only cervical injection for the SLN mapping, which is not ideal to identify PaLNs. In a review of SLNs in endometrial cancer, Delpech et al 2008, reported a lower rate of para-aortic SLN detection using cervical injection alone compared with cervical and subserosal or subendometrial injection of patent blue. Additionally, in the SENTI-ENDO study, PaLND was not done if the PLND did not identify metastasis. This means that the incidence of para-aortic metastases could have been underestimated, as about 10% to 16% of lymph node metastases occur exclusively in the para-aortic region.

An experimental study on female cadavers by Lecuru et al 1997, had identified that one of the main routes of lymphatic drainage from the uterus ran along the infundibulo-pelvic ligament to the para-aortic area. Furthermore, when sentinel lymph node were identified using hysteroscopic injection to the tumor base, the para-aortic region was shown to be an important site of sentinel nodes in endometrial cancer, with 14% of SLN being exclusively in the para-aortic region and 47% of para-aortic sentinel nodes located above the inferior mesenteric artery (Nijkura et al., 2004). This method is technically more demanding. Nevertheless, if sentinel lymph node mapping is to replace surgical staging for endometrial cancer, we are obliged to investigate and adopt the most accurate rather than the most expedient method of identifying the sentinel lymph node.

10. Conclusion

Patients who have Grade I/II, endometrioid adenocarinoma with minimal myometrial invasion have very low risk of lymph node metastasis and do not benefit from LND. However, only a thoroughly detailed intra-operative frozen section can identify this subgroup. All high-risk patients need a systematic PLND as well as a PaLND up to the renal vessels. Such dissection needs considerable technical skills on the part of surgeons, and has risk for patients; but confers a significant survival advantage. Analysis of numerous nodes, particularly when they are small, is tedious for the pathologist. Therefore, SLN mapping has the potential to identify the subset of low-/intermediate-risk patients who do not need lymph node dissection. Research needs to be directed at finding the most accurate method of identifying the sentinel lymph node/nodes in endometrial cancer. This will allow the judicious use of resources, including time, cost and energy, to recover the appropriate number of lymph nodes in high-risk patients who will benefit from this procedure.

11. References

Abu-Rustum, NR; Alektiar, K; Iasonos, A; Lev, G; Sonoda, Y; Aghajanian, C; Chi, DS & Barakat, RR (2006). The incidence of symptomatic lower-extremity lymphedema following treatment of uterine corpus malignancies: a 12-year experience at Memorial Sloan-Kettering Cancer Center. *Gynecologic Oncology*, Vol. 103, No. 2 (Nov 2006), pp. 714-718, 0090-8258 (Print) 0090-8258 (Linking)

Abu-Rustum, NR; Gomez, JD; Alektiar, KM; Soslow, RA; Hensley, ML; Leitao, MM, Jr.; Gardner, GJ; Sonoda, Y; Chi, DS & Barakat, RR (2009). The incidence of isolated paraaortic nodal metastasis in surgically staged endometrial cancer patients with negative pelvic lymph nodes. *Gynecologic Oncology*, Vol. 115, No. 2 (Nov 2009), pp. 236-238, 1095-6859 (Electronic) 0090-8258 (Linking)

Abu-Rustum, NR; Khoury-Collado, F; Pandit-Taskar, N; Soslow, RA; Dao, F; Sonoda, Y; Levine, DA; Brown, CL; Chi, DS; Barakat, RR & Gemignani, ML (2009). Sentinel lymph node mapping for grade 1 endometrial cancer: is it the answer to the surgical staging dilemma? *Gynecologic Oncology,* Vol. 113, No. 2 (May 2009), pp. 163-169, 1095-6859 (Electronic) 0090-8258 (Linking)

Alektiar, KM (2006). When and how should adjuvant radiation be used in early endometrial cancer? *Seminars in Radiation Oncology,* Vol. 16, No. 3 (Jul 2006), pp. 158-163, 1053-4296 (Print) 1053-4296 (Linking)

Altgassen, C; Hertel, H; Brandstadt, A; Kohler, C; Durst, M & Schneider, A (2008). Multicenter validation study of the sentinel lymph node concept in cervical cancer: AGO Study Group. *Journal of Clinical Oncology: Official Journal of the American Society of Clinical Oncology,* Vol. 26, No. 18 (Jun 20 2008), pp. 2943-2951, 1527-7755 (Electronic) 0732-183X (Linking)

Altgassen, C; Pagenstecher, J; Hornung, D; Diedrich, K & Hornemann, A (2007). A new approach to label sentinel nodes in endometrial cancer. *Gynecologic Oncology,* Vol. 105, No. 2 (May 2007), pp. 457-461, 0090-8258 (Print) 0090-8258 (Linking)

Arango, HA; Hoffman, MS; Roberts, WS; DeCesare, SL; Fiorica, JV & Drake, J (2000). Accuracy of lymph node palpation to determine need for lymphadenectomy in gynecologic malignancies. *Obstetrics and Gynecology,* Vol. 95, No. 4 (Apr 2000), pp. 553-556, 0029-7844 (Print) 0029-7844 (Linking)

Ballester, M; Dubernard, G; Lecuru, F; Heitz, D; Mathevet, P; Marret, H; Querleu, D; Golfier, F; Leblanc, E; Rouzier, R & Darai, E (2011). Detection rate and diagnostic accuracy of sentinel-node biopsy in early stage endometrial cancer: a prospective multicentre study (SENTI-ENDO). *The Lancet Oncology,* Vol. 12, No. 5 (May 2011), pp. 469-476, 1474-5488 (Electronic) 1470-2045 (Linking)

Benedetti Panici, P; Basile, S; Maneschi, F; Alberto Lissoni, A; Signorelli, M; Scambia, G; Angioli, R; Tateo, S; Mangili, G; Katsaros, D; Garozzo, G; Campagnutta, E; Donadello, N; Greggi, S; Melpignano, M; Raspagliesi, F; Ragni, N; Cormio, G; Grassi, R; Franchi, M; Giannarelli, D; Fossati, R; Torri, V; Amoroso, M; Croce, C & Mangioni, C (2008). Systematic pelvic lymphadenectomy vs. no lymphadenectomy in early-stage endometrial carcinoma: randomized clinical trial. *Journal of the National Cancer Institute,* Vol. 100, No. 23 (Dec 3, 2008), pp. 1707-1716, 1460-2105 (Electronic) 0027-8874 (Linking)

Berney, DM; Wheeler, TM; Grignon, DJ; Epstein, JI; Griffiths, DF; Humphrey, PA; van der Kwast, T; Montironi, R; Delahunt, B; Egevad, L & Srigley, JR (2011). International Society of Urological Pathology (ISUP) Consensus Conference on Handling and Staging of Radical Prostatectomy Specimens. Working group 4: seminal vesicles and lymph nodes. *Modern pathology: An Official Journal of the United States and Canadian Academy of Pathology, Inc,* Vol. 24, No. 1 (Jan 2011), pp. 39-47, 1530-0285 (Electronic) 0893-3952 (Linking)

Bijen, CB; Briet, JM; de Bock, GH; Arts, HJ; Bergsma-Kadijk, JA & Mourits, MJ (2009). Total laparoscopic hysterectomy versus abdominal hysterectomy in the treatment of patients with early stage endometrial cancer: a randomized multi center study. *BMC Cancer,* Vol. 9 (2009), pp. 23, 1471-2407 (Electronic) 1471-2407 (Linking)

Bijen, CB; Vermeulen, KM; Mourits, MJ; Arts, HJ; Ter Brugge, HG; van der Sijde, R; Wijma, J; Bongers, MY; van der Zee, AG & de Bock, GH (2011). Cost effectiveness of laparoscopy versus laparotomy in early stage endometrial cancer: a randomised trial. *Gynecologic Oncology,* Vol. 121, No. 1 (Apr 2011), pp. 76-82, 1095-6859 (Electronic) 0090-8258 (Linking)

Boggess, JF; Gehrig, PA; Cantrell, L; Shafer, A; Ridgway, M; Skinner, EN & Fowler, WC (2008). A comparative study of 3 surgical methods for hysterectomy with staging for endometrial cancer: robotic assistance, laparoscopy, laparotomy. *American Journal of Obstetrics and Gynecology*, Vol. 199, No. 4 (Oct 2008), pp. 360 e361-369, 1097-6868 (Electronic) 0002-9378 (Linking)

Bottke, D; Wiegel, T; Kreienberg, R; Kurzeder, C & Sauer, G (2007). Stage IB endometrial cancer. Does lymphadenectomy replace adjuvant radiotherapy? *Strahlentherapie und Onkologie : Organ der Deutschen Rontgengesellschaft* ... [et al], Vol. 183, No. 11 (Nov 2007), pp. 600-604, 0179-7158 (Print) 0179-7158 (Linking)

Celik, C; Ozdemir, S; Kiresi, D; Emlik, D; Tazegul, A & Esen, H (2010). Evaluation of cervical involvement in endometrial cancer by transvaginal sonography, magnetic resonance imaging and frozen section. *Journal of Obstetrics and Gynaecology: the Journal of the Institute of Obstetrics and Gynaecology*, Vol. 30, No. 3 (Apr 2010), pp. 302-307, 1364-6893 (Electronic) 0144-3615 (Linking)

Chan, JK & Kapp, DS (2007). Role of complete lymphadenectomy in endometrioid uterine cancer. *The Lancet Oncology*, Vol. 8, No. 9 (Sep 2007), pp. 831-841, 1470-2045 (Print) 1470-2045 (Linking)

Chan, JK; Urban, R; Cheung, MK; Shin, JY; Husain, A; Teng, NN; Berek, JS; Walker, JL; Kapp, DS & Osann, K (2007). Lymphadenectomy in endometrioid uterine cancer staging: how many lymph nodes are enough? A study of 11,443 patients. *Cancer*, Vol. 109, No. 12 (Jun 15 2007), pp. 2454-2460, 0008-543X (Print) 0008-543X (Linking)

Chan, JK; Wu, H; Cheung MK, et al. The outcomes of 27 063 women with unstaged endometrioid uterine cancer. *Gyncologic Oncology*, Vol. 106 (2007), pp. 282-288.

Chan, JK; Cheung, MK; Huh, WK; Osann, K; Husain, A; Teng, NN & Kapp, DS (2006). Therapeutic role of lymph node resection in endometrioid corpus cancer: a study of 12,333 patients. *Cancer*, Vol. 107, No. 8 (Oct 15 2006), pp. 1823-1830

Chung, HH; Kim, JW; Park, NH; Song, YS; Kang, SB & Lee, HP (2006). Use of preoperative serum CA-125 levels for prediction of lymph node metastasis and prognosis in endometrial cancer. *Acta obstetricia et gynecologica Scandinavica*, Vol. 85, No. 12, 2006, pp. 1501-1505, 0001-6349 (Print) 0001-6349 (Linking)

Clarke, BA & Gilks, CB (2010). Endometrial carcinoma: controversies in histopathological assessment of grade and tumor cell type. *Journal of Clinical Pathology*, Vol. 63, No. 5 (May 2010), pp. 410-415, 1472-4146 (Electronic) 0021-9746 (Linking)

Cragun, JM; Havrilesky, LJ; Calingaert, B; Synan, I; Secord, AA; Soper, JT; Clarke-Pearson, DL & Berchuck, A (2005). Retrospective analysis of selective lymphadenectomy in apparent early-stage endometrial cancer. *Journal of Clinical Oncology: Official Journal of the American Society of Clinical Oncology*, Vol. 23, No. 16 (Jun 1 2005), pp. 3668-3675, 0732-183X (Print) 0732-183X (Linking)

Creasman, WT; Morrow, CP; Bundy, BN; Homesley, HD; Graham, JE & Heller, PB (1987). Surgical pathologic spread patterns of endometrial cancer. A Gynecologic Oncology Group Study. *Cancer*, Vol. 60, No. 8 Suppl. (Oct 15 1987), pp. 2035-2041, 0008-543X (Print) 0008-543X (Linking)

Creasman, WT; Mutch, DE & Herzog, TJ (2010). ASTEC lymphadenectomy and radiation therapy studies: are conclusions valid? *Gynecologic Oncology*, Vol. 116, No. 3 (Mar 2010), pp. 293-294, 1095-6859 (Electronic) 0090-8258 (Linking)

Creasman, WT; Odicino, F; Maisonneuve, P; Quinn, MA; Beller, U; Benedet, JL; Heintz, AP; Ngan, HY & Pecorelli, S (2006). Carcinoma of the corpus uteri. FIGO 26th Annual Report on the Results of Treatment in Gynecological Cancer. *International Journal of Gynaecology and Obstetrics: The Official Organ of the International Federation of Gynaecology and Obstetrics,* Vol. 95 Suppl 1 (Nov 2006), pp. S105-143, 0020-7292 (Print) 0020-7292 (Linking)

Creutzberg, CL; van Putten, WL; Koper, PC; Lybeert, ML; Jobsen, JJ; Warlam-Rodenhuis, CC; De Winter, KA; Lutgens, LC; van den Bergh, AC; van de Steen-Banasik, E; Beerman, H & van Lent, M (2000). Surgery and postoperative radiotherapy versus surgery alone for patients with stage-1 endometrial carcinoma: multicentre randomised trial. PORTEC Study Group. Post Operative Radiation Therapy in Endometrial Carcinoma. *Lancet,* Vol. 355, No. 9213 (Apr 22 2000), pp. 1404-1411, 0140-6736 (Print) 0140-6736 (Linking)

Delpech Y, Coutant C, Darai E, Barranger E (2008). Sentinel lymph node evaluation in endometrial cancer and the importance of micrometastases. Surg Oncol 2008; 17: 237–45.

Delpech, Y & Barranger, E (2010). Management of lymph nodes in endometrioid uterine cancer. *Current Opinion in Oncology,* Vol. 22, No. 5 (Sep 2010), pp. 487-491, 1531-703X (Electronic) 1040-8746 (Linking)

Denschlag, D; Tan, L; Patel, S; Kerim-Dikeni, A; Souhami, L & Gilbert, L (2007). Stage III endometrial cancer: preoperative predictability, prognostic factors, and treatment outcome. *American Journal of Obstetrics and Gynecology,* Vol. 196, No. 6 (June 2007), pp. 546.e1-546.e7

Dijkhuizen, FP; Mol, BW; Brolmann, HA & Heintz, AP (2000). The accuracy of endometrial sampling in the diagnosis of patients with endometrial carcinoma and hyperplasia: a meta-analysis. *Cancer,* Vol. 89, No. 8 (Oct 15 2000), pp. 1765-1772, 0008-543X (Print) 0008-543X (Linking)

Dubinsky, TJ (2004). Value of sonography in the diagnosis of abnormal vaginal bleeding. *Journal of Clinical Ultrasound: JCU,* Vol. 32, No. 7 (Sep 2004), pp. 348-353, 0091-2751 (Print) 0091-2751 (Linking)

Dotters, DJ (2000). Preoperative CA 125 in endometrial cancer: is it useful? *American Journal of Obstetrics and Gynecology,* Vol. 182 (2000), pp. 1328-1334.

Fleischer, AC (1997). Optimizing the accuracy of transvaginal ultrasonography of the endometrium. *The New England Journal of Medicine,* Vol. 337, No. 25 (Dec 18 1997), pp. 1839-1840, 0028-4793 (Print) 0028-4793 (Linking)

Frumovitz, M; Slomovitz, BM; Singh, DK; Broaddus, RR; Abrams, J; Sun, CC; Bevers, M & Bodurka, DC (2004). Frozen section analyses as predictors of lymphatic spread in patients with early-stage uterine cancer. *Journal of the American College of Surgeons,* Vol. 199, No. 3 (Sep 2004), pp. 388-393, 1072-7515 (Print) 1072-7515 (Linking)

Fujimoto, T; Fukuda, J & Tanaka, T (2009). Role of complete para-aortic lymphadenectomy in endometrial cancer. *Current Opinion in Obstetrics & Gynecology,* Vol. 21, No. 1 (Feb 2009), pp. 10-14, 1473-656X (Electronic) 1040-872X (Linking)

Gehrig, PA; Cantrell, LA; Shafer, A; Abaid, LN; Mendivil, A & Boggess, JF (2008). What is the optimal minimally invasive surgical procedure for endometrial cancer staging in the obese and morbidly obese woman? *Gynecologic Pncology,* Vol. 111, No. 1 (Oct 2008), pp. 41-45, 1095-6859 (Electronic) 0090-8258 (Linking)

Giovagnorio, F; Drudi, FM; Fanelli, G; Flecca, D & Francioso, A (2005). Fatty changes as a misleading factor in the evaluation with ultrasound of superficial lymph nodes. *Ultrasound in Medicine & Biology,* Vol. 31, No. 8 (Aug 2005), pp. 1017-1022, 0301-5629 (Print) 0301-5629 (Linking)

Gortzak-Uzan, L; Jimenez, W; Nofech-Mozes, S; Ismiil, N; Khalifa, MA; Dube, V; Rosen, B; Murphy, J; Laframboise, S & Covens, A (2010). Sentinel lymph node biopsy vs. pelvic lymphadenectomy in early stage cervical cancer: is it time to change the gold standard? *Gynecologic Oncology,* Vol. 116, No. 1 (Jan 2010), pp. 28-32, 1095-6859 (Electronic) 0090-8258 (Linking)

Han, SS; Lee, SH; Kim, DH; Kim, JW; Park, NH; Kang, SB & Song, YS (2010). Evaluation of preoperative criteria used to predict lymph node metastasis in endometrial cancer. *Acta obstetricia et gynecologica Scandinavica,* Vol. 89, No. 2 (2010), pp. 168-174, 1600-0412 (Electronic) 0001-6349 (Linking)

Hauspy, J; Beiner, M; Harley, I; Ehrlich, L; Rasty, G & Covens, A (2007a). Sentinel lymph node in vulvar cancer. *Cancer,* Vol. 110, No. 5 (Sep 1 2007), pp. 1015-1023, 0008-543X (Print) 0008-543X (Linking)

Hauspy, J; Beiner, M; Harley, I; Ehrlich, L; Rasty, G & Covens, A (2007b). Sentinel lymph nodes in early stage cervical cancer. *Gynecologic Oncology,* Vol. 105, No. 2 (May 2007), pp. 285-290, 0090-8258 (Print) 0090-8258 (Linking)

Hsieh, CH; ChangChien, CC; Lin, H; Huang, EY; Huang, CC; Lan, KC & Chang, SY (2002). Can a preoperative CA 125 level be a criterion for full pelvic lymphadenectomy in surgical staging of endometrial cancer? *Gynecologic Oncology,* Vol. 86, No. 1 (Jul 2002), pp. 28-33, 0090-8258 (Print) 0090-8258 (Linking)

Janda, M; Gebski, V; Brand, A; Hogg, R; Jobling, TW; Land, R; Manolitsas, T; McCartney, A; Nascimento, M; Neesham, D; Nicklin, JL; Oehler, MK; Otton, G; Perrin, L; Salfinger, S; Hammond, I; Leung, Y; Walsh, T; Sykes, P; Ngan, H; Garrett, A; Laney, M; Ng, TY; Tam, K; Chan, K; Wrede, CD; Pather, S; Simcock, B; Farrell, R & Obermair, A (2010). Quality of life after total laparoscopic hysterectomy versus total abdominal hysterectomy for stage I endometrial cancer (LACE): a randomised trial. *The Lancet Oncology,* Vol. 11, No. 8 (Aug 2010), pp. 772-780, 1474-5488 (Electronic) 1470-2045 (Linking)

Ju, W; Myung, SK; Kim, Y; Choi, HJ; Kim, SC; Korean Meta-Analysis Study Group (2009). Comparison of laparoscopy and laparotomy for management of endometrial carcinoma: a meta-analysis. *International Journal of Gynecological Cancer,* Vol. 19, No. 3 (Apr 2009), pp. 400-406.

Jemal, A; Siegel, R; Xu, J & Ward, E (2010). Cancer statistics, 2010. *CA: A Cancer Journal for Clinicians,* Vol. 60, No. 5 (Sep-Oct 2010), pp. 277-300, 1542-4863 (Electronic) 0007-9235 (Linking)

Kadar, N; Malfetano, JH & Homesley, HD (1992). Determinants of survival of surgically staged patients with endometrial carcinoma histologically confined to the uterus: implications for therapy. *Obstetrics and Gynecology,* Vol. 80, No. 4 (Oct 1992), pp. 655-659, 0029-7844 (Print) 0029-7844 (Linking)

Keys, HM; Roberts, JA; Brunetto, VL; Zaino, RJ; Spirtos, NM; Bloss, JD; Pearlman, A; Maiman, MA & Bell, JG (2004). A phase III trial of surgery with or without adjunctive external pelvic radiation therapy in intermediate risk endometrial adenocarcinoma: a Gynecologic Oncology Group study. *Gynecologic Oncology,* Vol. 92, No. 3 (Mar 2004), pp. 744-751, 0090-8258 (Print) 0090-8258 (Linking)

Kitchener, H; Swart, AM; Qian, Q; Amos, C & Parmar, MK (2009). Efficacy of systematic pelvic lymphadenectomy in endometrial cancer (MRC ASTEC trial): a randomised study. *Lancet,* Vol. 373, No. 9658 (Jan 10 2009), pp. 125-136, 1474-547X (Electronic) 0140-6736 (Linking)

Koper, NP; Massuger, LF; Thomas, CM; Kiemeney, LA & Verbeek, AL (1998). Serum CA 125 measurements to identify patients with endometrial cancer who require lymphadenectomy. Anticancer Research, Vol. 18, No. 3B (May 1998), pp. 1897-1902.

Kornblith, AB; Huang, HQ; Walker, JL; Spirtos, NM; Rotmensch, J & Cella, D. Quality of life of patients with endometrial cancer undergoing laparoscopic FIGO staging compared to laparotomy: a Gynecologic Oncology Group Study. *Journal of Clinical Oncology,* Vol. 27, No. 32 (Nov 2009), pp. 5337-5342

Larson, DM & Johnson, KK (1993). Pelvic and para-aortic lymphadenectomy for surgical staging of high-risk endometrioid adenocarcinoma of the endometrium. *Gynecologic oncology,* Vol. 51, No. 3 (Dec 1993), pp. 345-348, 0090-8258 (Print) 0090-8258 (Linking)

Lécuru, F; Neji, K; Robin, F; Darles, C; de Bièvre, P & Taurelle, R (1997). Lymphatic drainage of the uterus. Preliminary results of an experimental study. *Journal de gynécologie, obstétrique et biologie de la reproduction,* Vol. 26, No. 4 (1997), pp. 418-423

Lee, JH; Dubinsky, T; Andreotti, RF; Cardenes, HR; Dejesus Allison, SO; Gaffney, DK; Glanc, P; Horowitz, NS; Jhingran, A; Lee, SI; Puthawala, AA; Royal, HD; Scoutt, LM; Small, W, Jr.; Varia, MA & Zelop, CM (2011). ACR Appropriateness Criteria(R) Pretreatment Evaluation and Follow-Up of Endometrial Cancer of the Uterus. *Ultrasound Quarterly,* Vol. 27, No. 2 (Jun 2011), pp. 139-145, 1536-0253 (Electronic) 0894-8771 (Linking)

Leitao, MM, Jr.; Kehoe, S; Barakat, RR; Alektiar, K; Gattoc, LP; Rabbitt, C; Chi, DS; Soslow, RA & Abu-Rustum, NR (2009). Comparison of D&C and office endometrial biopsy accuracy in patients with FIGO grade 1 endometrial adenocarcinoma. *Gynecologic Oncology,* Vol. 113, No. 1 (Apr 2009), pp. 105-108, 1095-6859 (Electronic) 0090-8258 (Linking)

Loubeyre, P; Undurraga, M; Bodmer, A & Petignat, P (2011). Non-invasive modalities for predicting lymph node spread in early stage endometrial cancer? *Surgical Oncology,* Vol. 20, No. 2 (Jun 2011), pp. e102-108, 1879-3320 (Electronic) 0960-7404 (Linking)

Lutman, CV; Havrilesky, LJ; Cragun, JM; Secord, AA; Calingaert, B; Berchuck, A; Clarke-Pearson, DL & Soper, JT (2006). Pelvic lymph node count is an important prognostic variable for FIGO stage I and II endometrial carcinoma with high-risk histology. *Gynecologic Oncology,* Vol. 102, No. 1 (Jul 2006), pp. 92-97, 0090-8258 (Print) 0090-8258 (Linking)

Mariani, A; Dowdy, SC; Cliby, WA; Gostout, BS; Jones, MB; Wilson, TO & Podratz, KC (2008). Prospective assessment of lymphatic dissemination in endometrial cancer: a paradigm shift in surgical staging. *Gynecologic Oncology,* Vol. 109, No. 1 (Apr 2008), pp. 11-18, 1095-6859 (Electronic) 0090-8258 (Linking)

Mariani, A; Dowdy, SC; Keeney, GL; Haddock, MG; Lesnick, TG & Podratz, KC (2005). Predictors of vaginal relapse in stage I endometrial cancer. *Gynecologic Oncology,* Vol. 97, No. 3 (Jun 2005), pp. 820-827, 0090-8258 (Print) 0090-8258 (Linking)

Mariani, A; Webb, MJ; Galli, L & Podratz, KC (2000). Potential therapeutic role of para-aortic lymphadenectomy in node-positive endometrial cancer. *Gynecologic Oncology*, Vol. 76, No. 3 (Mar 2000), pp. 348-356, 0090-8258 (Print) 0090-8258 (Linking)

Mariani, A; Webb, MJ; Keeney, GL; Haddock, MG; Calori, G & Podratz, KC (2000). Low-risk corpus cancer: is lymphadenectomy or radiotherapy necessary? *American Journal of Obstetrics and Gynecology*, Vol. 182, No. 6 (Jun 2000), pp. 1506-1519, 0002-9378 (Print) 0002-9378 (Linking)

May, K; Bryant, A; Dickinson, HO; Kehoe, S & Morrison, J (2010). Lymphadenectomy for the management of endometrial cancer. *Cochrane Database of Systematic Reviews*, No. 1 (2010), pp. CD007585, 1469-493X (Electronic) 1361-6137 (Linking)

Morrow, CP; Bundy, BN; Kurman, RJ; Creasman, WT; Heller, P; Homesley, HD & Graham, JE (1991). Relationship between surgical-pathological risk factors and outcome in clinical stage I and II carcinoma of the endometrium: a Gynecologic Oncology Group study. *Gynecologic Oncology*, Vol. 40, No. 1 (Jan 1991), pp. 55-65, 0090-8258 (Print) 0090-8258 (Linking)

Niikura, H; Okamura, C; Utsunomiya, H; Yoshinaga, K; Akahira, J; Ito, K & Yaegashi, N (2004). Sentinel lymph node detection in patients with endometrial cancer. *Gynecologic Oncology*, Vol. 92, No. 2 (Feb 2004), pp. 669-674, 0090-8258 (Print) 0090-8258 (Linking)

Obermair, A; Geramou, M; Gucer, F; Denison, U; Graf, AH; Kapshammer, E; Medl, M; Rosen, A; Wierrani, F; Neunteufel, W; Frech, I; Speiser, P; Kainz, C & Breitenecker, G (1999). Endometrial cancer: accuracy of the finding of a well differentiated tumor at dilatation and curettage compared to the findings at subsequent hysterectomy. *International Journal of Gynecological Cancer: Official Journal of the International Gynecological Cancer Society*, Vol. 9, No. 5 (Sep 1999), pp. 383-386, 1525-1438 (Electronic) 1048-891X (Linking)

Obermair, A; Manolitsas, TP; Leung, Y; Hammond, IG & McCartney, AJ (2005). Total laparoscopic hysterectomy versus total abdominal hysterectomy for obese women with endometrial cancer. *International Journal of Gynecological Cancer: Official Journal of the International Gynecological Cancer Society*, Vol. 15, No. 2 (Mar-Apr 2005), pp. 319-324, 1048-891X (Print) 1048-891X (Linking)

Palomba, S; Falbo, A; Mocciaro, R; Russo, T & Zullo, F (2009). Laparoscopic treatment for endometrial cancer: a meta-analysis of randomized controlled trials (RCTs). *Gynecologic Oncology*, Vol. 112, No. 2 (February 2009), pp. 415-421

Papadia, A; Azioni, G; Brusaca, B; Fulcheri, E; Nishida, K; Menoni, S; Simpkins, F; Lucci, JA, 3rd & Ragni, N (2009). Frozen section underestimates the need for surgical staging in endometrial cancer patients. *International Journal of Gynecological Cancer: Official Journal of the International Gynecological Cancer Society*, Vol. 19, No. 9 (Dec 2009), pp. 1570-1573, 1525-1438 (Electronic) 1048-891X (Linking)

Prat, J; Gallardo, A; Cuatrecasas, M & Catasus, L (2007). Endometrial carcinoma: pathology and genetics. *Pathology*, Vol. 39, No. 1 (Feb 2007), pp. 72-87, 0031-3025 (Print) 0031-3025 (Linking)

Querleu, D; Leblanc, E; Cartron, G; Narducci, F; Ferron, G & Martel, P (2006). Audit of preoperative and early complications of laparoscopic lymph node dissection in 1000 gynecologic cancer patients. *American Journal of Obstetrics and Gynecology*, Vol. 195, No. 5 (Nov 2006), pp. 1287-1292, 1097-6868 (Electronic) 0002-9378 (Linking)

Schink, JC; Lurain, JR; Wallemark, CB & Chmiel, JS (1987). Tumor size in endometrial cancer: a prognostic factor for lymph node metastasis. *Obstetrics and Gynecology,* Vol. 70, No. 2 (Aug 1987), pp. 216-219, 0029-7844 (Print) 0029-7844 (Linking)

Scholten, AN; van Putten, WL; Beerman, H; Smit, VT; Koper, PC; Lybeert, ML; Jobsen, JJ; Warlam-Rodenhuis, CC; De Winter, KA; Lutgens, LC; van Lent, M & Creutzberg, CL (2005). Postoperative radiotherapy for Stage 1 endometrial carcinoma: long-term outcome of the randomized PORTEC trial with central pathology review. *International journal of radiation oncology, biology, physics,* Vol. 63, No. 3 (Nov 1 2005), pp. 834-838, 0360-3016 (Print) 0360-3016 (Linking)

Scribner, DR, Jr.; Walker, JL; Johnson, GA; McMeekin, SD; Gold, MA & Mannel, RS (2001). Surgical management of early-stage endometrial cancer in the elderly: is laparoscopy feasible? *Gynecologic Oncology,* Vol. 83, No. 3 (Dec 2001), pp. 563-568, 0090-8258 (Print) 0090-8258 (Linking)

Smith-Bindman, R; Kerlikowske, K; Feldstein, VA; Subak, L; Scheidler, J; Segal, M; Brand, R & Grady, D (1998). Endovaginal ultrasound to exclude endometrial cancer and other endometrial abnormalities. *JAMA: The Journal of the American Medical Association,* Vol. 280, No. 17 (Nov 4 1998), pp. 1510-1517, 0098-7484 (Print) 0098-7484 (Linking)

Sood, AK; Buller, RE; Burger, RA; Dawson, JD; Sorosky, JI & Berman, M (1997). Value of preoperative CA 125 level in the management of uterine cancer and prediction of clinical outcome. *Obstetrics and Gynecology,* Vol. 90, No. 3 (Sep 1997), pp. 441-447, 0029-7844 (Print) 0029-7844 (Linking)

Todo, Y; Kato, H; Kaneuchi, M; Watari, H; Takeda, M & Sakuragi, N (2010). Survival effect of para-aortic lymphadenectomy in endometrial cancer (SEPAL study): a retrospective cohort analysis. *Lancet,* Vol. 375, No. 9721 (Apr 3 2010), pp. 1165-1172, 1474-547X (Electronic) 0140-6736 (Linking)

Tozzi, R; Malur, S; Koehler, C & Schneider, A (2005). Laparoscopy versus laparotomy in endometrial cancer: first analysis of survival of a randomized prospective study. *Journal of Minimally Invasive Surgery and Gyncology,* Vol. 12, No. 2 (Apr 2005), pp. 12: 130-136

Walker, JL; Piedmonte, MR; Spirtos, NM; Eisenkop, SM; Schlaerth, JB; Mannel, RS; Spiegel, G; Barakat, R; Pearl, ML & Sharma, SK (2009). Laparoscopy compared with laparotomy for comprehensive surgical staging of uterine cancer: Gynecologic Oncology Group Study LAP2. *Journal of Clinical Oncology,* Vol. 27, No. 32 (Nov 10 2009), pp. 5331-5336

Watari, H; Todo, Y; Takeda, M; Ebina, Y; Yamamoto, R & Sakuragi, N (2005). Lymph-vascular space invasion and number of positive para-aortic node groups predict survival in node-positive patients with endometrial cancer. *Gynecologic Oncology,* Vol. 96, No. 3 (Mar 2005), pp. 651-657, 0090-8258 (Print) 0090-8258 (Linking)

Weingartner, K; Ramaswamy, A; Bittinger, A; Gerharz, EW; Voge, D & Riedmiller, H (1996). Anatomical basis for pelvic lymphadenectomy in prostate cancer: results of an autopsy study and implications for the clinic. *The Journal of Urology,* Vol. 156, No. 6 (Dec 1996), pp. 1969-1971, 0022-5347 (Print) 0022-5347 (Linking)

Yanazume, S; Saito, T; Eto, T; Yamanaka, T; Nishiyama, K; Okadome, M & Ariyoshi, K (2011). Reassessment of the utility of frozen sections in endometrial cancer surgery using tumor diameter as an additional factor. *American Journal of Obstetrics and Gynecology,* Vol. 204, No. 6 (June 2011), pp. 531.e1-531.e7, 1097-6868 (Electronic) 0002-9378 (Linking)

Part 4

Therapeutic Strategies

8

Treatment Strategies and Prognosis of Endometrial Cancer

Gunjal Garg and David G. Mutch
Department of Obstetrics and Gynecology, Division of Gynecologic Oncology, Washington University School of Medicine, St. Louis, Missouri USA

1. Introduction

Endometrial cancer is the fourth most common cancer and the most common gynecological cancer diagnosed in the women in the United States. The lifetime risk of developing endometrial cancer is 2.58% in US women. The American Cancer Society estimates approximately 47,000 new cases and 8,120 deaths due to endometrial cancer in 2011 (Siegel et al. 2011). There does appear to be a significant difference in prognosis based on race. The incidence of endometrial cancer is higher in white women compared to the black women (age adjusted incidence rate: 24.8 vs. 20.9 per 100,000 women), but the death rate from endometrial cancer in the black women is almost two times that of the white women (age adjusted death rate: 3.9 vs. 7.2 per 100,000 women) (Howlader N). Furthermore, the incidence and the death rate have remained stable in the white women; although it has been rising steadily in the black women (by 1.7% per year and 0.8% per year, respectively) (Howlader N).

The management strategies in endometrial cancer have evolved dramatically in the past two decades. Despite the advances in the treatment of endometrial cancer; the death rate from endometrial cancer remains high. Clearly, more effective treatment strategies are needed.

2. Histological classification

Endometrial cancer can be divided into two histologic subtypes: Type I and Type II. Type I endometrial cancers account for the majority of uterine cancer cases and occur more commonly in association with overexposure to estrogen. They are of endometrioid histology, diagnosed in early stages, and are commonly associated with K-ras, PTEN, and/or mismatch repair gene mutations. They are also associated with obesity. Type II endometrial cancers, on the other hand, are typically of aggressive non endometrioid histology and are therefore more commonly diagnosed in advanced stages. They often develop in a background of atrophic endometrium (Bokhman 1983) and have a greater probability of having p53 mutations and/or HER2/neu over expression (Prat et al. 2007).

3. Management of endometrial cancer

The primary treatment of endometrial cancer is surgical. Following tissue diagnosis, most patients are offered surgical staging. Routine preoperative work-up includes complete blood count, serum electrolytes/ creatinine, liver function tests, urinalysis, and a CXR. Further evaluation with CT/MRI/PET-CT (with or without CA-125) may be performed, if extrauterine disease is suspected on initial assessment. In patients with suspected cervical involvement, MRI or cervical biopsy may be helpful to confirm the diagnosis (Akin et al. 2007).

3.1 Surgical staging and related issues

In 1988 the FIGO staging committee replaced the clinical staging system for endometrial cancer with a surgical staging system. This transition from clinical to surgical staging was mainly due to the seminal findings of a large gynecologic oncology group trial (GOG 33), which evaluated the surgical-pathologic patterns in apparent early stage endometrial cancer with particular emphasis on pelvic and para-aortic lymph node involvement (Creasman et al. 1987). A significant number (25%) of patients with clinical stage I in this study were found to have extrauterine disease upon comprehensive surgical staging.

The 1988 FIGO staging system was recently modified (Pecorelli et al. 2009). These two staging criteria are shown in Tables 1 and 2 respectively.

Stage IA G123	Tumor limited to the endometrium
Stage IB G123	Invasion to less than half of the myometrium
Stage IC G123	Invasion equal to or more than half of the myometrium
Stage IIA G123	Endocervical glandular involvement only
Stage IIB G123	Cervical stromal invasion
Stage IIIA G123	Tumor invades serosa and/or adnexa and/or positive peritoneal cytology
Stage IIIB G123	Vaginal metastasis
Stage IIIC G123	Metastasis to pelvic and/or para-aortic lymph nodes
Stage IVA G123	Tumor invasion of bladder and/or bowel mucosa
Stage IVB G123	Distant metastasis including intra-abdominal metastasis and/or inguinal lymph nodes

Table 1. 1988 FIGO Surgical Staging for Endometrial Cancer.

Stage IA G123	Invasion to less than half of the myometrium
Stage IB G123	Invasion equal to or more than half of the myometrium
Stage II G123	Cervical stromal invasion
Stage IIIA G123	Tumor invades serosa and/or adnexa
Stage IIIB G123	Vaginal metastasis
Stage IIIC1 G123	Metastasis to pelvic lymph nodes
Stage IIIC2 G123	Metastasis to para-aortic lymph nodes
Stage IVA G123	Tumor invasion of bladder and/or bowel mucosa
Stage IVB G123	Distant metastasis including intra-abdominal metastasis and/or inguinal lymph nodes

Table 2. 2009 FIGO Surgical Staging for Endometrial Cancer.

The current standard surgical staging procedure includes total abdominal hysterectomy, bilateral salpingo-oophorectomy, pelvic and para-aortic lymphadenectomy, peritoneal washings for cytology, and meticulous exploration of the abdomen and pelvis with biopsy of any suspicious lesions (NCCN guidelines for uterine neoplams, V.2.2011) (NCCN Clinical Practice Guidelines in Oncology (NCCN Guidelines™) for Uterine Neoplasms V.2.2011. © 2011 National Comprehensive Cancer Network). This procedure has been shown feasible by laparoscopy. In LAP-2 trial; the pelvic and para-aortic lymph nodes were obtained in 96% patients undergoing laparotomy compared to 92% of those who had laparoscopy (p<0.001). The detection rate of advanced stage was also comparable between the groups (17% vs. 17%, p=0.841) (Walker et al. 2009).

GOG 33 identified that depth of myometrial invasion, and tumor grade were predictive of lymph node metastasis (Creasman et al. 1987) and that all were predictive of recurrence. The preoperative and intra-operative evaluation of these high-risk features is often inaccurate, and surgical staging is therefore recommended in most patients diagnosed with endometrial cancer (NCCN guidelines for uterine neoplasms, V.2.2011).

The preoperative tumor grade was upgraded on final pathology in approximately 18% patients in different studies (Goudge et al. 2004) (Ben-Shachar et al. 2005). Neither imaging nor frozen section is very accurate for assessing the depth of myometrial invasion. In a recent study by Case et al, concordance between frozen and final pathology was noted only in 67% patients for depth of myometrial invasion and 58% patients for tumor grade (Case et al. 2006). The sensitivity of MRI has similarly been found to be only 54%-75% in this regard (Hricak et al. 1991; Nakao et al. 2006).

The use of imaging (CT, MRI, and PET-CT) has been evaluated for the pre-operative assessment of lymph node metastasis in endometrial cancer. Park et al showed that the sensitivity and specificity of MRI and PET-CT was only modest (46% and 88%; and 69% and 90%, respectively) (Park et al. 2008). Palpation of lymph nodes is also not reliable, with a false negative rate of over 35% in some studies (Girardi et al. 1993; Arango et al. 2000). Intra-operative frozen section evaluation was found to miss nearly 2/3rds of endometrial cancer patients with positive lymph nodes, in a recent study (Pristauz et al. 2009).

Several retrospective studies have shown an improvement in survival following pelvic and para-aortic lymphadenectomy (Kilgore et al. 1995; Mohan et al. 1998; Trimble et al. 1998; Cragun et al. 2005; Chan et al. 2006). In contrast, no survival benefit could be demonstrated in either of the two recent prospective randomized controlled trials (Kitchener et al. 2009; Panici et al. 2008). The ASTEC trial recruited 1,408 women with early stage endometrial cancer from 85 centers across four countries (U.K., Poland, New Zealand, and South Africa) (Kitchener et al. 2009). These women were randomized to undergo surgery either with or without lymphadenectomy. To control for postsurgical treatment, women with intermediate or high risk of recurrence were randomized into the ASTEC radiotherapy trial. No survival benefit was observed from pelvic lymphadenectomy in this trial. The 5-year overall survival was 81% in the surgery only group and 80% in the surgery plus lymphadenectomy group (HR: 1.04, CI: 0.74-1.45, p=0.83). The corresponding 5-year recurrence free survival was 79% and 73%, respectively (HR: 1.25, CI: 0.93-1.66, p=0.14). In another randomized study from Italy, 514 patients with preoperative FIGO stage I endometrial carcinoma were evaluated (Panici et al. 2008). At a median follow-up of 49 months, the rates of disease free survival

(81.0% vs. 81.7%, HR: 1.20, CI: 0.75-1.91) and overall survival (85.9% vs. 90.0%; HR: 1.16, CI: 0.67-2.02) were not significantly different between the lymphadenectomy and the no-lymphadenectomy arms. Although, these trials have been criticized for various shortcomings (Amant et al. 2009; Uccella et al. 2009; Uccella et al. 2009); they constitute level one evidence and indicate that lymphadenectomy by itself does not provide survival advantage in endometrial cancer.

The morbidity associated with surgical staging has been reported in several studies (Moore et al. 1989; Larson and Johnson 1993; Franchi et al. 2001). In a study of 168 patients with endometrial cancer; the short term complications after complete surgical staging included fever (31.5%), surgical site infection (4.7%), embolic events (1.3%), and death (0.7%). The late complications in this series were leg edema (0.7%), intestinal obstruction (0.7%), and lymphocysts (1.3%) (Larson et al. 1993). In another study by Cragun et al, adverse events were noted in 18% patients. The most common complications were illeus (2.6%), deep venous thrombosis (2.6%), lymphocysts (2.4%), and small bowel obstruction (1.8%) (Cragun et al. 2005). The postoperative morbidity after surgical staging was significantly less in patients undergoing laparoscopy compared to those who had the procedure performed via laparotomy (14% vs. 21%, $p<0.001$) in the LAP-2 trial (Walker et al. 2009). To further limit the morbidity associated with complete lymph node dissection; sentinel lymph node detection is being evaluated in endometrial cancer (Gien et al. 2005; Delaloye et al. 2007; Frumovitz et al. 2007). Though controversial worldwide, FIGO staging remains the standard at this time as it allows for more accurate post surgical treatment.

3.2 Treatment after surgical staging

Treatment after initial staging depends on the final stage assigned after regarding different surgical-pathologic risk factors. It is discussed here under three broad headings: treatment of stage I endometrial cancer; treatment of endometrial cancer with cervical involvement (stage II); and treatment of advanced stage endometrial cancer(stages III and IV) (Table 3).

3.2.1 Treatment of stage I endometrial cancer

3.2.1.1 Low-risk patients

Patients with no myometrial invasion and grade 1/2 disease have particularly low risk of recurrence (2-10%) (Creasman et al. 1987). Neither pelvic external beam radiotherapy nor vaginal brachytherapy is recommended for these patients. In a recent study, no vaginal recurrences were reported in these patients after surgery alone (Straughn et al. 2002).

3.2.1.2 Intermediate risk

Intermediate risk endometrial cancer is divided into low-intermediate risk and high-intermediate risk disease. Low-intermediate risk group includes patients with no myometrial invasion and grade 3 disease; patients with less than 50% myometrial invasion and grade 1/2 disease. High-intermediate risk group includes patients with less than 50% myometrial invasion and grade 3 disease; patients with myometrial invasion ≥50% and grade 1/2 disease; and patients with stage IIA disease and grade 1/2 disease.

Stage	Adverse risk factors	Adjuvant Treatment		
		G1	G2	G3
Stage IA	Absent	Observe	Observe or Vaginal brachytherapy	Observe or Vaginal brachytherapy
	Present	Observe or Vaginal brachytherapy	Observe or Vaginal brachytherapy and/or Pelvic RT	Observe or Vaginal brachytherapy and/or Pelvic RT
Stage IB	Absent	Observe or Vaginal brachytherapy	Observe or Vaginal brachytherapy	Observe or Vaginal brachytherapy and/or Pelvic RT
	Present	Observe or Vaginal brachytherapy and/or Pelvic RT	Observe or Vaginal brachytherapy and/or Pelvic RT	Observe or Pelvic RT and/or Vaginal brachytherapy ± Chemotherapy
Stage II	---	Vaginal brachytherapy and/or Pelvic RT	Pelvic RT + Vaginal brachytherapy	Pelvic RT + Vaginal brachytherapy ± Chemotherapy
Stage IIIA	---	Chemotherapy ± RT or Tumor-directed RT± Chemotherapy or Pelvic RT ± Vaginal brachytherapy	Chemotherapy ± RT or Tumor-directed RT± Chemotherapy or Pelvic RT ± Vaginal brachytherapy	Chemotherapy ± RT or Tumor-directed RT± Chemotherapy or Pelvic RT ± Vaginal brachytherapy
Stage IIIB	---	Chemotherapy and/or Tumor-directed RT	Chemotherapy and/or Tumor-directed RT	Chemotherapy and/or Tumor-directed RT
Stage IIIC1, IIIC2	---	Chemotherapy and/or Tumor-directed RT	Chemotherapy and/or Tumor-directed RT	Chemotherapy and/or Tumor-directed RT
Stage IVA, IVB	---	Chemotherapy ± RT	Chemotherapy ± RT	Chemotherapy ± RT

1: All staging is based on updated 2009 FIGO staging.
2: Adapted with permission from the NCCN Clinical Practice Guidelines in Oncology (NCCN Guidelines™) for Uterine Neoplasms V.2.2011. To view the most recent and complete version of the NCCN Guidelines, go online to NCCN.org.

Table 3. NCCN Guidelines for Adjuvant Treatment in Endometrial Cancer.

Patients in intermediate risk group have been the subjects of different randomized controlled trials (Table 4). The Norwegian trial led by Aalders et al recruited 540 stage I patients between 1968-1974 (Aalders et al. 1980). All patients underwent surgery and subsequently received vaginal brachytherapy at the dose of 60 Gy. Patients were then randomized to receive either external beam radiotherapy (EBRT) or no further treatment (NFT). The vaginal and pelvic recurrence rate was higher in the observation arm compared to the radiotherapy arm (7% vs. 2%, p=0.01). Interestingly, the distant failure rate was higher in the radiotherapy group than the control group (10% vs. 5%, p=0.05). The 5-year overall survival was not different between the groups. A distinct survival advantage was observed

on subgroup analysis among patients with grade 3 tumor and deep myometrial invasion who had received RT (Aalders et al. 1980).
PORTEC-1 included stage I endometrial cancer patients with either: grade I disease and deep myometrial invasion (≥50%); grade II disease with any myoinvasion; or grade III disease with superficial (<50%) myometrial invasion (Creutzberg et al. 2000). A total of 715 patients were enrolled. All patients underwent a total abdominal hysterectomy and bilateral salpingo-oophorectomy without lymph node dissection. Subsequently, these patients were randomized to external beam radiotherapy or no further treatment. The loco-regional recurrence rate was significantly lower in the EBRT arm compared to the NFT arm (4% vs. 14%, p<0.001). The distant recurrence rate, the 5-year overall survival rate, and the endometrial cancer related death rate were however comparable (p≥0.05). Treatment related complications were more common in the radiotherapy group compared to the control group (25% vs. 6%, p<0.001). Scholten et al published a 10-year follow-up of PORTEC-1, which excluded cases downgraded after central pathology review (Scholten et al. 2005). Similar to the original study, the 10-year loco-regional relapse rate was significantly higher in the no further treatment group compared to the RT group (14% vs. 5%, p>0.001). Radiation was particularly effective in patients with two out of the following three high-risk features (age >60 years, > 50% myometrial invasion, and grade III)--loco-regional recurrence rate 4% in the RT group vs. 23% in the control group. Most loco-regional recurrences however were isolated vaginal recurrences, with higher salvage rate in control group versus the RT group (70% vs. 38%).
The Gynecologic Oncology Group also evaluated the role of adjuvant pelvic radiotherapy in patients with early stage endometrial cancer (GOG 99) (Keys et al. 2004). This trial included patients with stage IB, IC, and stage II (occult) disease. Patients with clear cell and papillary serous endometrial cancers were excluded. All patients were required to undergo a complete surgical staging procedure. Afterwards, patients were randomized to either no further treatment or external beam radiation. Based on the following risk factors: age, lymphovascular space invasion, grade III tumors, and outer third myometrial invasion; a high intermediate risk group was defined including patients aged ≥70 years with ≥1 risk factor; 50-70 years with ≥ 2 risk factors; or <50 years with all three risk factors. All other patients were considered low-intermediate risk. The median follow up was 69 months. The two year cumulative incidence of recurrence was 12% in the no additional treatment arm and 3% in the RT arm (relative hazard=0.42, p=0.007). Majority of the difference between the two groups could be explained on the basis of disparity in the occurrence of vaginal recurrences (13 in the NFT arm and 2 in the RT arm). The overall survival was not significantly different between the RT and the NFT groups (p=0.56). On subgroup analysis, RT resulted in statistically significant improvement in the incidence of recurrence in the high intermediate risk group (2 year CIR: 6% VS. 26%; relative hazard 0.42, 90% CI: 0.21-0.83), but not in the low-intermediate risk group (2 year CIR: 2% VS. 6%; relative hazard: 0.46, 90% CI: 0.19-1.11). However, patients in the RT group experienced more frequent and more severe toxicities, and the difference was particularly significant for hematologic, gastrointestinal, genitourinary, and cutaneous toxicities.
ASTEC/EN.5 trial enrolled 905 women between 1996-2005 with node negative early stage endometrial cancer (stages I-IIA) and intermediate or high risk features (IA grade 3, IB all grades, papillary serous or clear cell histology all stages and grades) (Blake et al. 2009). After

surgery, brachytherapy was allowed to all patients according to the local policy. Patients were then randomized to either EBRT or observation. There was no difference between groups in regards to either overall survival (5-year OS: 84% in both groups; HR 1.05 CI: 0.75-1.48, p=0.77) or recurrence free survival (84.7% NFT vs. 85.3% EBRT; HR: 0.92 CI: 0.66-1.31). The 5-year cumulative incidence of isolated vaginal or pelvic recurrence was 6.1% in the NFT arm and 3.2% in the EBRT arm (HR 0.46 CI: 0.24-0.89, p=0.02). Both acute (57% vs. 27%) and late toxicity (61% vs. 45%) was significantly more in the EBRT group compared to the observation group.

Based on the results of these trials, it appears that radiotherapy decreases the incidence of loco-regional recurrence but does not improve survival. The reduction of loco-regional recurrences is mainly due to a decrease in the incidence of vaginal recurrences which accounted for almost 75% of all locoregional recurrences in the control arm. Given the adverse effects noted with radiation, a randomized PORTEC-2 trial was opened to investigate if vaginal brachytherapy would be as effective as EBRT (Nout et al. 2010). Patients at high-intermediate risk for recurrence were eligible for enrollment (age >60 years and IC grade 1/2 disease or stage IB grade 3 disease; stage IIA any age (apart from grade 3 with >50% myometrial invasion). All patients underwent a total abdominal hysterectomy and bilateral salpingo-oophorectomy without lymphadenecetomy. Subsequently, patients were randomized to receive either pelvic RT or vaginal brachytherapy. The 5-year vaginal recurrence rate was 1.8% in the vaginal brachytherapy group (VBT) and 1.6% in the EBRT group (HR=0.78 CI: 0.17-3.49; p=0.74). Although, pelvic recurrence rate was higher in the VBT arm (3.8% vs. 0.5%; p=0.02); there was no difference between groups regarding the incidence of either locoregional recurrence (EBRT: 2.1% vs. VBT: 5.1%; p=0.17), distant recurrence (EBRT: 5.7% vs. VBT: 8.3%; p=0.46), or survival (5-year overall survival: 79.6% in EBRT vs. 84.8% in VBT; p=0.57). The gastrointestinal side effects were however significantly more common in the EBRT group compared to the VBT group (53.8% v12.6%, respectively) with resultant poorer quality of life (Nout et al. 2009).

First Author, yr (Reference study)	N	Stages	LND	Treatment	LRR	DRR	5-yr OS
1. Aalders et al, 1980 (Norwegian)	540	I	No	Sx + VBT	7%[1]	5%	91%
				Sx + VBT + EBRT	2%[1]	10%	89%
2. Creutzberg et al, 2000 (PORTEC-1)	715	I	No	Sx	14%[1]	7%	85%
				Sx + EBRT	4%[1]	8%	81%
3. Keys et al, 2004 (GOG 99)	342	I-II	Yes	Sx	7%[1]	8%	86%[2]
				Sx + EBRT	2%[1]	5%	92%[2]
4. Blake et al, 2009 (ASTEC/EN.5)	905	I-II	No	Sx	6%	--	84%
				Sx + EBRT	3%	--	84%
5. Nout et al, 2010 (PORTEC-2)	427	I-II	No	Sx + VBT	5%	8%	85%
				Sx + EBRT	2%	6%	80%

1: Statistically significant difference; 2: 4-yr OS
LND: Lymph Node Dissection; LRR: Locoregional Recurrence Rate; DRR: Distant Recurrence Rate
Sx: Surgery; VBT: Vaginal Brachytherapy; EBRT: External Beam Radiotherapy
GOG: Gynecologic Oncology Group

Table 4. Randomized Controlled Trials of Adjuvant Radiotherapy in Early Stage Endometrial Cancer.

These data suggest that vaginal brachytherapy could be used as effectively as external beam RT to optimize local control in patients deemed to be at high-intermediate risk, and with less morbidity and better quality of life.

3.2.1.3 High risk patients

High risk endometrial cancer includes patients with 1988 FIGO stage IC with grade 3 disease and/or lymphovascular space invasion; 1988 FIGO stage IIA with grade 3 disease, deep myometrial invasion, and/or lymphovascular space invasion; stages IIB, III and IV; clear cell or papillary serous histologies. Creutzberg et al compared 104 patients with stage IC grade 3 endometrial cancer against the PORTEC patients who received RT (Creutzberg et al. 2004). The locoregional recurrence rate was 1-3% among the PORTEC patients, and 14% for stage IC grade 3 patients. The 5-year distant metastasis rates were 3-8% for grade 1/2 patients, 20% for stage IB grade III patients, and 31% for stage IC grade III patients. The high-risk patients remain at significant risk for distant failure despite EBRT. In an attempt to improve distant failure rate and survival in these patients, the use of adjuvant chemotherapy has been explored in several clinical trials (Table 5). The results of most of these trials have been negative with the exception of two trials (Randall et al. 2006 and Hogberg et al. 2010).

First Author, yr (Reference Study)	N	Stages	Treatment	5-yr PFS	5-yr OS
1. Morrow et al, 1990	181	I-II	Sx + XRT	--	60%
(GOG 34)			Sx + XRT + A	--	60%
2. Maggi et al, 2006	345	I-III	Sx + CAP	63%	66%
			Sx + XRT	63%	69%
3. Susumu et al, 2008	385	I-III	Sx + CAP	82%	87%
(JGOG)			Sx + XRT	84%	85%
4. Kuoppala et al, 2008	156	I-III	Sx + XRT	---	85%
(Finnish)			Sx + XRT + CAP	---	82%
5. Hogberg et al, 2010	534	I-III	Sx + XRT	69%[1]	75%
(Combined NSGO/EORTC and MaNGO/ILIADE III)			Sx + XRT + CT	78%[1]	82%

1: Statistically significant difference.
Sx: Surgery; XRT: Radiotherapy; A: Doxorubicin; CAP: Cyclophosphamide + Doxorubicin + Cisplatin; CT: Chemotherapy
GOG: Gynecologic Oncology Group; JGOG: Japanese Gynecologic Oncology Group; NSGO-EORTC: The Nordic Society of Gynecologic Oncology- European Organization for Research and Treatment of Cancer; MaNGO: Mario Negri Institute.

Table 5. Randomized Controlled Trials of Adjuvant Chemotherapy in Early Stage Endometrial Cancer.

Morrow et al included patients diagnosed with stages IC-IIIC (Morrow et al. 1990). All patients underwent a complete staging followed by the administration of pelvic RT. Patients were then randomized to either doxorubicin (45 mg/m2) or no further treatment. There was no significant difference with regards to either overall survival or progression free survival between the chemotherapy group and the observation group. There was a trend towards fewer extrapelvic recurrences in the doxorubicin arm compared to the control arm (16.3% vs. 22.5%).

In an Italian trial, patients were randomized to either chemotherapy with cyclophosphamide (600 mg/m2), doxorubicin (45 mg/m2), and cisplatin (50 mg/m2) [CAP] or radiation treatment after the initial staging (Maggi et al. 2006). Only one third of the patients in this trial were stage I/II, remaining 2/3 had stage III disease. There was no difference between the CT arm and the RT arm with regards to either overall survival (5year OS: 66% vs. 69%; p=0.78) or progression free survival (5-year PFS: 63% vs. 63%; p=0.45). There were more local recurrences in the CT group compared to the RT group (11% vs. 7%); but distant recurrences were higher in the RT group than the CT group (21% vs. 16%).

In a similar study design; Susumu et al evaluated patients with stages IC-IIIC with > 50% myometrial invasion and no residual tumor after surgery (Susumu et al. 2008). Patients received either pelvic RT (45-50 Gy) or chemotherapy with cyclyophosphamide (333 mg/m2), doxorubicin (40 mg/m2), and cisplatin (50 mg/m2). Patients were divided into low-intermediate risk group (IC plus age <70 years plus grade I/II) and high-intermediate risk group (IC plus age >70 years plus grade III or stage II/IIIA with > 50% myometrial invasion). The 5-year progression free survival for low-intermediate risk patients was 94.5% in the RT group and 87.6% in the CT group (p=0.11). The corresponding 5-year overall survival rates were 95.1% and 90.8%, respectively (p=0.28). The survival was however significantly better in the CT group compared to the RT group among the high-intermediate risk patients (5-year PFS: 83.8% vs. 66.2%, p=0.024; 5-year OS: 89.7% vs. 73.6%, p=0.006). The overall incidence of G3/G4 complications was 1.6% in the RT group and 4.7% in the CT group.

Kuoppala et al randomized high-risk patients after surgery to either radiotherapy alone or radiation plus chemotherapy with cisplatin(50 mg/m2), doxorubicin(60 mg/m2), and cyclophosphamide (500 mg/m2) (Kuoppala et al. 2008). Adjuvant chemotherapy failed to improve overall survival or the recurrence rate in their study [5-year disease specific survival: 84.7% RT vs. 82.1% RT +CT, p=0.148; median disease free survival: 18 months for RT vs. 25 months for RT+ CT, p=0.134).

The Nordic society for gynecologic oncology 9501/ European Organization for Research and Treatment of Cancer Group 55991 and MaNGO/ILIADE-III trial compared radiation alone to radiation followed by CT (Hogberg et al. 2010). The combination of radiation and chemotherapy was associated with a superior progression free survival (HR: 0.63, CI: 0.44-0.89; p=0.009) and cancer specific survival (HR: 0.55, CI: 0.35-0.88; p=0.01) compared to the radiation only arm. Recently, the Cochrane review group led by Johnson et al reported (presented in abstract form at the 2010 annual meeting of the International Gynecological Cancer Society) data from 7 randomized trials and 1,919 women showing a survival advantage in favor of adjuvant chemotherapy (RR: 0.85 CI: 0.75-0.96) (Lai et al. 2011).

While, there is little doubt as to the usefulness of chemotherapy in the treatment of high-risk patients; its role in the treatment of these patients will be further clarified with the results of PORTEC-3 trial (comparing EBRT+CT vs. EBRT alone). It is debatable whether patients receiving adjuvant radiotherapy should receive pelvic RT or vaginal brachytherapy alone. The exclusion of RT in these patients has been shown to increase the risk of pelvic failure in

some studies (Mundt et al. 2001; Klopp et al. 2009). GOG 249 is currently evaluating outcomes in high-intermediate risk and high risk endometrial cancer patients treated with 3 cycles of carboplatin/taxol followed by either VBT or EBRT.
The role of hormone therapy in early stage endometrial cancer has been studied in different randomized trials (Table 6). Only patients with stage I endometrial cancer were included in four trials (Lewis et al. 1974; Malkasian and Bures 1978; Macdonald et al. 1988; De Palo et al. 1993). Other trials also included patients with more advanced disease (COSA-NZ-UK Endometrial Cancer Study Group ; Vergote et al. 1989; Urbanski et al. 1993). A meta-analysis of four of these trials was recently reported by Martin-Hirsch et al. There was no significant difference in the risk of death between patients who received progestogen compared to those who did not receive progestogen (RR: 1.00, CI: 0.85-1.18)(Martin-Hirsch et al. 2011). Although, the risk of relapse was lower in patients receiving progestogen compared to those who did not receive progestogen (RR: 0.71, CI: 0.52-0.97) (Urbanski et al. 1993); this effect was not reproduced in another trial (RR 1.34, CI: 0.79-2.27) (De Palo et al. 1993). The authors concluded that there is no evidence to support the routine use of progestogens in the primary treatment of endometrial cancer.

First Author, yr	N	Stages	Treatment	Risk of Death at 5-yrs Hazard Ratio [95% CI]
1.Lewis et al, 1974	956	I	Progestogen Control	1.63 [1.00-2.67]
2.Malkasian et al, 1978	35	I	Progestogen Control	1.89[0.40-9.01]
3.MacDonald et al, 1988	429	I	Progestogen Control	1.09 [0.70-1.72]
4.Vergote et al, 1989	1048	I-II	Progestogen Control	1.00 [0.74-1.34]
5.Urbanski et al, 1993	205	I-III	Progestogen Control	0.10 [0.03-0.30][1]
6.De Palo et al, 1993	771	I	Progestogen Control	1.48 [0.82-2.66]
7.COSA-NZ-UK, 1998	1012	I-III	Progestogen Control	0.91 [0.74-1.12]

1: Favors progestogen.

Table 6. Randomized Controlled Trials of Adjuvant Hormonal Therapy in Early Stage Endometrial Cancer.

3.2.2 Treatment of endometrial cancer with cervical involvement

In the past, one of the most commonly employed procedure for the treatment of these patients was preoperative RT followed by total abdominal hysterectomy. The 5-year actuarial survival rate reported among patients treated with pre or postoperative radiation therapy has been reported to range from 57% to 85% and 52% to 87%, respectively (Menczer 2005). Calais et al performed a retrospective comparison of outcomes among 184 patients who received vaginal brachytherapy before or after radical hysterectomy (Calais et al. 1990). There was no significant difference in survival between patients treated with either preoperative or postoperative radiation therapy (87% and 91%, respectively). Similarly, the incidence of local recurrence (13% vs. 9%) and distant recurrence (12% and 9%) was also comparable between the two groups. Although, not statistically significant, a trend towards more late complications was observed in patients treated with preoperative radiation (14% vs. 7.9%). Similar results have been reported by others (Lanciano et al. 1990). Additionally, preoperative RT can confound the pathological determination of grade, depth of myometrial invasion, and pelvic lymph node involvement.

The role of radical hysterectomy in endometrial cancer with cervical involvement has been investigated by several authors. A series by Sartori et al included 203 patients with stage II endometrial cancer (Sartori et al. 2001). Of these; 66% underwent a simple TAH, whereas RH was performed in the remaining 34% patients. The 5-year survival rates were significantly better in the RH group compared to the TAH group (94% vs. 79%, $p<0.05$). The local and distant recurrences were also fewer in the RH group. Cornelison et al also demonstrated a superior survival among stage II endometrial cancer patients treated with RH compared to TAH (surgery only group: 93% vs. 84%, $p<0.05$; surgery plus radiation group: 88% vs. 82.7%, $p<0.05$)(Cornelison et al. 1999).

The schema for risk-stratification for stage II patients and results of clinical trials have been discussed elsewhere in this chapter. The NCCN recommendations for management of this group of patients are as shown in figure 1. Although, both pelvic RT and brachytherapy are recommended; observation or vaginal brachytherapy is also an option for stage II patients who have undergone a RH with negative surgical margins and no evidence of extrauterine disease (NCCN guidelines for uterine neoplams, V.2.2011). In a small study by Ng et al, no recurrences were observed in stage II patients undergoing extended surgical staging followed by vaginal vault brachytherapy (Ng et al. 2001).

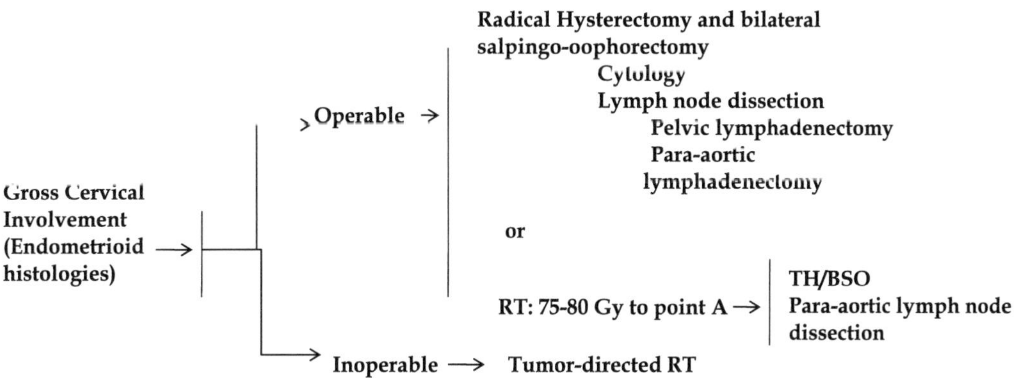

Fig. 1. Schematic representation of primary management of endometrial cancer with cervical involvement.

3.2.3 Treatment of advanced stage endometrial carcinoma (stages III and IV)

Although, most endometrial cancers are diagnosed in early stages due to symptoms; those who are diagnosed in advanced stages do poorly on available treatments. Generally, a multimodality approach involving surgery ± radiation ± chemotherapy ± hormonal agents is required. NCCN guidelines for the management of these patients are shown in Figure 2.

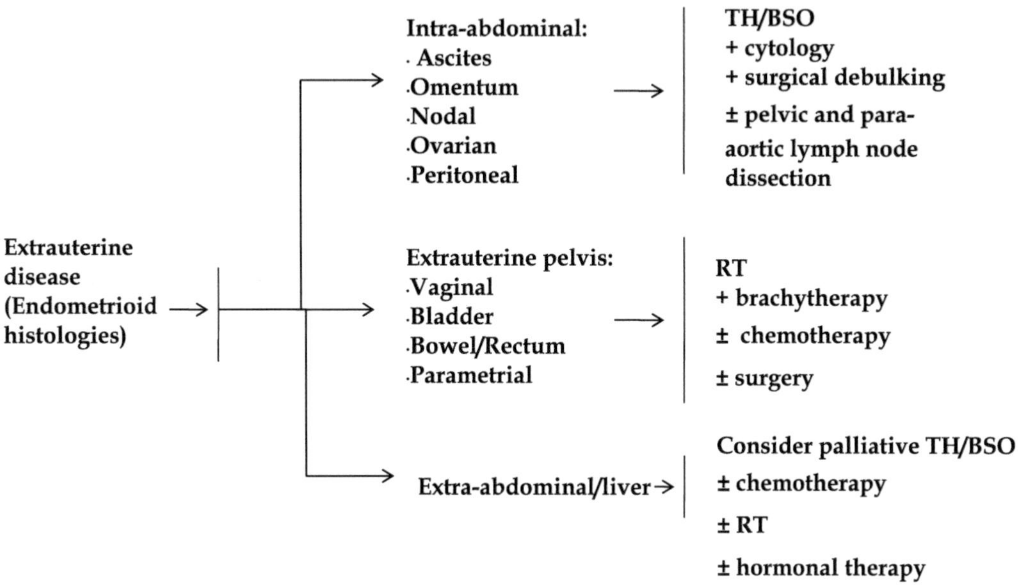

Fig. 2. Schematic representation of primary management of endometrial cancer with extrauterine disease.

3.2.3.1 Role of cytoreductive surgery

The role of cytoreductive surgery in patients diagnosed with advanced stage endometrial cancer is debatable. Goff et al showed that survival was significantly better in patients that were cytoreduced (18 months) compared to those that did not undergo surgery (8 months) (Goff et al. 1994). In another study, Chi et al compared the outcomes among those stage IV endometrial cancer patients that underwent either optimal cytoreduction (residual disease ≤2 cm), suboptimal cytoreduction (gross residual disease >2cm), or no cytoreduction (Chi et al. 1997). The median survival recorded for patients in these groups was 31 months , 13 months, and 3 months, respectively ($p<0.01$). Only the extent of cytoreduction was a significant predictor of survival on multivariate analysis. Similar findings have been reported by other investigators (Bristow et al. 2000; Ayhan et al. 2002). Although, data from these small retrospective studies appear encouraging, it is important to note that there has been no randomized trial to date to validate this beneficial effect.

3.2.3.2 Role of radiotherapy

Pelvic radiotherapy with or without vaginal brachytherapy has been used to prevent local and/or lymph node metastasis in patients with advanced stage endometrial cancer. In a study by Mariani et al, the incidence of pelvic side wall recurrences at 5 years was 57% among those node positive stage III/IV endometrial cancer patients that underwent inadequate node dissection and/or no radiotherapy compared to 10% for those receiving both adequate lymphadenectomy and postoperative radiotherapy ($p<0.001$)(Mariani et al. 2006). While the 5-year para-aortic failure rate was 34% among patients undergoing para-aortic lymphadenectomy and no adjuvant radiation; there were no failures among those 11 patients who received both para-aortic lymphadenectomy and para-aortic radiation. Similarly, in a study, by Mundt et al, there was a trend towards improved local failure rate among those stage IIIC endometrial cancer patients who received vaginal brachytherapy compared to those who did not (vaginal recurrence: 0/10 vs. 4/20; $p=0.12$)(Mundt et al. 2001).

Due to the risk of abdominal recurrence in advanced stage endometrial cancer and/or high-risk histologies; the use of whole abdominal radiation has been proposed. Smith et al reported a 3-year estimated progression free survival of 79% and overall survival of 89% in 22 patients with stage III/IV adenocarcinoma using postoperative whole abdominal radiation(Smith et al. 2000). All four failures in these patients were extra-abdominal. The 3 year actuarial major complication rate was 7% in their series, and there were no treatment related deaths. In another report by Gibbons et al; the 7-year disease specific survival after WAI was 57.8% for stage III and 25.0% for stage IV disease ($p=0.006$)(Gibbons et al. 1991). Although, acute toxicity was common, the complications were generally mild.

In the GOG study, the 3-year recurrence free survival was 29% and overall survival was 31% in patients with endometrial adenocarcinoma (Sutton et al. 2005). The corresponding rates in papillary serous/clear cell carcinoma were 27% and 35%, respectively. The incidence of different types of severe toxicities was as follows: myelosuppression (12.6%), gastrointestinal toxicity (15%), and hepatic toxicity (2.2%). Although these results look promising, GOG 122 emphatically established the superiority of chemotherapy over whole abdominal radiation in the treatment of patients with advanced stage endometrial cancer(Randall et al. 2006). The progression free survival and overall survival were both higher in the chemotherapy arm compared to the whole abdominal radiation arm. There were more pelvic failures in the group receiving chemotherapy compared to those treated with WAI (18% vs. 13%). Others have similarly reported high pelvic failure rate with chemotherapy alone (Mundt et al. 2001; Klopp et al. 2009; Barrena Medel et al. 2011). These data lend support to the use of combined modality therapy in the treatment of patients with advanced stage endometrial cancer. Several studies have shown improved outcomes with combination of radiation and chemotherapy (Schorge et al. 1996; Onda et al. 1997; Hoskins et al. 2001; Bruzzone et al. 2004) and it is currently being further evaluated on a Gynecologic Oncology Group study (GOG 258: A Randomized Phase III trial of Cisplatin and Tumor Volume Directed Irradiation Followed by Carboplatin and Paclitaxel vs. Carboplatin and Paclitaxel for Optimally Debulked Advanced Endometrial Carcinoma).

3.2.3.3 Role of chemotherapy

In advanced stage endometrial cancer, chemotherapy may be administered in various settings: as primary systemic therapy, adjuvant therapy, or neoadjuvant therapy. Response rates have been over 20% in phase II studies with anthracyclines, platinum compounds, alkylating agents, and taxanes (Humber et al. 2007). The Gynecologic Oncology Group has undertaken several trials over the last three decades to evaluate the effectiveness of various single agents and combinations in the treatment of advanced/recurrent endometrial cancer (Table 7).

Thigpen et al evaluated those patients with advanced stage (stages III/IV) and recurrent endometrial cancer who were chemonaive and had measurable disease after prior surgery or radiotherapy on GOG 107(Thigpen et al. 2004). A total of 281 patients were eligible. Patients were randomized to receive either doxorubicin alone or a combination of doxorubicin and cisplatin. The overall response rate was significantly higher in the combination arm compared to the doxorubicin alone arm (42% vs. 25%, p=0.004). The median progression free survival was also significantly longer in patients receiving doxorubicin plus cisplatin compared to those who received doxorubicin alone (5.7 months vs. 3.8 months; HR: 0.74 CI: 0.58-0.94). The toxicity was significantly greater in patients treated with the doxorubicin and cisplatin doublet.

Randall et al included patients with stage III/IV endometrial cancer on GOG 122 (Randall et al. 2006). All patients underwent an optimal cytoreduction (residual disease ≤ 2 cm). Patients were then randomized to either whole abdominal irradiation (WAI) or chemotherapy with cisplatin and doxorubicin (AP). Between 1992 and 2000, 422 patients were accrued. The median follow up was 74 months. The 5-year PFS was 50% in the AP arm and 38% in the WAI arm (HR: 0.71 CI: 0.55-0.91, p<0.01). The 5-year overall survival was 55% in the AP arm and 42% in the WAI arm (HR: 0.68 CI: 0.52-0.89, p<0.01). Analysis of the site of recurrence revealed 18% pelvic, 14% abdominal, and 18% extra-abdominal recurrence in the AP arm, and 13% pelvic, 16% abdominal, and 22% extra-abdominal recurrence in the WAI arm. Administration of AP was associated with significantly more acute toxicity (treatment related deaths 4% in AP arm and 2% in the WAI arm).

Homesley et al compared outcomes between stage III/IV endometrial cancer patients treated with combination of cisplatin plus doxorubicin (AP) or cisplatin plus doxorubicin plus taxol (TAP)(Homesley et al. 2009). All patients had previously undergone a cytoreductive surgery followed by tumor volume directed radiation. The 3-year PFS was not significantly different between the two groups (64% vs. 62%; HR: 0.90, CI: 0.69-1.17). Subgroup analysis revealed a significant reduction in the risk of recurrence and death among patients with gross residual disease treated with TAP compared to AP (RR: 0.50, CI: 0.27-0.92). Toxicity was also more frequent and more severe in the TAP arm (p<0.01). Similarly, both median progression free survival (8.3 months vs. 5.3 months; HR: 0.60, CI: 0.46-0.78) and median overall survival (15.3 months vs. 12.3 months; HR: 0.75, CI: 0.57-0.99) were found to be significantly longer in another GOG study among advanced stage patients treated with (TAP) compared to those treated with (AP) (Fleming et al. 2004). Neurotoxicity was worse in the TAP arm compared to the AP arm (40% vs. 5%) and there were 5 treatment related deaths in the TAP arm and none in the AP arm.

The combination of carboplatin and taxol has shown efficacy in phase II setting for the primary treatment of advanced and recurrence endometrial cancer (Hoskins et al. 2001). The 3-year overall survival was 39% and toxicity was acceptable. Many practitioners are already administering this combination despite the lack of evidence from a randomized controlled trial. GOG 209 randomized patients with measurable and non-measurable stage III/IV or recurrent endometrial cancer to either TAP or carboplatin/Taxol. This trial has finished accrual and its results will be crucial in regards to identifying the most efficacious and safe chemotherapy regimen for treatment of patients with high-risk or advanced endometrial cancer. This combination is also being evaluated in 2 other ongoing GOG trials (GOG 249 and GOG 258, described elsewhere).

First Author, yr (Reference Study)	N	Stages	Regimen	5-yr PFS/ Median PFS	5-yr OS/ Median OS
1. Thigpen et al, 2004	281	III/IV/R	A	3.8 months[1]	9.2 months
(GOG 107)			AP	5.7 months[1]	9.0 months
2. Randall et al, 2006	396	III/IV	AP	50%[1]	55%[1]
(GOG 122)			WAI	38%[1]	42%[1]
3. Fleming et al, 2008	273	III/IV/R	TAP	8.3 months[1]	15.3 months[1]
(GOG 177)			AP	5.3 months[1]	12.3 months[1]
4. Homesley et al, 2009	552	III/IV	Sx + XRT + TAP	64%[2]	---
(GOG 184)			Sx + XRT + AP	62%[2]	---

1: Statistically significant; 2: 3-yr PFS
R: Recurrent; Sx: Surgery; XRT: Radiotherapy; A: Doxorubicin; AP: Doxorubicin + Cisplatin; TAP: Paclitaxel + Doxorubicin + Cisplatin;
GOG: Gynecologic Oncology Group.

Table 7. Randomized Controlled Trials of Adjuvant Chemotherapy in Advanced Endometrial Cancer.

The role of hormonal treatment in advanced endometrial cancer is discussed with recurrent endometrial cancer.

3.3 Papillary serous and clear cell carcinoma

Patients diagnosed with these histotypes should undergo comprehensive surgical staging. In a study by Thomas et al, 52% of patients with clear cell cancer confined to the uterus on clinical assessment were found to have extrauterine disease on surgical staging (Thomas et al. 2008). In another study by Goff et al, high incidence of lymph node metastasis and intraperitoneal metastasis was noted in patients with papillary serous cancer even in the absence of high risk features found significant on GOG 33 (Goff et al. 1994).

Surgical staging should include peritoneal cytology, total abdominal hysterectomy, bilateral salpingo-oophorectomy, pelvic and para-aortic lymphadenectomy, omentectomy, and biopsies of peritoneal surfaces including the underside of diaphragm(NCCN Clinical Practice Guidelines in Oncology (NCCN Guidelines™) for Uterine Neoplasms V.2.2011. © 2011 National Comprehensive Cancer Network). This is due to the propensity for omental involvement(Sherman et al. 1992; Saygili et al. 2001) and spread to the peritoneal surfaces (Geisler et al. 1999; Chan et al. 2003) in women diagnosed with papillary serous or clear cell

endometrial cancer. Maximum cytoreductive effort is recommended in the presence of extrauterine disease due to the associated survival advantage(Olawaiye and Boruta 2009).
The majority of patients with papillary serous or clear cell cancer relapse outside of pelvis, and distant recurrences are common even in patients with early stage disease. As a result, adjuvant chemotherapy with or without tumor volume directed radiotherapy is widely recommended in all patients, even those in whom the disease is confined to the uterus at the time of diagnosis(NCCN Clinical Practice Guidelines in Oncology (NCCN Guidelines™) for Uterine Neoplasms V.2.2011. © 2011 National Comprehensive Cancer Network).

3.4 Recurrent endometrial cancer

The risk of endometrial cancer recurrence ranges from 2-15% in early stage disease and 50-60% in advanced stages or aggressive histologies (Salani et al. 2011). The treatment options depend on previous radiation exposure, location and extent of disease, and goals of therapy (curative vs. palliative).
Isolated vaginal recurrence may be treated with surgery, radiotherapy, or a combination of both. For unresectable or disseminated metastases, systemic treatment with hormone therapy, chemotherapy with or without tumor directed radiation is generally employed. Local/regional recurrence can be treated with radiation ± surgical resection in patients with no prior radiation exposure. In the event of prior RT administration, surgical exploration, chemotherapy, or hormonal therapy is preferred (NCCN Clinical Practice Guidelines in Oncology (NCCN Guidelines™) for Uterine Neoplasms V.2.2011. © 2011 National Comprehensive Cancer Network). An analysis of survival after relapse in patients included in the PORTEC-trial, revealed 3-year survival rates of 73% after vaginal relapse, 8% after pelvic relapse, and 14% after distant relapse. There was no significant difference in survival between patients with pelvic and distant relapse (Creutzberg et al. 2003).
Historically, total pelvic exenteration has been performed in select patients who have failed the standard surgery and radiation treatment with reported long term survival rates of 20-45% and complication rates of 60-80% (Morris et al. 1996; Barakat et al. 1999). For patients who are not candidates for pelvic exenteration, the existing options are not very effective. In order to enhance the response to salvage therapies; the role of cytoreductive surgery has been explored. Scarabelli et al reported a complete macroscopic resection of disease in 65% patients with recurrent endometrial cancer, with significant improvement in survival ($p<0.01$)(Scarabelli et al. 1998). In another series by Bristow et al, 61 patients with recurrent endometrial cancer were evaluated (Bristow et al. 2006). The median post recurrence survival was significantly longer in the optimally cytoreduced patients compared to those left with gross residual disease (39 months vs. 14 months, $p=0.0005$). Similar results have been reported by others (Campagnutta et al. 2004; Awtrey et al. 2006).
Hormonal agents have been found valuable in patients with advanced/recurrent disease. They are generally associated with fewer side effects (compared to systemic chemotherapy) making them particularly suitable for use in patients with poor performance status and/or multiple co-morbidities. Various hormonal agents have been used (progestins, selective estrogen receptor modulators, aromatase inhibitors, synthetic steroid derivatives, and gonadotropin-releasing (GN-RH) hormone analogs) with a response rate of 9% to 55% in different studies(Kokka et al. 2010). Cochrane Database Systematic Review of hormonal

therapy in advanced or recurrent endometrial cancer assessed 542 patients from 6 different randomized trials(Stolyarova I ; Rendina et al. 1984; Ayoub et al. 1988; Urbanski et al. 1993; Thigpen et al. 1999; Pandya et al. 2001) (Table 8). The results indicated that hormonal therapy did not prolong overall survival or progression free survival in women with advanced or recurrent endometrial cancer (Kokka et al. 2010). Low-dose hormonal therapy was more effective than high-dose hormonal therapy (Thigpen et al. 1999). Despite the lack of survival advantage, hormonal agents may be used to alleviate symptoms and prevent progression.

First Author, yr	N	Stages	Treatment	Risk of Death or Recurrence Hazard Ratio [95% CI]
1.Rendina et al, 1984	93	III/IV	TMX MPA	1.00 [0.77-1.29]
2. Ayoub et al, 1988	43	IV/R	CAF CAF + MPA + TMX	0.80 [0.48-1.33]
3. Urbanski et al, 1993	31[1]	III	Progestogen Control	0.08 [0.01-1.28]
4. Thigpen et al, 1999	299	III/IV/R	MPA (200 mg/day) MPA (1000 mg/day)	1.31 [1.04-1.66]
5. Stolyarova et al, 2001	14[1]	III	XRT XRT + OPC	1.00 [0.40-2.48][2]
6. Pandya et al, 2001	62	III/IV	Megestrol Megestrol + TMX	1.03 [0.87-1.22]

1: Sub-group analysis; 2: Risk of recurrence
R: Recurrent
TMX: Tamoxifen; MPA:Medroxyprogesterone Acetate; CAF: Cyclophosphamide + Adriamycin + 5-Fluorouracil; XRT: Radiotherapy; OPC : 17-Oxyprogesterone Caproate.

Table 8. Randomized Controlled Trials of Adjuvant Hormonal Therapy in Advanced Endometrial Cancer.

4. Post treatment surveillance

The current NCCN guidelines recommend physical examination every 3-6 months for 2 years and then 6 months or annually thereafter(NCCN Clinical Practice Guidelines in

Oncology (NCCN Guidelines™) for Uterine Neoplasms V.2.2011. © 2011 National Comprehensive Cancer Network). A review of symptoms and physical examination is recommended at each visit. The yield of vaginal cytology (0-7%) and CXR (0-20%)for detection of recurrence has been shown to be very low in asymptomatic patients and therefore not currently recommended for routine use(Salani et al. 2011). Although, monitoring CA-125 levels may be beneficial in select patients (advanced stage disease, serous histology, pretreatment elevated CA-125); its routine use is also not supported by the available evidence (Salani et al. 2011).

5. Prognosis

The data concerning survival are provided in the Annual Report on the Results of Treatment in Gynecological Cancer (Creasman et al. 2006)and are shown in Table 9.

Strata	Patients	1-Year OS	3-Year OS	5-Year OS
Stage IA	1,054	98.2%	95.3%	90.8%
Stage IB	2,833	98.7%	94.6%	91.1%
Stage IC	1,426	97.5%	89.7%	85.4%
Stage IIA	430	95.2%	89.0%	83.3%
Stage IIB	543	93.5%	80.3%	74.2%
Stage IIIA	612	89.0%	73.3%	66.2%
Stage IIIB	80	73.5%	56.7%	49.9%
Stage IIIC	356	89.9%	66.3%	57.3%
Stage IVA	49	63.4%	34.4%	25.5%
Stage IVB	206	59.5%	29.0%	20.1%

Data taken from Creasman et al, 2006.

Table 9. Carcinoma of the Corpus Uteri: Patients Treated from 1999-2001; Survival Rates by FIGO Surgical Stage.

6. References

Aalders, J., V. Abeler, P. Kolstad and M. Onsrud (1980). "Postoperative external irradiation and prognostic parameters in stage I endometrial carcinoma: clinical and histopathologic study of 540 patients." *Obstet Gynecol* 56(4): 419-427.

Akin, O., S. Mironov, N. Pandit-Taskar and L. E. Hann (2007). "Imaging of uterine cancer." *Radiol Clin North Am* 45(1): 167-182.

Amant, F., P. Neven and I. Vergote (2009). "Lymphadenectomy in endometrial cancer." *Lancet* 373(9670): 1169-1170; author reply 1170-1161.

Arango, H. A., M. S. Hoffman, W. S. Roberts, S. L. DeCesare, J. V. Fiorica and J. Drake (2000). "Accuracy of lymph node palpation to determine need for lymphadenectomy in gynecologic malignancies." *Obstet Gynecol* 95(4): 553-556.

Awtrey, C. S., M. G. Cadungog, M. M. Leitao, K. M. Alektiar, C. Aghajanian, A. J. Hummer, R. R. Barakat and D. S. Chi (2006). "Surgical resection of recurrent endometrial carcinoma." *Gynecol Oncol* 102(3): 480-488.

Ayhan, A., C. Taskiran, C. Celik, K. Yuce and T. Kucukali (2002). "The influence of cytoreductive surgery on survival and morbidity in stage IVB endometrial cancer." *Int J Gynecol Cancer* 12(5): 448-453.

Ayoub, J., P. Audet-Lapointe, Y. Methot, J. Hanley, R. Beaulieu, R. Chemaly, A. Cormier, J. P. Dery, P. Drouin, P. Gauthier and et al. (1988). "Efficacy of sequential cyclical hormonal therapy in endometrial cancer and its correlation with steroid hormone receptor status." *Gynecol Oncol* 31(2): 327-337.

Barakat, R. R., N. A. Goldman, D. A. Patel, E. S. Venkatraman and J. P. Curtin (1999). "Pelvic exenteration for recurrent endometrial cancer." *Gynecol Oncol* 75(1): 99-102.

Barrena Medel, N. I., T. J. Herzog, I. Deutsch, W. M. Burke, X. Sun, S. N. Lewin and J. D. Wright (2011). "Comparison of the prognostic significance of uterine factors and nodal status for endometrial cancer." *Am J Obstet Gynecol* 204(3): 248 e241-247.

Blake, P., A. M. Swart, J. Orton, H. Kitchener, T. Whelan, H. Lukka, E. Eisenhauer, M. Bacon, D. Tu, M. K. Parmar, C. Amos, C. Murray and W. Qian (2009). "Adjuvant external beam radiotherapy in the treatment of endometrial cancer (MRC ASTEC and NCIC CTG EN.5 randomised trials): pooled trial results, systematic review, and meta-analysis." *Lancet* 373(9658): 137-146.

Bokhman, J. V. (1983). "Two pathogenetic types of endometrial carcinoma." *Gynecol Oncol* 15(1): 10-17.

Bristow, R. E., A. Santillan, M. L. Zahurak, G. J. Gardner, R. L. Giuntoli, 2nd and D. K. Armstrong (2006). "Salvage cytoreductive surgery for recurrent endometrial cancer." *Gynecol Oncol* 103(1): 281-287.

Bristow, R. E., M. J. Zerbe, N. B. Rosenshein, F. C. Grumbine and F. J. Montz (2000). "Stage IVB endometrial carcinoma: the role of cytoreductive surgery and determinants of survival." *Gynecol Oncol* 78(2): 85-91.

Bruzzone, M., L. Miglietta, P. Franzone, A. Gadducci and F. Boccardo (2004). "Combined treatment with chemotherapy and radiotherapy in high-risk FIGO stage III-IV endometrial cancer patients." *Gynecol Oncol* 93(2): 345-352.

Calais, G., L. Vitu, P. Descamps, G. Body, A. Reynaud-Bougnoux, J. Lansac, P. Bougnoux and O. Le Floch (1990). "Preoperative or postoperative brachytherapy for patients with endometrial carcinoma stage I and II." *Int J Radiat Oncol Biol Phys* 19(3): 523-527.

Campagnutta, E., G. Giorda, G. De Piero, F. Sopracordevole, M. C. Visentin, L. Martella and C. Scarabelli (2004). "Surgical treatment of recurrent endometrial carcinoma." *Cancer* 100(1): 89-96.

Case, A. S., R. P. Rocconi, J. M. Straughn, Jr., M. Conner, L. Novak, W. Wang and W. K. Huh (2006). "A prospective blinded evaluation of the accuracy of frozen section for the surgical management of endometrial cancer." *Obstet Gynecol* 108(6): 1375-1379.

Chan, J. K., M. K. Cheung, W. K. Huh, K. Osann, A. Husain, N. N. Teng and D. S. Kapp (2006). "Therapeutic role of lymph node resection in endometrioid corpus cancer: a study of 12,333 patients." *Cancer* 107(8): 1823-1830.

Chan, J. K., V. Loizzi, M. Youssef, K. Osann, J. Rutgers, S. A. Vasilev and M. L. Berman (2003). "Significance of comprehensive surgical staging in noninvasive papillary serous carcinoma of the endometrium." *Gynecol Oncol* 90(1): 181-185.

Chi, D. S., M. Welshinger, E. S. Venkatraman and R. R. Barakat (1997). "The role of surgical cytoreduction in Stage IV endometrial carcinoma." *Gynecol Oncol* 67(1): 56-60.

Cornelison, T. L., E. L. Trimble and C. L. Kosary (1999). "SEER data, corpus uteri cancer: treatment trends versus survival for FIGO stage II, 1988-1994." *Gynecol Oncol* 74(3): 350-355.

COSA-NZ-UK Endometrial Cancer Study Group (1998). Adjuvant medroxy progesterone acetate in high risk endometrial cancer. "Int J Gyn Cancer 8: 387-391.

Cragun, J. M., L. J. Havrilesky, B. Calingaert, I. Synan, A. A. Secord, J. T. Soper, D. L. Clarke-Pearson and A. Berchuck (2005). "Retrospective analysis of selective lymphadenectomy in apparent early-stage endometrial cancer." *J Clin Oncol* 23(16): 3668-3675.

Creasman, W. T., C. P. Morrow, B. N. Bundy, H. D. Homesley, J. E. Graham and P. B. Heller (1987). "Surgical pathologic spread patterns of endometrial cancer. A Gynecologic Oncology Group Study." *Cancer* 60(8 Suppl): 2035-2041.

Creasman, W. T., F. Odicino, P. Maisonneuve, M. A. Quinn, U. Beller, J. L. Benedet, A. P. Heintz, H. Y. Ngan and S. Pecorelli (2006). "Carcinoma of the corpus uteri. FIGO 26th Annual Report on the Results of Treatment in Gynecological Cancer." *Int J Gynaecol Obstet* 95 Suppl 1: S105-143.

Creutzberg, C. L., W. L. van Putten, P. C. Koper, M. L. Lybeert, J. J. Jobsen, C. C. Warlam-Rodenhuis, K. A. De Winter, L. C. Lutgens, A. C. van den Bergh, E. van de Steen-Banasik, H. Beerman and M. van Lent (2000). "Surgery and postoperative radiotherapy versus surgery alone for patients with stage-1 endometrial carcinoma: multicentre randomised trial. PORTEC Study Group. Post Operative Radiation Therapy in Endometrial Carcinoma." *Lancet* 355(9213): 1404-1411.

Creutzberg, C. L., W. L. van Putten, P. C. Koper, M. L. Lybeert, J. J. Jobsen, C. C. Warlam-Rodenhuis, K. A. De Winter, L. C. Lutgens, A. C. van den Bergh, E. van der Steen-Banasik, H. Beerman and M. van Lent (2003). "Survival after relapse in patients with endometrial cancer: results from a randomized trial." *Gynecol Oncol* 89(2): 201-209.

Creutzberg, C. L., W. L. van Putten, C. C. Warlam-Rodenhuis, A. C. van den Bergh, K. A. de Winter, P. C. Koper, M. L. Lybeert, A. Slot, L. C. Lutgens, M. C. Stenfert Kroese, H. Beerman and M. van Lent (2004). "Outcome of high-risk stage IC, grade 3, compared with stage I endometrial carcinoma patients: the Postoperative Radiation Therapy in Endometrial Carcinoma Trial." *J Clin Oncol* 22(7): 1234-1241.

De Palo, G., C. Mangioni, P. Periti, M. Del Vecchio and E. Marubini (1993). "Treatment of FIGO (1971) stage I endometrial carcinoma with intensive surgery, radiotherapy and hormonotherapy according to pathological prognostic groups. Long-term results of a randomised multicentre study." *Eur J Cancer* 29A(8): 1133-1140.

Delaloye, J. F., S. Pampallona, E. Chardonnens, M. Fiche, H. A. Lehr, P. De Grandi and A. B. Delaloye (2007). "Intraoperative lymphatic mapping and sentinel node biopsy using hysteroscopy in patients with endometrial cancer." *Gynecol Oncol* 106(1): 89-93.

Fleming, G. F., V. L. Brunetto, D. Cella, K. Y. Look, G. C. Reid, A. R. Munkarah, R. Kline, R. A. Burger, A. Goodman and R. T. Burks (2004). "Phase III trial of doxorubicin plus cisplatin with or without paclitaxel plus filgrastim in advanced endometrial carcinoma: a Gynecologic Oncology Group Study." *J Clin Oncol* 22(11): 2159-2166.

Franchi, M., F. Ghezzi, C. Riva, M. Miglierina, M. Buttarelli and P. Bolis (2001). "Postoperative complications after pelvic lymphadenectomy for the surgical staging of endometrial cancer." *J Surg Oncol* 78(4): 232-237; discussion 237-240.

Frumovitz, M., D. C. Bodurka, R. R. Broaddus, R. L. Coleman, A. K. Sood, D. M. Gershenson, T. W. Burke and C. F. Levenback (2007). "Lymphatic mapping and sentinel node biopsy in women with high-risk endometrial cancer." *Gynecol Oncol* 104(1): 100-103.

Geisler, J. P., H. E. Geisler, M. E. Melton and M. C. Wiemann (1999). "What staging surgery should be performed on patients with uterine papillary serous carcinoma?" *Gynecol Oncol* 74(3): 465-467.

Gibbons, S., A. Martinez, M. Schray, K. Podratz, R. Stanhope, G. Garton, S. Weiner, D. Brabbins and G. Malkasian (1991). "Adjuvant whole abdominopelvic irradiation for high risk endometrial carcinoma." *Int J Radiat Oncol Biol Phys* 21(4): 1019-1025.

Gien, L. T., J. S. Kwon and M. S. Carey (2005). "Sentinel node mapping with isosulfan blue dye in endometrial cancer." *J Obstet Gynaecol Can* 27(12): 1107-1112.

Girardi, F., E. Petru, M. Heydarfadai, J. Haas and R. Winter (1993). "Pelvic lymphadenectomy in the surgical treatment of endometrial cancer." *Gynecol Oncol* 49(2): 177-180.

Goff, B. A., A. Goodman, H. G. Muntz, A. F. Fuller, Jr., N. Nikrui and L. W. Rice (1994). "Surgical stage IV endometrial carcinoma: a study of 47 cases." *Gynecol Oncol* 52(2): 237-240.

Goff, B. A., D. Kato, R. A. Schmidt, M. Ek, J. A. Ferry, H. G. Muntz, J. M. Cain, H. K. Tamimi, D. C. Figge and B. E. Greer (1994). "Uterine papillary serous carcinoma: patterns of metastatic spread." *Gynecol Oncol* 54(3): 264-268.

Goudge, C., S. Bernhard, N. G. Cloven and P. Morris (2004). "The impact of complete surgical staging on adjuvant treatment decisions in endometrial cancer." *Gynecol Oncol* 93(2): 536-539.

Hogberg, T., M. Signorelli, C. F. de Oliveira, R. Fossati, A. A. Lissoni, B. Sorbe, H. Andersson, S. Grenman, C. Lundgren, P. Rosenberg, K. Boman, B. Tholander, G. Scambia, N. Reed, G. Cormio, G. Tognon, J. Clarke, T. Sawicki, P. Zola and G. Kristensen (2010). "Sequential adjuvant chemotherapy and radiotherapy in endometrial cancer--results from two randomised studies." *Eur J Cancer* 46(13): 2422-2431.

Homesley, H. D., V. Filiaci, S. K. Gibbons, H. J. Long, D. Cella, N. M. Spirtos, R. T. Morris, K. DeGeest, R. Lee and A. Montag (2009). "A randomized phase III trial in advanced endometrial carcinoma of surgery and volume directed radiation followed by cisplatin and doxorubicin with or without paclitaxel: A Gynecologic Oncology Group study." *Gynecol Oncol* 112(3): 543-552.

Hoskins, P. J., K. D. Swenerton, J. A. Pike, F. Wong, P. Lim, C. Acquino-Parsons and N. Lee (2001). "Paclitaxel and carboplatin, alone or with irradiation, in advanced or recurrent endometrial cancer: a phase II study." *J Clin Oncol* 19(20): 4048-4053.

Howlader N, N. A., Krapcho M, Neyman N, Aminou R, Waldron W, Altekruse SF, Kosary CL, Ruhl J, Tatalovich Z, Cho H, Mariotto A, Eisner MP, Lewis DR, Chen HS, Feuer EJ, Cronin KA, Edwards BK (eds). SEER Cancer Statistics Review, 1975-2008, National Cancer Institute. Bethesda, MD, http://seer.cancer.gov/csr/1975_2008/, based on November 2010 SEER data submission, posted to the SEER web site, 2011.

Hricak, H., L. V. Rubinstein, G. M. Gherman and N. Karstaedt (1991). "MR imaging evaluation of endometrial carcinoma: results of an NCI cooperative study." *Radiology* 179(3): 829-832.

Humber, C. E., J. F. Tierney, R. P. Symonds, M. Collingwood, J. Kirwan, C. Williams and J. A. Green (2007). "Chemotherapy for advanced, recurrent or metastatic endometrial cancer: a systematic review of Cochrane collaboration." *Ann Oncol* 18(3): 409-420.

Keys, H. M., J. A. Roberts, V. L. Brunetto, R. J. Zaino, N. M. Spirtos, J. D. Bloss, A. Pearlman, M. A. Maiman and J. G. Bell (2004). "A phase III trial of surgery with or without adjunctive external pelvic radiation therapy in intermediate risk endometrial adenocarcinoma: a Gynecologic Oncology Group study." *Gynecol Oncol* 92(3): 744-751.

Kilgore, L. C., E. E. Partridge, R. D. Alvarez, J. M. Austin, H. M. Shingleton, F. Noojin, 3rd and W. Conner (1995). "Adenocarcinoma of the endometrium: survival comparisons of patients with and without pelvic node sampling." *Gynecol Oncol* 56(1): 29-33.

Klopp, A. H., A. Jhingran, L. Ramondetta, K. Lu, D. M. Gershenson and P. J. Eifel (2009). "Node-positive adenocarcinoma of the endometrium: outcome and patterns of recurrence with and without external beam irradiation." *Gynecol Oncol* 115(1): 6-11.

Kokka, F., E. Brockbank, D. Oram, C. Gallagher and A. Bryant (2010). "Hormonal therapy in advanced or recurrent endometrial cancer." *Cochrane Database Syst Rev*(12): CD007926.

Kuoppala, T., J. Maenpaa, E. Tomas, U. Puistola, T. Salmi, S. Grenman, P. Lehtovirta, M. Fors, T. Luukkaala and P. Sipila (2008). "Surgically staged high-risk endometrial cancer: randomized study of adjuvant radiotherapy alone vs. sequential chemo-radiotherapy." *Gynecol Oncol* 110(2): 190-195.

Lai, C. H., A. Chao, F. Amant and I. Vergote (2011). "The 13th Biennial Meeting of the International Gynecologic Cancer Society (IGCS 2010)." *Gynecol Oncol* 120(1): 3-4.

Lanciano, R. M., W. J. Curran, Jr., K. M. Greven, J. Fanning, P. Stafford, M. E. Randall and G. E. Hanks (1990). "Influence of grade, histologic subtype, and timing of radiotherapy on outcome among patients with stage II carcinoma of the endometrium." *Gynecol Oncol* 39(3): 368-373.

Larson, D. M. and K. K. Johnson (1993). "Pelvic and para-aortic lymphadenectomy for surgical staging of high-risk endometrioid adenocarcinoma of the endometrium." *Gynecol Oncol* 51(3): 345-348.

Lewis, G. C., Jr., N. H. Slack, R. Mortel and I. D. Bross (1974). "Adjuvant progestogen therapy in the primary definitive treatment of endometrial cancer." *Gynecol Oncol* 2(2-3): 368-376.

Macdonald, R. R., J. Thorogood and M. K. Mason (1988). "A randomized trial of progestogens in the primary treatment of endometrial carcinoma." *Br J Obstet Gynaecol* 95(2): 166-174.

Maggi, R., A. Lissoni, F. Spina, M. Melpignano, P. Zola, G. Favalli, A. Colombo and R. Fossati (2006). "Adjuvant chemotherapy vs radiotherapy in high-risk endometrial carcinoma: results of a randomised trial." *Br J Cancer* 95(3): 266-271.

Malkasian, G. D., Jr. and J. Bures (1978). "Adjuvant progesterone therapy for stage I endometrial carcinoma." *Int J Gynaecol Obstet* 16(1): 48-49.

Mariani, A., S. C. Dowdy, W. A. Cliby, M. G. Haddock, G. L. Keeney, T. G. Lesnick and K. C. Podratz (2006). "Efficacy of systematic lymphadenectomy and adjuvant radiotherapy in node-positive endometrial cancer patients." *Gynecol Oncol* 101(2): 200-208.

Martin-Hirsch, P. P., A. Bryant, S. L. Keep, H. C. Kitchener and R. Lilford (2011). "Adjuvant progestagens for endometrial cancer." *Cochrane Database Syst Rev* 6: CD001040.

Menczer, J. (2005). "Management of endometrial carcinoma with cervical involvement. An unsettled issue." *Eur J Gynaecol Oncol* 26(3): 245-255.

Mohan, D. S., M. A. Samuels, M. A. Selim, A. D. Shalodi, R. J. Ellis, J. R. Samuels and H. J. Yun (1998). "Long-term outcomes of therapeutic pelvic lymphadenectomy for stage I endometrial adenocarcinoma." *Gynecol Oncol* 70(2): 165-171.

Moore, D. H., W. C. Fowler, Jr., L. A. Walton and W. Droegemueller (1989). "Morbidity of lymph node sampling in cancers of the uterine corpus and cervix." *Obstet Gynecol* 74(2): 180-184.

Morris, M., R. D. Alvarez, W. K. Kinney and T. O. Wilson (1996). "Treatment of recurrent adenocarcinoma of the endometrium with pelvic exenteration." *Gynecol Oncol* 60(2): 288-291.

Morrow, C. P., B. N. Bundy, H. D. Homesley, W. T. Creasman, N. B. Hornback, R. Kurman and J. T. Thigpen (1990). "Doxorubicin as an adjuvant following surgery and radiation therapy in patients with high-risk endometrial carcinoma, stage I and occult stage II: a Gynecologic Oncology Group Study." *Gynecol Oncol* 36(2): 166-171.

Mundt, A. J., R. McBride, J. Rotmensch, S. E. Waggoner, S. D. Yamada and P. P. Connell (2001). "Significant pelvic recurrence in high-risk pathologic stage I--IV endometrial carcinoma patients after adjuvant chemotherapy alone: implications for adjuvant radiation therapy." *Int J Radiat Oncol Biol Phys* 50(5): 1145-1153.

Mundt, A. J., K. T. Murphy, J. Rotmensch, S. E. Waggoner, S. D. Yamada and P. P. Connell (2001). "Surgery and postoperative radiation therapy in FIGO Stage IIIC endometrial carcinoma." *Int J Radiat Oncol Biol Phys* 50(5): 1154-1160.

Nakao, Y., M. Yokoyama, K. Hara, Y. Koyamatsu, M. Yasunaga, Y. Araki, Y. Watanabe and T. Iwasaka (2006). "MR imaging in endometrial carcinoma as a diagnostic tool for the absence of myometrial invasion." *Gynecol Oncol* 102(2): 343-347.

NCCN Clinical Practice Guidelines in Oncology (NCCN Guidelines™) for Uterine Neoplasms V.2.2011. © 2011 National Comprehensive Cancer Network, Inc. NCCN.org (Accessed 08/01/2011).

Ng, T. Y., J. L. Nicklin, L. C. Perrin, R. Cheuk and A. J. Crandon (2001). "Postoperative vaginal vault brachytherapy for node-negative Stage II (occult) endometrial carcinoma." *Gynecol Oncol* 81(2): 193-195.

Nout, R. A., H. Putter, I. M. Jurgenliemk-Schulz, J. J. Jobsen, L. C. Lutgens, E. M. van der Steen-Banasik, J. W. Mens, A. Slot, M. C. Stenfert Kroese, B. N. van Bunningen, V. T. Smit, H. W. Nijman, P. P. van den Tol and C. L. Creutzberg (2009). "Quality of life after pelvic radiotherapy or vaginal brachytherapy for endometrial cancer: first results of the randomized PORTEC-2 trial." *J Clin Oncol* 27(21): 3547-3556.

Nout, R. A., V. T. Smit, H. Putter, I. M. Jurgenliemk-Schulz, J. J. Jobsen, L. C. Lutgens, E. M. van der Steen-Banasik, J. W. Mens, A. Slot, M. C. Kroese, B. N. van Bunningen, A. C. Ansink, W. L. van Putten and C. L. Creutzberg (2010). "Vaginal brachytherapy versus pelvic external beam radiotherapy for patients with endometrial cancer of high-intermediate risk (PORTEC-2): an open-label, non-inferiority, randomised trial." *Lancet* 375(9717): 816-823.

Olawaiye, A. B. and D. M. Boruta, 2nd (2009). "Management of women with clear cell endometrial cancer: a Society of Gynecologic Oncology (SGO) review." *Gynecol Oncol* 113(2): 277-283.

Onda, T., H. Yoshikawa, K. Mizutani, M. Mishima, H. Yokota, H. Nagano, Y. Ozaki, A. Murakami, K. Ueda and Y. Taketani (1997). "Treatment of node-positive endometrial cancer with complete node dissection, chemotherapy and radiation therapy." *Br J Cancer* 75(12): 1836-1841.

Pandya, K. J., B. Y. Yeap, L. M. Weiner, J. E. Krook, J. K. Erban, R. A. Schinella and T. E. Davis (2001). "Megestrol and tamoxifen in patients with advanced endometrial cancer: an Eastern Cooperative Oncology Group Study (E4882)." *Am J Clin Oncol* 24(1): 43-46.

Park, J. Y., E. N. Kim, D. Y. Kim, D. S. Suh, J. H. Kim, Y. M. Kim, Y. T. Kim and J. H. Nam (2008). "Comparison of the validity of magnetic resonance imaging and positron emission tomography/computed tomography in the preoperative evaluation of patients with uterine corpus cancer." *Gynecol Oncol* 108(3): 486-492.

Pecorelli, S., L. Zigliani and F. Odicino (2009). "Revised FIGO staging for carcinoma of the cervix." *Int J Gynaecol Obstet* 105(2): 107-108.

Prat, J., A. Gallardo, M. Cuatrecasas and L. Catasus (2007). "Endometrial carcinoma: pathology and genetics." *Pathology* 39(1): 72-87.

Pristauz, G., A. A. Bader, P. Regitnig, J. Haas, R. Winter and K. Tamussino (2009). "How accurate is frozen section histology of pelvic lymph nodes in patients with endometrial cancer?" *Gynecol Oncol* 115(1): 12-17.

Randall, M. E., V. L. Filiaci, H. Muss, N. M. Spirtos, R. S. Mannel, J. Fowler, J. T. Thigpen and J. A. Benda (2006). "Randomized phase III trial of whole-abdominal irradiation versus doxorubicin and cisplatin chemotherapy in advanced endometrial carcinoma: a Gynecologic Oncology Group Study." *J Clin Oncol* 24(1): 36-44.

Rendina, G. M., C. Donadio, M. Fabri, P. Mazzoni and P. Nazzicone (1984). "Tamoxifen and medroxyprogesterone therapy for advanced endometrial carcinoma." *Eur J Obstet Gynecol Reprod Biol* 17(4): 285-291.

Salani, R., F. J. Backes, M. Fung Kee Fung, C. H. Holschneider, L. P. Parker, R. E. Bristow and B. A. Goff (2011). "Posttreatment surveillance and diagnosis of recurrence in women with gynecologic malignancies: Society of Gynecologic Oncologists recommendations." *Am J Obstet Gynecol* 204(6): 466-478.

Sartori, E., A. Gadducci, F. Landoni, A. Lissoni, T. Maggino, P. Zola and V. Zanagnolo (2001). "Clinical behavior of 203 stage II endometrial cancer cases: the impact of primary surgical approach and of adjuvant radiation therapy." *Int J Gynecol Cancer* 11(6): 430-437.

Saygili, U., S. Kavaz, S. Altunyurt, T. Uslu, M. Koyuncuoglu and O. Erten (2001). "Omentectomy, peritoneal biopsy and appendectomy in patients with clinical stage I endometrial carcinoma." *Int J Gynecol Cancer* 11(6): 471-474.

Scarabelli, C., E. Campagnutta, G. Giorda, G. DePiero, F. Sopracordevole, M. Quaranta and L. DeMarco (1998). "Maximal cytoreductive surgery as a reasonable therapeutic alternative for recurrent endometrial carcinoma." *Gynecol Oncol* 70(1): 90-93.

Scholten, A. N., W. L. van Putten, H. Beerman, V. T. Smit, P. C. Koper, M. L. Lybeert, J. J. Jobsen, C. C. Warlam-Rodenhuis, K. A. De Winter, L. C. Lutgens, M. van Lent and C. L. Creutzberg (2005). "Postoperative radiotherapy for Stage 1 endometrial carcinoma: long-term outcome of the randomized PORTEC trial with central pathology review." *Int J Radiat Oncol Biol Phys* 63(3): 834-838.

Schorge, J. O., K. L. Molpus, A. Goodman, N. Nikrui and A. F. Fuller, Jr. (1996). "The effect of postsurgical therapy on stage III endometrial carcinoma." *Gynecol Oncol* 63(1): 34-39.

Sherman, M. E., P. Bitterman, N. B. Rosenshein, G. Delgado and R. J. Kurman (1992). "Uterine serous carcinoma. A morphologically diverse neoplasm with unifying clinicopathologic features." *Am J Surg Pathol* 16(6): 600-610.

Siegel, R., E. Ward, O. Brawley and A. Jemal (2011). "Cancer statistics, 2011: The impact of eliminating socioeconomic and racial disparities on premature cancer deaths." *CA Cancer J Clin* 61(4): 212-236.

Smith, R. S., D. S. Kapp, Q. Chen and N. N. Teng (2000). "Treatment of high-risk uterine cancer with whole abdominopelvic radiation therapy." *Int J Radiat Oncol Biol Phys* 48(3): 767-778.

Stolyarova I, Minaev A. Effect of hormonotherapy on the results of radiation treatment in patients with endometrial carcinoma." Journal of B.U.On 6(3): 271-274.

Straughn, J. M., Jr., W. K. Huh, F. J. Kelly, C. A. Leath, 3rd, M. J. Kleinberg, J. Hyde, Jr., T. M. Numnum, Y. Zhang, S. J. Soong, J. M. Austin, Jr., E. E. Partridge, L. C. Kilgore and R. D. Alvarez (2002). "Conservative management of stage I endometrial carcinoma after surgical staging." *Gynecol Oncol* 84(2): 194-200.

Susumu, N., S. Sagae, Y. Udagawa, K. Niwa, H. Kuramoto, S. Satoh and R. Kudo (2008). "Randomized phase III trial of pelvic radiotherapy versus cisplatin-based combined chemotherapy in patients with intermediate- and high-risk endometrial cancer: a Japanese Gynecologic Oncology Group study." *Gynecol Oncol* 108(1): 226-233.

Sutton, G., J. H. Axelrod, B. N. Bundy, T. Roy, H. D. Homesley, J. H. Malfetano, B. R. Mychalczak and M. E. King (2005). "Whole abdominal radiotherapy in the adjuvant treatment of patients with stage III and IV endometrial cancer: a gynecologic oncology group study." *Gynecol Oncol* 97(3): 755-763.

Thigpen, J. T., M. F. Brady, R. D. Alvarez, M. D. Adelson, H. D. Homesley, A. Manetta, J. T. Soper and F. T. Given (1999). "Oral medroxyprogesterone acetate in the treatment of advanced or recurrent endometrial carcinoma: a dose-response study by the Gynecologic Oncology Group." *J Clin Oncol* 17(6): 1736-1744.

Thigpen, J. T., M. F. Brady, H. D. Homesley, J. Malfetano, B. DuBeshter, R. A. Burger and S. Liao (2004). "Phase III trial of doxorubicin with or without cisplatin in advanced endometrial carcinoma: a gynecologic oncology group study." *J Clin Oncol* 22(19): 3902-3908.

Thomas, M., A. Mariani, J. D. Wright, E. O. Madarek, M. A. Powell, D. G. Mutch, K. C. Podratz and S. C. Dowdy (2008). "Surgical management and adjuvant therapy for patients with uterine clear cell carcinoma: a multi-institutional review." *Gynecol Oncol* 108(2): 293-297.

Trimble, E. L., C. Kosary and R. C. Park (1998). "Lymph node sampling and survival in endometrial cancer." *Gynecol Oncol* 71(3): 340-343.

Uccella, S., K. C. Podratz, G. D. Aletti and A. Mariani (2009). "Lymphadenectomy in endometrial cancer." *Lancet* 373(9670): 1170; author reply 1170-1171.

Uccella, S., K. C. Podratz, G. D. Aletti and A. Mariani (2009). "Re: Systematic pelvic lymphadenectomy vs no lymphadenectomy in early-stage endometrial carcinoma: randomized clinical trial." *J Natl Cancer Inst* 101(12): 897-898; author reply 898-899.

Urbanski, K., K. Karolewski, Z. Kojs, M. Klimek and T. Dyba (1993). "Adjuvant progestagen therapy improves survival in patients with endometrial cancer after hysterectomy. Results of one-institutional prospective clinical trial." *Eur J Gynaecol Oncol* 14 Suppl: 98-104.

Vergote, I., K. Kjorstad, V. Abeler and P. Kolstad (1989). "A randomized trial of adjuvant progestagen in early endometrial cancer." *Cancer* 64(5): 1011-1016.

Walker, J. L., M. R. Piedmonte, N. M. Spirtos, S. M. Eisenkop, J. B. Schlaerth, R. S. Mannel, G. Spiegel, R. Barakat, M. L. Pearl and S. K. Sharma (2009). "Laparoscopy compared with laparotomy for comprehensive surgical staging of uterine cancer: Gynecologic Oncology Group Study LAP2." *J Clin Oncol* 27(32): 5331-5336.

9

Reducing the Risk of Endometrial Cancer in Patients Receiving Selective Estrogen Receptor Modulator (SERM) Therapy

Victor G Vogel
Geisinger Health System
USA

1. Introduction

Selective Estrogen Receptor Modulators (SERMs) are synthetic compounds originally designed as oral contraceptives in the 1960s. During the ensuing decades, they have been shown to be effective for the prevention of both invasive and *in situ* breast cancer, for the treatment and prevention of osteoporosis, and for the primary prevention of breast cancer. This chapter will review the most important agents focusing on their uterine effect derived from dozens of clinical trials that have explored their efficacy for the listed indications. We will compare and contrast the agents and highlight recent development of newer, more efficacious SERMs that have an improved safety profile.

2. Tamoxifen

The finding of a decrease in contralateral breast cancer incidence following tamoxifen administration for adjuvant therapy led to the concept that the drug might play a role in breast cancer prevention. To test this hypothesis, the National Surgical Adjuvant Breast and Bowel Project initiated the Breast Cancer Prevention Trial (P-1) in 1992. Women at increased risk for breast cancer were randomly assigned to receive placebo or 20 mg/day tamoxifen for 5 years (Fisher et al. 1998). Gail's algorithm, based on a multivariate logistic regression model using combinations of risk factors, was used to estimate the risk of occurrence of breast cancer over time.

Tamoxifen reduced the risk of invasive breast cancer by 49%, with cumulative incidence through 69 months of follow-up of 43.4 versus 22.0 per 1000 women in the placebo and tamoxifen groups, respectively. The decreased risk occurred in women aged 49 years or younger (44%), 50–59 years (51%), and 60 years or older (55%); risk was also reduced in women with a history of lobular carcinoma in situ (56%) or atypical hyperplasia (86%) and in those with any category of predicted 5-year risk. Tamoxifen reduced the risk of noninvasive breast cancer by 50% (two-sided $P<.002$). Tamoxifen reduced the occurrence of estrogen receptor-positive tumors by 69%, but no difference in the occurrence of estrogen receptor-negative tumors was seen. Tamoxifen administration did not alter the average annual rate of ischemic heart disease; however, a reduction in hip, radius (Colles'), and spine fractures was observed.

2.1 Endometrial cancer

The rate of endometrial cancer was increased in the tamoxifen group by more than 2.5-fold (risk ratio = 2.53; 95% confidence interval = 1.35–4.97); this increased risk occurred predominantly in women aged 50 years or older. All endometrial cancers in the tamoxifen group were stage I (localized disease); no endometrial cancer deaths have occurred in this group. No liver cancers or increase in colon, rectal, ovarian, or other tumors was observed in the tamoxifen group. The rates of stroke, pulmonary embolism, and deep-vein thrombosis were elevated in the tamoxifen group; these events occurred more frequently in women aged 50 years or older.

	No. of events		**Rate per 1000 women**				
Type of cancer	**Placebo**	**Tam**	**Placebo**	**Tam**	**Diff**	**RR‡**	**95% CI**
Invasive	17	53	0.68	2.24	−1.56	3.28	1.87 to 6.03
≤49 y at entry	9	12	0.82	1.16	−0.34	1.42	0.55 to 3.81
≥50 y at entry	8	41	0.58	3.08	−2.50	5.33	2.47 to 13.17
In situ cancer	3	1	0.12	0.04	0.08	0.35	0.01 to 4.36

Table 1. Events and incidence rates of invasive and *in situ* endometrial cancer in the placebo and tamoxifen groups by age at study entry in the BCPT.

The average annual rate of invasive endometrial cancer per 1000 participants was 2.30 in the tamoxifen group and 0.91 in the placebo group. The increased risk was predominantly in women 50 years of age or older. The relative risk of endometrial cancer was 4.01 (95% CI 4 1.70–10.90) in women aged 50 years or older, and increase in incidence after tamoxifen administration was observed early in the follow-up period. Through 66 months of follow-up, the cumulative incidence was 5.4 per 1000 women and 13.0 per 1000 women in the placebo and tamoxifen groups, respectively. Fourteen (93%) of the 15 invasive endometrial cancers that occurred in the placebo group were International Federation of Gynecology and Obstetrics (FIGO) stage I, and one (7%) was FIGO stage IV. All 36 invasive endometrial cancers that occurred in the group receiving tamoxifen were FIGO stage I. Four *in situ* endometrial cancers were reported; three of these occurred in the placebo group and one in the tamoxifen group. The cumulative incidence of invasive endometrial carcinoma along with other side effects in the trial through seven years of follow-up is shown in Figure 1.

Through 66 months of follow-up, the cumulative incidence was 5.4 per 1000 women and 13.0 per 1000 women in the placebo and tamoxifen groups, respectively. These rates are shown in Figure 2. Fourteen (93%) of the 15 invasive endometrial cancers that occurred in the placebo group were International Federation of Gynecology and Obstetrics (FIGO) stage I, and one (7%) was FIGO stage IV. All 36 invasive endometrial cancers that occurred in the group receiving tamoxifen were FIGO stage I. Four in situ endometrial cancers were reported; three of these occurred in the placebo group and one in the tamoxifen group.

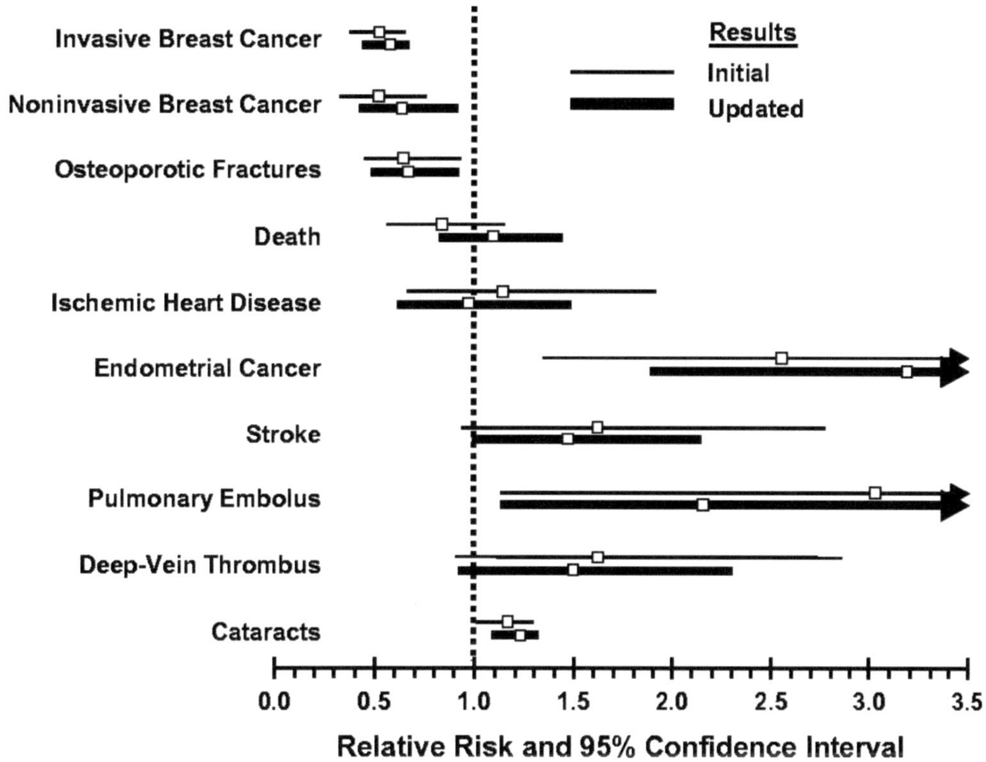

Fig. 1. Comparison of relative risks (with 95% confidence intervals) of benefits and undesirable effects of tamoxifen from the initial and updated results of NSABP P-1. (Fisher 2005).

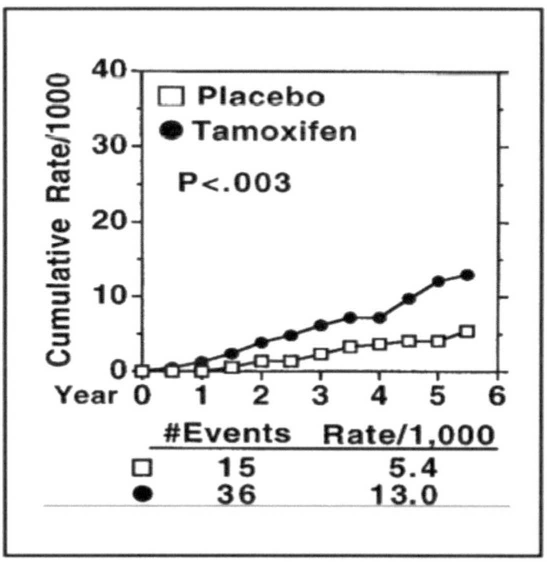

Fig. 2. Cumulative incidence of invasive endometrial carcinoma through seven years of follow-up.

After 7 years of follow-up, women who received tamoxifen still had a statistically significantly increased risk of invasive endometrial cancer (RR = 3.28, 95% CI = 1.87 to 6.03) (Fisher et al. 2005). Again, the risk was not increased in women aged 49 years or younger (RR = 1.42, 95% CI = 0.55 to 3.81), but there was a statistically significant increase in risk in women aged 50 years or older (RR = 5.33, 95% CI = 2.47 to 13.17). The cumulative rate of invasive endometrial cancer through 7 years of follow-up was 4.68 per 1000 women in the placebo group and 15.64 per 1000 women in the tamoxifen group, respectively ($P<.001$). Of the 70 cases of endometrial cancer (17 in the placebo group and 53 in the tamoxifen group), 67 cases (15 in the placebo group and 52 in the tamoxifen group) were International Federation of Gynecology and Obstetrics (FIGO) stage I. Of the remaining two cases in the placebo group, one was stage III and one was stage IV. The remaining case in the tamoxifen group was stage III. Four cases of endometrial cancer *in situ* were observed: three in the placebo group and one in the tamoxifen group. In addition to these cases of endometrial cancer, there were four cases of uterine sarcoma, one in the placebo group and three in the tamoxifen group.

2.2 Gynecologic and vasomotor symptoms

Vaginal discharge was reported in almost 55% of women on tamoxifen in the NSABP-P1 trial, and 78% of women on tamoxifen reported bothersome hot flashes during treatment. Results from the Italian trial, which included only women who had a hysterectomy, also showed a statistically significant increase in vaginal discharge for women taking tamoxifen (RR = 3.44; 95% CI, 2.90 to 4.09).17

3. Raloxifene

Raloxifene was the first of a benzothiophene series of antiestrogens to be labeled a SERM. Raloxifene has the ability to bind to and activate the estrogen receptor while exhibiting tissue-specific effects distinct from estradiol (Vogel 2007). As a result, raloxifene was specifically developed to maintain beneficial estrogenic activity on bone and lipids and antiestrogenic activity on endometrial and breast tissue. In December 1997, the U.S. Food and Drug Administration (FDA) labeled raloxifene for the prevention of osteoporosis. These agents work by inducing conformational changes in the estrogen receptor resulting in differential expression of specific estrogen-regulated genes in different tissues. Activation of the estrogen receptor by raloxifene may involve multiple molecular pathways that may result in gene expression of ligand-, tissue- and/or gene-specific receptors

Raloxifene undergoes extensive systemic biotransformation, but it does not appear to be metabolized by the cytochrome P450 pathway. Clinically significant interactions are unlikely to occur with drugs typically eliminated by this route. Raloxifene has a plasma elimination half-life of approximately 27 hours. This prolonged elimination half-life has been attributed to the drug's reversible systemic metabolism and significant enterohepatic cycling.

Raloxifene appears to lack proliferative effects on endometrial tissue. Data from both animal and human studies demonstrate that raloxifene has minimal effects on the uterus and causes no significant changes in the histologic appearance of the endometrium (Boss et al. 1997). Two six-month studies involving a total of 969 postmenopausal women showed that endometrial thickness did not differ between women receiving raloxifene (30 to 150 mg per day) and those receiving placebo (Delmas et al. 1997).

In healthy, postmenopausal women raloxifene (200 to 600 mg per day given over eight weeks) does not induce endometrial proliferation as measured by endometrial biopsies. By comparison, 77 percent of the women who receive unopposed estrogen (0.625 mg per day of conjugated estrogen) have moderate to marked estrogenic proliferation of endometrial tissue. Women who received conjugated estrogen were also noted to have a much higher incidence of vaginitis than those who received raloxifene or placebo.

A trial in 136 healthy postmenopausal women compared the stimulatory effects on the uterus of raloxifene (150 mg per day) and continuous hormone replacement therapy (0.625 mg per day of conjugated estrogen with 2.5 mg per day of medroxyprogesterone). After a period of 12 months, the women who received estrogen replacement therapy experienced significant changes in endometrial thickness and uterine volume. In contrast, the women who were treated with raloxifene exhibited no changes in either parameter. Additional short-term trials appear to support the view that raloxifene does not produce endometrial stimulation.

3.1 MORE/CORE trials uterine events

The MORE trial randomized 7,705 postmenopausal women younger than 81 years (mean age= 66.5 years) with osteoporosis to raloxifene or placebo (Cummings et al. 1999). The primary aim of the MORE study was to test whether 3 years of raloxifene reduced the risk of fracture in postmenopausal women with osteoporosis, and the occurrence of breast cancer was a secondary end point. Women were excluded if they took estrogens within 6 months of randomization and were not permitted to take concomitant estrogen replacement therapy with the study drug. With a median follow-up of 40 months, raloxifene reduced the risk of invasive breast cancer by 76% in postmenopausal women with osteoporosis, largely accounted for by a 90% reduction in ER-positive breast cancer. Raloxifene did not reduce the risk of ER-negative breast cancer. There was no apparent decrease in ER-negative cancers. In addition, raloxifene decreased the risk of vertebral fractures and decreased low-density lipoprotein cholesterol levels. Raloxifene did not increase the risk of endometrial cancer, endometrial hyperplasia or vaginal bleeding (Table 2) but was associated with a threefold increase in thromboembolic events. More women in the raloxifene group reported increased rates of hot flashes, leg cramps, and peripheral edema.

The Continuing Outcomes Relevant to Evista (CORE) trial was designed to evaluate the efficacy of an additional 4 years of raloxifene therapy in preventing invasive breast cancer in women who participated in the MORE trial (Martino et al. 2004). CORE was a multicenter, double-blind, placebo-controlled clinical trial. The CORE trial was conducted in the subset of the MORE women who agreed to participate in what was an extension of the MORE trial, with a change in the primary endpoint from vertebral fracture incidence to invasive breast cancer. A secondary objective of the CORE trial was to examine the effect of raloxifene (at 60 mg/day) on the incidence of invasive ER-positive breast cancer. Women who had been randomly assigned to receive raloxifene (either 60 or 120 mg/day) in MORE were assigned to receive raloxifene (60 mg/day) in CORE (n= 3510), and women who had been assigned to receive placebo in MORE continued on placebo in CORE (n=1703). Women in the raloxifene group had a 59% reduction in the incidence of all invasive breast cancer compared with women in the placebo group and a 66% reduction in the incidence of invasive ER-positive breast cancers compared with women in the placebo group. By contrast, the incidence of invasive ER-negative breast cancer in women who received raloxifene was not statistically significantly different from that in women who received placebo. The overall incidence of breast cancer, regardless of invasiveness, was reduced by 50% in the raloxifene group compared with the placebo group. Again, there was no observed increase in the risk of endometrial cancer attributable to raloxifene.

	CORE enrollees, % (No.)					
	4 years beginning at visit 1 of the CORE trial			8 years beginning at randomization in the MORE trial		
Adverse event	Placebo group (N = 1286)	Raloxifene group† (N = 2725)	P ‡	Placebo group (N = 1286)	Raloxifene group§ (N = 2725)	P ‡
Vaginal bleeding[ǀ]	0.20 (2)	0.19 (4)	>.99	1.36 (14)	1.25 (27)	.87
Endometrial hyperplasia[ǀ]	0.20 (2)	0.05 (1)	.24	0.29 (3)	0.37 (8)	>.99
Endometrial cancer[ǀ]	0.30 (3)	0.19 (4)	.69	0.39 (4)	0.32 (7)	.75

* CORE = Continuing Outcomes of Relevant to Evista; MORE = Multiple Outcomes of Raloxifene Evaluation.

† Dose of 60 mg of raloxifene per day during the CORE trial.

‡ Based on two-sided Fisher's exact test.

§ Doses of 60 mg or 120 mg of raloxifene per day during the MORE trial and 60 mg of raloxifene per day during the CORE trial.

ǀ Includes only women who had an intact uterus at baseline of the MORE trial. For 4 years beginning at visit 1 of CORE, n = 1008 and n = 2138 for the placebo and raloxifene groups, respectively. For 8 years beginning at randomization in MORE, n = 1026 and n = 2167 for the placebo and raloxifene groups, respectively.

Table 2. Rates of adverse events among the CORE enrollees*.

3.2 RUTH Trial

The Raloxifene Use and the Heart (RUTH) trial randomly assigned 10,101 postmenopausal women (mean age, 67.5 years) with CHD or multiple risk factors for coronary heart disease (CHD) to 60 mg of raloxifene daily or placebo and followed them for a median of 5.6 years (Barrett-Connor et al. 2006). The two primary outcomes were coronary events (i.e., death from coronary causes, myocardial infarction, or hospitalization for an acute coronary syndrome) and invasive breast cancer.

As compared with placebo, raloxifene had no significant effect on the risk of primary coronary events, and it reduced the risk of invasive breast cancer (40 vs. 70 events; hazard ratio, 0.56; 95 percent confidence interval, 0.38 to 0.83; absolute risk reduction, 1.2 invasive breast cancers per 1000 women treated for one year); the benefit was primarily due to a reduced risk of estrogen-receptor–positive invasive breast cancers. There was no significant difference in the rates of death from any cause or total stroke according to group assignment, but raloxifene was associated with an increased risk of fatal stroke. Raloxifene reduced the risk of clinical vertebral fractures. Raloxifene did not significantly affect the risk of CHD. There was no significant difference between the treatment groups in the number of women with one or more reported adverse events. More women in the raloxifene group than in the placebo group permanently discontinued use of the study drug because of an adverse event.

Four common adverse events (an acute coronary syndrome, anxiety, constipation, and osteoporosis) were reported more frequently in the placebo group than in the raloxifene group, and seven (arthritis, cholelithiasis, dyspepsia, hot flush, intermittent claudication, muscle spasm, and peripheral edema) were reported more frequently in the raloxifene group than in the placebo group (P≤0.05). Hot flushes, leg cramps, peripheral edema, and gallbladder disease, all special search categories, were more common in women assigned to raloxifene than to placebo. The rates of cholecystectomy did not differ significantly between the treatment groups (P=0.25). The incidences of endometrial cancer and all cancers other than breast cancer did not differ significantly between treatment groups. Few details were provided about the endometrial cancers that were observed.

3.3 STAR Trial

The Study of Tamoxifen and Raloxifene (STAR Trial) was conducted to compare the relative effects and safety of raloxifene and tamoxifen on the risk of developing invasive breast cancer and other disease outcomes (Vogel et al. 2006). It was carried out by The National Surgical Adjuvant Breast and Bowel Project Study and was a prospective, double-blind, randomized clinical trial conducted in nearly 200 clinical centers throughout North America. Patients were 19,747 postmenopausal women of mean age 58.5 years who had increased 5-year breast cancer risk. Women received either oral tamoxifen (20 mg/d) or raloxifene (60 mg/d) daily over 5 years. Outcome measures included the incidence of invasive breast cancer, uterine cancer, noninvasive breast cancer, bone fractures, and thromboembolic events.

At the time of the planned, initial analysis, there were 163 cases of invasive breast cancer in women assigned to tamoxifen and 168 in those assigned to raloxifene (incidence, 4.30 per 1000 vs. 4.41 per 1000; RR = 1.02; 95% confidence interval [CI], 0.82-1.28). There were 36 cases of uterine cancer with tamoxifen and 23 with raloxifene (RR = 0.62; 95% CI, 0.35-1.08).

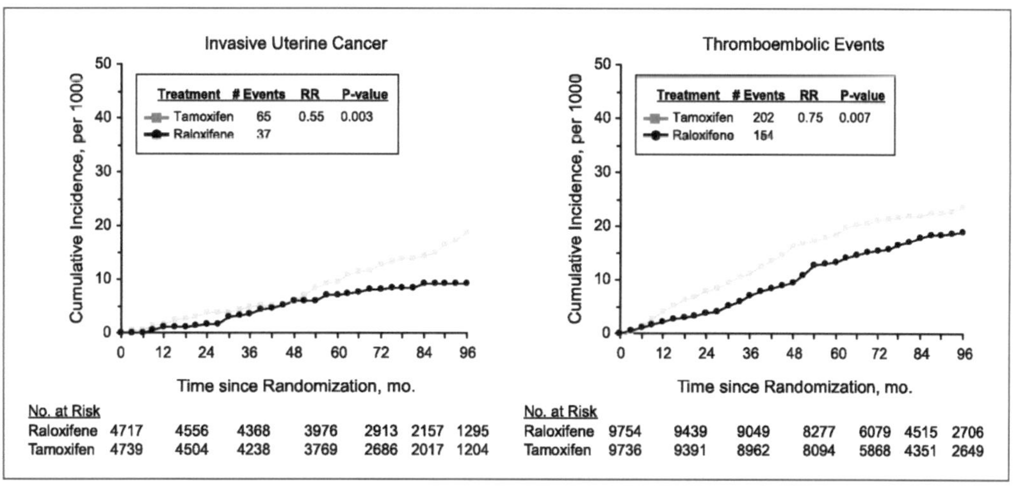

Fig. 3. Invasive uterine cancer and thromboembolic events in the STAR Trial.

After a median of 47 months of follow-up, there was a trend toward a decreased incidence of uterine cancer in the raloxifene group, but the difference was not statistically significant—36 cases (tamoxifen) vs. 23 (raloxifene). Annual incidence rates were 2.00 per 1000 (tamoxifen) and 1.25 per 1000 women (raloxifene) (RR = 0.62; 95% CI, 0.35-1.08). Cumulative incidence rates through 7 years were 14.7 per 1000 (tamoxifen) and 8.1 per 1000 (raloxifene) (P = .07,). These events are shown in Figure 3. Only 1 case of uterine cancer occurred among women younger than 50 years, in a participant in the tamoxifen group. The majority of women who developed uterine cancer (56 [91%]) were diagnosed with stage I disease. Of the remaining cases, there was 1 case of stage II disease in each of the treatment groups, 2 with stage III disease in the raloxifene group, and 1 with stage IV disease in the raloxifene group. Two of these cases were mixed Mullerian cell type; both were in the tamoxifen group.

Table 3 shows that while there were no statistically significant differences with respect to risk of uterine cancer, there were differences between the treatment groups indicating that the effect of raloxifene on the uterus is less than that of tamoxifen. Among those who did not have a diagnosis of uterine cancer, there was a statistically significant difference between the groups in the incidence of uterine hyperplasia. The rates were 84% less in the raloxifene-treated group (14 cases) than in the tamoxifen-treated group (84 cases) (RR, 0.16; 95% CI, 0.09-0.29). This magnitude of difference between treatment groups was evident for hyperplasia both with and without atypia. For the tamoxifen and raloxifene groups, respectively, there were 12 cases and 1 case with atypia (RR, 0.08; 95% CI, 0.00-0.55) and 72 and 13 cases without atypia (RR, 0.18; 95% CI, 0.09-0.32). There also was a statistically significant difference between the treatment groups in the number of hysterectomies performed during the course of follow-up. Among women who were not diagnosed with endometrial cancer, there were 244 hysterectomies performed in those assigned to tamoxifen compared with 111 in those assigned to raloxifene (RR, 0.44; 95% CI, 0.35-0.56).

After 81 months of follow-up, the incidence of invasive uterine cancer was significantly lower in the raloxifene group (Vogel et al. 2010). The annual average rate per 1,000 was 2.25 in the tamoxifen group compared with 1.23 in the raloxifene group (RR = 0.55; 95% CI, 0.36–0.83). In the original report, the difference between treatment groups for the rate of invasive uterine cancer was not statistically significant. The average annual incidence rate of uterine hyperplasia, the majority of which was hyperplasia without atypia, was 5 times higher in the tamoxifen group (4.40 per 1,000) than in the raloxifene group (0.84 per 1,000; RR = 0.19; 95% CI, 0.12–0.29). The number of hysterectomies performed in the tamoxifen group, including those done for benign disease, was more than double that performed in the raloxifene group (RR = 0.45; 95% CI, 0.37–0.54).

Disease/uterine event	Events, *n*		Rate per 1,000			RR*	RR (95% CI)
	Tam	Ralox	Tam	Ralox	Diff		
Uterine disease and hysterectomy							
Invasive Cancer	65	37	2.25	1.23	1.02	0.55	0.36–0.83
Hyperplasia	126	25	4.40	0.84	3.56	0.19	0.12–0.29
Without atypia	104	21	3.63	0.70	2.93	0.19	0.11–0.31
With atypia	22	4	0.77	0.13	0.64	0.17	0.04–0.51
Hysterectomy during follow-up	349	162	12.08	5.41	6.67	0.45	0.37–0.54

Table 3. Uterine Events in the Study of Tamoxifen and Raloxifene (STAR Trial).

Previous studies had shown that raloxifene does not increase the risk of uterine malignancy when compared with placebo. In the STAR trial, only 59 invasive uterine cancers were diagnosed in both study groups during more than 76,000 woman-years of follow-up. As noted above, approximately 25% fewer cases of uterine cancer were diagnosed in the raloxifene than in the tamoxifen group. Although uterine cancer of the mixed Mullerian type occurred in only 2 cases in the tamoxifen group of the STAR trial, there have been isolated case reports of this tumor associated with raloxifene. The rates of uterine cancer were 2.00 per 1000 (tamoxifen) and 1.25 per 1000 (raloxifene), but this difference did not reach statistical significance. Endometrial hyperplasia, however, a risk factor for endometrial cancer, was far more common in the tamoxifen-treated group than in the raloxifene group (RR, 0.16; 95% CI, 0.09-0.29). The number of participants undergoing a hysterectomy for non–cancer-related reasons was significantly reduced 56% in the raloxifene group. It is important to note that the difference between the treatment groups in non–cancer-related hysterectomies has likely caused an underestimate of the true magnitude of endometrial cancer risk associated with tamoxifen and an underestimate of the true magnitude of difference between the two treatment groups for this end point.

These data demonstrate that raloxifene is nearly as effective as tamoxifen in reducing the risk of invasive breast cancer and has a lower risk of thromboembolic events and cataracts but a non-statistically significant higher risk of noninvasive breast cancer.

3.3.1 Summary for uterine cancer, uterine hyperplasia, and hysterectomy for raloxifene and tamoxifen in the STAR Trial

In the STAR Trial, there was a trend toward a decreased incidence of uterine cancer in the raloxifene group, but the difference was not statistically significant—36 cases (tamoxifen) vs. 23 (raloxifene). Annual incidence rates were 2.00 per 1000 (tamoxifen) and 1.25 per 1000 women (raloxifene) (RR, 0.62; 95% CI, 0.35-1.08). Cumulative incidence rates through 7 years were 14.7 per 1000 (tamoxifen) and 8.1 per 1000 (raloxifene) (P = 0.07,). Only 1 case of uterine cancer occurred among women younger than 50 years, in a participant in the tamoxifen group. At the time of analysis, clinicopathological stage was unknown for 3 cases (1 in the tamoxifen group, 2 in the raloxifene group). The majority of the others who developed uterine cancer (56 [91%]) were diagnosed with stage I disease. Of the remaining cases, there was 1 case of stage II disease in each of the treatment groups, 2 with stage III disease in the raloxifene group, and 1 with stage IV disease in the raloxifene group. As noted, two of these cases were mixed Mullerian cell type; both were in the tamoxifen group.

While there were no significant differences with respect to risk of uterine cancer in the STAR trial, there were differences between the treatment groups indicating that the effect of raloxifene on the uterus is less than that of tamoxifen. Among those who did not have a diagnosis of uterine cancer, there was a statistically significant difference between the groups in the incidence of uterine hyperplasia. The rates were 84% less in the raloxifene-treated group (14 cases) than in the tamoxifen-treated group (84 cases). This magnitude of difference between treatment groups was evident for hyperplasia both with and without atypia. For the tamoxifen and raloxifene groups, respectively, there were 12 cases and 1 case with atypia (RR, 0.08; 95% CI, 0.00-0.55) and 72 and 13 cases without atypia (RR, 0.18; 95% CI, 0.09-0.32). There also was a statistically significant difference between the treatment groups in the number of hysterectomies performed during the course of follow-up. Among women who were not diagnosed with endometrial cancer, there were 244 hysterectomies performed in those assigned to tamoxifen compared with 111 in those assigned to raloxifene (RR, 0.44; 95% CI, 0.35-0.56).

3.3.2 STAR quality of life

No significant differences existed between the tamoxifen and raloxifene groups in patient-reported outcomes for physical health, mental health, and depression, although the tamoxifen group reported better sexual function (Land et al. 2006). Although mean symptom severity was low among these postmenopausal women, those in the tamoxifen group reported more gynecological problems, vasomotor symptoms, leg cramps, and bladder control problems, whereas women in the raloxifene group reported more musculoskeletal problems, dyspareunia, and weight gain.

3.4 Raloxifene summary

The selective estrogen-receptor modulator (SERM) tamoxifen became the first U.S. Food and Drug Administration (FDA)–approved agent for reducing breast cancer risk but did not gain wide acceptance for prevention, largely because it increased the risk of endometrial cancer and thromboembolic events. The FDA approved the SERM raloxifene for breast cancer risk reduction following its demonstrated effectiveness in preventing invasive breast cancer in the Study of Tamoxifen and Raloxifene (STAR). Raloxifene caused less toxicity (versus tamoxifen), including reduced thromboembolic events and endometrial cancer. The risk ratio (RR; raloxifene:tamoxifen) for invasive breast cancer was 1.24 (95% confidence interval [CI], 1.05–1.47) and for noninvasive disease, 1.22 (95% CI, 0.95–1.59). Compared with initial results, the RRs widened for invasive and narrowed for noninvasive breast cancer.

With follow-up extended to 81 months in the STAR Trial, toxicity relative risks (raloxifene:tamoxifen) were 0.55 (95% CI, 0.36–0.83; P = 0.003) for endometrial cancer (this difference was not significant in the initial results), 0.19 (95% CI, 0.12–0.29) for uterine hyperplasia, and 0.75 (95% CI, 0.60–0.93) for thromboembolic events. There were no significant mortality differences. Long-term raloxifene retained 76% of the effectiveness of tamoxifen in preventing invasive disease and grew closer over time to tamoxifen in preventing noninvasive disease, with far less toxicity (e.g., highly significantly less endometrial cancer). These results have important public health implications and clarify that both raloxifene and tamoxifen are good preventive choices for postmenopausal women with elevated risk for breast cancer.

Invasive uterine cancer and uterine hyperplasia are well-established toxicities associated with tamoxifen treatment. When compared with tamoxifen, raloxifene does not have such a profile. The incidence of invasive uterine cancer is significantly lower in the raloxifene group (P = 0.003). The annual average rate per 1,000 was 2.25 in the tamoxifen group compared with 1.23 in the raloxifene group (RR = 0.55; 95% CI, 0.36–0.83). In the original report of the STAR trial (Vogel et al. 2006), the difference between treatment groups for the rate of invasive uterine cancer was not statistically significant. The average annual incidence rate of uterine hyperplasia, the majority of which was hyperplasia without atypia, was 5 times higher in the tamoxifen group (4.40 per 1,000) than in the raloxifene group (0.84 per

1,000; RR = 0.19; 95% CI, 0.12–0.29). The number of hysterectomies performed in the tamoxifen group (349), including those done for benign disease, was more than double that performed in the raloxifene group (162; RR = 0.45; 95% CI, 0.37–0.54).

4. Lasofoxifene

Lasofoxifene is a nonsteroidal selective estrogen-receptor modulator that decreases bone resorption, bone loss, and low-density- lipoprotein (LDL) cholesterol in postmenopausal women. It is a potent third-generation SERM that was developed because of its potentially attractive pharmacological profile as an agent for risk reduction of fractures, breast cancer, and heart disease in postmenopausal women at increased risk of osteoporotic fractures. Preclinical laboratory evidence showed that lasofoxifene reduced bone loss and cholesterol, prevented experimental breast cancers, and did not cause endometrial hyperplasia (Cummings et al. 2010). Early clinical studies confirmed its potency relative to raloxifene in reducing bone loss and serum cholesterol, whereas neither agent increased the risk for endometrial hyperplasia.

As we have seen, currently available selective estrogen receptor modulators reduce the risk of breast cancer, but they are not widely used. In the Postmenopausal Evaluation and Risk-Reduction with Lasofoxifene (PEARL) trial, lasofoxifene reduced the risk of estrogen receptor–positive breast cancer, non-vertebral and vertebral fractures, coronary artery disease, and stroke.

The effects on total breast cancer (invasive and ductal carcinoma in situ, ER- positive and estrogen receptor–negative) and ER- positive invasive breast cancer were also assessed. Postmenopausal women (n = 8556) aged 59–80 years with low bone density and normal mammograms were randomly assigned to two doses of lasofoxifene (0.25 and 0.5 mg) or placebo. The primary endpoints of the PEARL trial were incidence of ER+ breast cancer and non-vertebral fractures at 5 years (LaCroix et al. 2010). A nested case–control study of 49 incident breast cancer case patients and 156 unaffected control subjects from the PEARL trial was performed to evaluate treatment effects on risk of total and ER- positive invasive breast cancer by baseline serum estradiol and sex hormone–binding globulin levels. Breast cancer was confirmed in 49 women. Compared with placebo, 0.5 mg of lasofoxifene significantly reduced the risk of total breast cancer by 79% (hazard ratio = 0.21; 95% confidence interval [CI] = 0.08 to 0.55) and ER+ invasive breast cancer by 83% (hazard ratio = 0.17; 95% CI = 0.05 to 0.57). The effects of 0.5 mg of lasofoxifene on total breast cancer were similar regardless of Gail breast cancer risk score, whereas the effects were markedly stronger for women with baseline estradiol levels greater than the median (odds ratio = 0.11; 95% CI = 0.02 to 0.51) vs. those with levels less than the median (odds ratio = 0.78; 95% CI = 0.16 to 3.79).

These data confirm that a 0.5-mg dose of lasofoxifene appears to reduce the risks of both total and ER-positive invasive breast cancer in postmenopausal women with osteoporosis.

Lasofoxifene at a dose of 0.5 mg per day, as compared with placebo, is associated with reduced risks of vertebral fracture, non-vertebral fracture, ER-positive breast cancer, coronary heart disease events, and stroke. Lasofoxifene at a dose of 0.25 mg per day, as compared with placebo, is associated with reduced risks of vertebral fracture and stroke. Both the lower and higher doses, as compared with placebo, were associated with an increase in venous thromboembolic events, respectively. Endometrial cancer occurred in three women in the placebo group, two women in the lower-dose lasofoxifene group, and two women in the higher-dose lasofoxifene group. Endometrial cancers were diagnosed in two women in each lasofoxifene group and three women in the placebo group. Endometrial hyperplasia was confirmed in two women in the higher-dose lasofoxifene group, three women in the lower-dose lasofoxifene group, and no women in the placebo group. This SERM may represent a much safer option than either tamoxifen or raloxifene for the prevention of both osteoporosis and invasive breast cancer.

A prospective study established the gynecological effects of 5 years of treatment with lasofoxifene versus placebo in postmenopausal osteoporotic women (Goldstein et al. 2011). The results are shown in Table 4. A total of 8,556 women aged 59 to 80 years with femoral neck or spine bone mineral density T scores of -2.5 or lower were randomly assigned to receive either lasofoxifene 0.25 mg/day, or lasofoxifene 0.5 mg/day, or placebo, for 5 years.

	Lasofoxifene 0.25 mg/day	**Lasofoxifene 0.50 mg/day**	**Placebo**
Endometrial cancer (number of cases)	2	2	3
Uterine hyperplasia (number of cases)	3	2	0
Vaginal bleeding (percent)	2.2%*	2.6%*	1.3%
Surgery for prolapsed or incontinence (percent)	1.9%*	1.6%	1.2%
Endometrial polyps (percent)	8.8%*	5.5*	3.3%

*Statistically significant difference from placebo.

Table 4. Rates of gynecological events among postmenopausal women taking lasofoxifene.

Endometrial cancer was confirmed for two women in each lasofoxifene group and for three women in the placebo group. Endometrial hyperplasia and vaginal bleeding occurred in more women treated with either 0.25 mg/day or 0.5 mg/day lasofoxifene than in women treated with placebo. Lasofoxifene treatment resulted in a small increase in endometrial thickness versus placebo. Similar numbers of women required surgery for pelvic organ prolapse or urinary incontinence in the placebo and 0.5 mg/day lasofoxifene groups. These findings indicate that 5 years of lasofoxifene treatment result in benign endometrial changes that do not increase the risk for endometrial cancer or hyperplasia in postmenopausal women.

5. Population risks and benefits of SERM therapy

The risks associated with tamoxifen therapy are shown in Table 5. Using the rates shown in the table, we can calculate that among the more than 65 million women aged 35–79 years without reported breast cancer in the United States in 2000, 10 million women (Freedman et al. 2003) would have been eligible for tamoxifen chemoprevention. The percentage of U.S. women who would be eligible varied dramatically by race, with 18.7% (95% CI = 17.8% to 19.7%) of white women, 5.7% (95% CI = 4.3% to 7.5%) of black women, and 2.9% (95% CI = 2.1% to 3.9%) of Hispanic women being eligible. Of the 50 million white U.S. women aged 35–79 years, more than 2.4 million (would have a positive benefit/risk index for tamoxifen chemoprevention. Of the 7 million black U.S. women aged 35–79 years, only 42,000 would have a positive benefit/risk index. Among white women, more than 28,000 breast cancers would be prevented or deferred if those women who have a positive net benefit index took tamoxifen over the next 5 years.: A substantial percentage of U.S. women are eligible for chemoprevention according to FDA criteria, and a percentage of them would have an estimated net benefit. Nevertheless, this latter percentage corresponds to more than two million women.

Revised estimates show that of the more than 9 million white U.S. women in 2010 who would be eligible for tamoxifen chemoprevention, about one-third would derive a net benefit from taking the drug on the basis of their age and breast cancer risk factors (Freedman et al. 2011). Among the white women who would benefit from tamoxifen, approximately more than 58,000 invasive breast cancers will develop over the next 5 years. If all 2 431 911 women in the US with an estimated net benefit/risk index took tamoxifen over the next 5 years, and if the risk reduction of 49% applies, then 28 492 of these breast cancers would be prevented, or deferred, which would be a substantial achievement.

Type of event	Age groups for white women (years)					Age groups for black women (years)				
	35-39	40-49	50-59	60-69	70-79	35-39	40-49	50-59	60-69	70-79
Life-threatening events										
Hip fracture	1	1	22	52	151	1	1	12	20	57
Endometrial cancer	−2	−16	−120	−206	−223	−1	−6	−52	−126	−119
(without uterus)	(0)	(0)	(0)	(0)	(0)	(0)	(0)	(0)	(0)	(0)
Stroke	−2	−13	−32	−91	−196	−8	−36	−90	−200	−228
Pulmonary embolism	−7	−15	−49	−85	−177	−20	−46	−145	−189	−273
Severe events										
Deep vein thrombosis	−13	−15	−16	−28	−44	−37	−45	−48	−63	−69
Other events										
Colles' fracture	11	11	19	25	25	9	9	10	10	9
Spine fracture	2	2	23	46	90	1	1	13	17	62
Cataracts	−35	−35	−101	−269	−384	−35	−35	−100	−264	−377

Table 5. Numbers of non-breast cancer events prevented (positive number) or caused (negative number) in 5 years among 10,000 women treated with tamoxifen (Gail et al. 1999).

For non-Hispanic white women age 50 years or older with a uterus, raloxifene displays a better benefit/risk profile than tamoxifen overall (Freedman et al. 2011). For tamoxifen, women age 50 to 59 years with a 5-year risk of invasive breast cancer of 4.5% to 6.5% showed moderate evidence of net positive benefit, and women with risk of 7.0% or higher showed strong evidence. For women age 50 to 59 years with a 5-year risk of invasive breast cancer less than 4.0%, the risks outweighed the benefits. The risks outweighed the benefits for women age 60 years or older, regardless of IBC risk. In contrast, for raloxifene, there was strong evidence that benefits outweighed risks, compared with placebo, for women age 50 to 59 years with a 5-year breast cancer risk of 3.5% or higher and for women age 60 to 69 years with an risk of 6.5% risk or higher. There was moderate evidence of a net benefit for women age 50 to 59 years with a 5-year risk of 2.0% to 3.0%, women age 60 to 69 years with a 5-year risk of 3.0% to 6.0%, and women age 70 to 79 years with a 5-year IBC risk of 4.0% or higher. For postmenopausal black and Hispanic women with a uterus, raloxifene also displayed a better benefit/risk profile than tamoxifen and in a similar pattern to that for whites. Net benefit indices tended to be larger in Hispanic women and smaller in black women than in white women, however.

6. American Society of Clinical Oncology (ASCO) recommendations for breast cancer risk reduction

In premenopausal women, tamoxifen for 5 years reduces the risk of breast cancer for at least 10 years, particularly estrogen receptor (ER) -positive invasive tumors. Women ≤ 50 years of age experience fewer serious side effects. Vascular and vasomotor events do not persist post-treatment across all ages. In postmenopausal women, raloxifene and tamoxifen reduce the risk of ER-positive invasive BC with equal efficacy. Raloxifene is associated with a lower risk of thromboembolic disease, benign and malignant uterine conditions, and cataracts than tamoxifen in postmenopausal women. No evidence exists establishing whether a reduction in risk of breast cancer from either agent translates into reduced BC mortality.

6.1 2009 Recommendation for the Use of tamoxifen to reduce the risk of developing breast cancer

Five years of tamoxifen (20 mg/d) may be offered to women at increased risk of breast cancer to reduce their risk of estrogen receptor (ER) -positive invasive breast cancers for up to 10 years (Visvanathan et al. 2009). Eligible women include those with a 5-year projected breast cancer risk ≥ 1.66% (according to the National Cancer Institute [NCI] Breast Cancer Risk Assessment Tool based on the Gail model23 —available at http://www.cancer.gov/bcrisktool) or women with LCIS. The benefit of taking tamoxifen for more than 5 years is unknown. The greatest clinical benefit and the fewest side effects were derived from the use of tamoxifen in younger (premenopausal) women 35 to 50 years of age who are unlikely to experience thromboembolic sequelae or uterine cancer, women without a uterus, and women at high risk of breast cancer (Newman and Vogel 2007). Vascular and vasomotor side effects were observed to decline post-treatment across all ages. Tamoxifen is not recommended in women with a prior history of deep vein thrombosis (DVT), pulmonary embolus (PE), stroke, or transient ischemic attack. Combined use of tamoxifen for breast cancer prevention and hormone therapy (HT) is currently not recommended. Follow-up should include a baseline gynecologic examination before initiation of treatment and annually thereafter, with a timely work-up for abnormal vaginal bleeding. The risks and benefits of tamoxifen should be given careful consideration during the decision-making process. There has been no mortality differences observed in the tamoxifen prevention trials so far, most likely because these trials were not powered to detect such outcomes. Nevertheless, a reduction in breast cancer incidence is considered to be an important health outcome in and of itself.

6.2 ASCO 2009 recommendation for the use of raloxifene to reduce the risk of developing breast cancer

For postmenopausal women at increased risk for breast cancer, raloxifene (60 mg/d) for 5 years may be offered as another option to reduce the risk of ER-positive invasive breast cancer. Raloxifene has been shown to be equally efficacious to tamoxifen in reducing breast cancer risk in postmenopausal women. However, raloxifene was not as effective in reducing the incidence of noninvasive breast cancer compared with tamoxifen, although the association was not statistically significant. In the STAR trial, raloxifene was associated with a more favorable side-effect profile compared with tamoxifen, including a statistically significant lower risk of thromboembolic disease, benign uterine complaints, and cataracts as compared with tamoxifen. Raloxifene, like tamoxifen, is not known to have an effect on overall or breast cancer–specific mortality in women at increased risk of breast cancer. However, the risk reduction trials were not powered to detect a reduction in breast cancer incidence rather than mortality, as it was felt to be an important end point in and of itself. Raloxifene may be used for longer than 5 years in women with osteoporosis in whom breast cancer risk reduction is an additional potential benefit. Raloxifene is not recommended in premenopausal women or in women with a prior history of DVT, PE, stroke, or transient ischemic attack. In postmenopausal women, the risks and benefits of both tamoxifen and raloxifene, including risks of noninvasive breast cancer, adverse events, and impact on quality of life, should be discussed in detail with women before coming to a decision about risk reduction strategies.

7. References

Barrett-Connor, E; Mosca, L; Collins, P; Geiger, MJ; Grady, D; Kornitzer, M; McNabb, MA; Wenger, NK & Raloxifene Use for The Heart (RUTH) Trial Investigators. (2006). Effects of raloxifene on cardiovascular events and breast cancer in postmenopausal women. *The New England Journal of Medicine* Vol.355, No.2, (Jul 13), pp. 125-37, ISSN 1533-4406; 0028-4793.

Boss, SM; Huster, WJ; Neild, JA; Glant, MD; Eisenhut, CC & Draper, MW. (1997). Effects of raloxifene hydrochloride on the endometrium of postmenopausal women. *American Journal of Obstetrics and Gynecology* Vol.177, No.6, (Dec), pp. 1458-64, ISSN 0002-9378; 0002-9378.

Cummings, SR; Eckert, S; Krueger, KA; Grady, D; Powles, TJ; Cauley, JA; Norton, L; Nickelsen, T; Bjarnason, NH; Morrow, M; Lippman, ME; Black, D; Glusman, JE; Costa, A & Jordan, VC. (1999). The effect of raloxifene on risk of breast cancer in postmenopausal women: Results from the MORE randomized trial. multiple outcomes of raloxifene evaluation. *JAMA : The Journal of the American Medical Association* Vol.281, No.23, (Jun 16), pp. 2189-97, ISSN 0098-7484; 0098-7484.

Cummings, SR; Ensrud, K; Delmas, PD; LaCroix, AZ; Vukicevic, S; Reid, DM; Goldstein, S; Sriram, U; Lee, A; Thompson, J; Armstrong, RA; Thompson, DD; Powles, T; Zanchetta, J; Kendler, D; Neven, P; Eastell, R & PEARL Study Investigators. (2010). Lasofoxifene in postmenopausal women with osteoporosis. *The New England Journal of Medicine* Vol.362, No.8, (Feb 25), pp. 686-96, ISSN 1533-4406; 0028-4793.

Delmas, PD; Bjarnason, NH; Mitlak, BH; Ravoux, AC; Shah, AS; Huster, WJ; Draper, M & Christiansen, C. (1997). Effects of raloxifene on bone mineral density, serum cholesterol concentrations, and uterine endometrium in postmenopausal women. *The New England Journal of Medicine* Vol.337, No.23, (Dec 4), pp. 1641-7, ISSN 0028-4793; 0028-4793.

Fisher, B; Costantino, JP; Wickerham, DL; Cecchini, RS; Cronin, WM; Robidoux, A; Bevers, TB; Kavanah, MT; Atkins, JN; Margolese, RG; Runowicz, CD; James, JM; Ford, LG & Wolmark, N. (2005). Tamoxifen for the prevention of breast cancer: Current status of the national surgical adjuvant breast and bowel project P-1 study. *Journal of the National Cancer Institute* Vol.97, No.22, (Nov 16), pp. 1652-62, ISSN 1460-2105; 0027-8874.

Fisher, B; Costantino, JP; Wickerham, DL; Redmond, CK; Kavanah, M; Cronin, WM; Vogel, V; Robidoux, A; Dimitrov, N; Atkins, J; Daly, M; Wieand, S; Tan-Chiu, E; Ford, L & Wolmark, N. (1998). Tamoxifen for prevention of breast cancer: Report of the national surgical adjuvant breast and bowel project P-1 study. *Journal of the National Cancer Institute* Vol.90, No.18, (Sep 16), pp. 1371-88, ISSN 0027-8874; 0027-8874.

Freedman, AN; Graubard, BI; Rao, SR; McCaskill-Stevens, W; Ballard-Barbash, R & Gail, MH. (2003). Estimates of the number of US women who could benefit from tamoxifen for breast cancer chemoprevention. *Journal of the National Cancer Institute* Vol.95, No.7, (Apr 2), pp. 526-32, ISSN 0027-8874; 0027-8874.

Freedman, AN; Yu, B; Gail, MH; Costantino, JP; Graubard, BI; Vogel, VG; Anderson, GL & McCaskill-Stevens, W. (2011). Benefit/Risk assessment for breast cancer chemoprevention with raloxifene or tamoxifen for women age 50 years or older. *Journal of Clinical Oncology : Official Journal of the American Society of Clinical Oncology* Vol.29, No.17, (Jun 10), pp. 2327-33, ISSN 1527-7755; 0732-183X.

Gail, MH; Costantino, JP; Bryant, J; Croyle, R; Freedman, L; Helzlsouer, K & Vogel, V. (1999). Weighing the risks and benefits of tamoxifen treatment for preventing breast cancer. *Journal of the National Cancer Institute* Vol.91, No.21, (Nov 3), pp. 1829-46, ISSN 0027-8874; 0027-8874.

Goldstein, SR; Neven, P; Cummings, S; Colgan, T; Runowicz, CD; Krpan, D; Proulx, J; Johnson, M; Thompson, D; Thompson, J & Sriram, U. (2011). Postmenopausal evaluation and risk reduction with lasofoxifene (PEARL) trial: 5-year gynecological outcomes. *Menopause (New York, N.Y.)* Vol.18, No.1, (Jan), pp. 17-22, ISSN 1530-0374; 1072-3714.

LaCroix, AZ; Powles, T; Osborne, CK; Wolter, K; Thompson, JR; Thompson, DD; Allred, DC; Armstrong, R; Cummings, SR; Eastell, R; Ensrud, KE; Goss, P; Lee, A; Neven, P; Reid, DM; Curto, M; Vukicevic, S & PEARL Investigators. (2010). Breast cancer incidence in the randomized PEARL trial of lasofoxifene in postmenopausal osteoporotic women. *Journal of the National Cancer Institute* Vol.102, No.22, (Nov 17), pp. 1706-15, ISSN 1460-2105; 0027-8874.

Land, SR; Wickerham, DL; Costantino, JP; Ritter, MW; Vogel, VG; Lee, M; Pajon, ER; Wade, JL,3rd; Dakhil, S; Lockhart, JB,Jr; Wolmark, N & Ganz, PA. (2006). Patient-reported symptoms and quality of life during treatment with tamoxifen or raloxifene for breast cancer prevention: The NSABP study of tamoxifen and raloxifene (STAR) P-2 trial. *JAMA : The Journal of the American Medical Association* Vol.295, No.23, (Jun 21), pp. 2742-51, ISSN 1538-3598; 0098-7484.

Martino, S; Cauley, JA; Barrett-Connor, E; Powles, TJ; Mershon, J; Disch, D; Secrest, RJ; Cummings, SR & CORE Investigators. (2004). Continuing outcomes relevant to evista: Breast cancer incidence in postmenopausal osteoporotic women in a randomized trial of raloxifene. *Journal of the National Cancer Institute* Vol.96, No.23, (Dec 1), pp. 1751-61, ISSN 1460-2105; 0027-8874.

Newman, LA & Vogel, VG. (2007). Breast cancer risk assessment and risk reduction. *The Surgical Clinics of North America* Vol.87, No.2, (Apr), pp. 307,16, vii-viii, ISSN 0039-6109; 0039-6109.

Visvanathan, K; Chlebowski, RT; Hurley, P; Col, NF; Ropka, M; Collyar, D; Morrow, M; Runowicz, C; Pritchard, KI; Hagerty, K; Arun, B; Garber, J; Vogel, VG; Wade, JL; Brown, P; Cuzick, J; Kramer, BS; Lippman, SM & American Society of Clinical Oncology. (2009). American society of clinical oncology clinical practice guideline update on the use of pharmacologic interventions including tamoxifen, raloxifene, and aromatase inhibition for breast cancer risk reduction. *Journal of Clinical Oncology : Official Journal of the American Society of Clinical Oncology* Vol.27, No.19, (Jul 1), pp. 3235-58, ISSN 1527-7755; 0732-183X.

Vogel, VG. (2007). Raloxifene: A selective estrogen receptor modulator for reducing the risk of invasive breast cancer in postmenopausal women. *Women's Health (London, England)* Vol.3, No.2, (Mar), pp. 139-53, ISSN 1745-5065; 1745-5057.

Vogel, VG; Costantino, JP; Wickerham, DL; Cronin, WM; Cecchini, RS; Atkins, JN; Bevers, TB; Fehrenbacher, L; Pajon, ER; Wade, JL,3rd; Robidoux, A; Margolese, RG; James, J; Runowicz, CD; Ganz, PA; Reis, SE; McCaskill-Stevens, W; Ford, LG; Jordan, VC; Wolmark, N & National Surgical Adjuvant Breast and Bowel Project. (2010). Update of the national surgical adjuvant breast and bowel project study of tamoxifen and raloxifene (STAR) P-2 trial: Preventing breast cancer. *Cancer Prevention Research (Philadelphia, Pa.)* Vol.3, No.6, (Jun), pp. 696-706, ISSN 1940-6215; 1940-6215.

Vogel, VG; Costantino, JP; Wickerham, DL; Cronin, WM; Cecchini, RS; Atkins, JN; Bevers, TB; Fehrenbacher, L; Pajon, ER,Jr; Wade, JL,3rd; Robidoux, A; Margolese, RG; James, J; Lippman, SM; Runowicz, CD; Ganz, PA; Reis, SE; McCaskill-Stevens, W; Ford, LG; Jordan, VC; Wolmark, N & National Surgical Adjuvant Breast and Bowel Project (NSABP). (2006). Effects of tamoxifen vs raloxifene on the risk of developing invasive breast cancer and other disease outcomes: The NSABP study of tamoxifen and raloxifene (STAR) P-2 trial. *JAMA : The Journal of the American Medical Association* Vol.295, No.23, (Jun 21), pp. 2727-41, ISSN 1538-3598; 0098-7484.

10

Adjuvant Chemotherapy for Endometrial Cancer

N. Susumu[1], H. Nomura[1], W. Yamagami[1], A. Hirasawa[1], K. Banno[1], H. Tsuda[1], S. Sagae[2] and D. Aoki[1]
[1]*School of Medicine, Keio University, Shinjyuku-ku, Tokyo*
[2]*JR Sapporo Hospital, Sapporo, Hokkaido*
Japan

1. Introduction

The prognosis of early-stage endometrial cancer is favorable, even when treated using surgery alone, whereas recurrent cases or advanced cases (stage III or IV) with progression beyond the uterus have a poor prognosis[1)], and therapy for such cancers is still in the exploratory stages. Stage I and II cases are sometimes treated with adjuvant therapy to prevent recurrence after surgical therapy; however, the treatment options for these cases remain controversial. The boundaries encompassing intermediate risk cases may be approached in several ways, and it would be difficult to say that any consensus has been reached, although examples often include stage IIB (FIGO stage 1988) and higher, stage IC endometrioid adenocarcinoma, all grade 3 (poorly-differentiated) endometrioid adenocarcinoma, non-endometrioid adenocarcinoma, and marked lymphovascular space invasion[2,3)]. Radiation therapy and chemotherapy are the two primary modalities of postoperative adjuvant therapy for patients with these types of endometrial cancer characterized by a poor prognosis or a risk of recurrence. In this chapter, we first refer briefly to adjuvant radiotherapy.

2. Radiation therapy for endometrial cancer

In Europe and the US, the postoperative therapy most commonly used for intermediate-risk patients with advanced endometrial cancer or early-stage cancer who are at risk of recurrence is mainly radiation therapy[4)]. In Japan, on the other hand, chemotherapy is often chosen as a postoperative therapy, and radiation therapy is performed only for limited cases. Radiation therapy is indicated as an option for initial treatment only when surgery would be difficult to perform from a practical perspective, such as in advanced cases that are considered inoperable, and in cases where surgery is considered a high-risk procedure because of serious complications, obesity, or other reasons[5)]. The following types of radiation therapy can be used for endometrial cancer following a hysterectomy. (1)Vaginal brachytherapy: A radioactive source for brachytherapy is inserted into the vagina and left there for two to three days. (2)External-beam radiation therapy (EBRT): Tumors are exposed to radiation from outside the body.

There are two kinds of EBRT: whole abdominal irradiation (WAI) and whole pelvic irradiation (WPI). WAI or WPI is usually carried out as postoperative radiation therapy and is sometimes accompanied by vaginal brachytherapy.

The effects of postoperative radiation therapy on intermediate-risk cases of early-stage endometrial cancer have been studied in comparison with groups observed over time in the absence of postoperative treatment in NRH[6)], PORTEC[7)], GOG-99[8)]. Although these reports are from different regions, they all showed the same results. Specifically, the effect in suppressing local recurrence was significantly better in the radiation therapy groups, but radiation did not significantly prolong progression-free survival (PFS) or overall survival (OS).

A study on the effects of postoperative (adjuvant) EBRT on outcome in patients with early-stage endometrial cancer was recently reported in The Lancet[9)]. Out of 905 patients with early-stage cancer in seven countries that had been enrolled in the ASTEC and EN.5 studies, intermediate to high-risk patients who had undergone surgery for endometrial cancer were randomly assigned to an observation or an EBRT group. The risk of developing distant metastasis based on the PORTEC and GOG99 data, where a high risk was defined as "all papillary serous and clear cell subtypes, all other subtypes in IC (grade 3) and IIA (grade 3), and all patients with stage IIB", and intermediate risk was defined as "subtypes other than papillary serous and clear cell histology within stage IA and IB (grade 3) and stage IC and IIA (grades 1 and 2)." The results of an analysis revealed that, after 58 months of follow up, the hazard ratio (HR) for death was 1.05 (95% CI, 0.75 to 1.48; P = 0.77) in 68 out of 453 subjects in the group observed over time and in 67 out of 452 subjects in the EBRT group, indicating no difference in OS. There was also no significant difference in terms of recurrence-free survival (RFS), with a HR of 0.93 (95% CI, 0.66 to 1.31; P = 0.68). The incidence of distant recurrence was also the same (8% in the observation group and 9% in the EBRT group), but the HR of 0.46 (95% CI, 0.24 to 0.89; P = 0.02) for vaginal or pelvic initial recurrence indicated that local recurrence was suppressed in the EBRT group. However, since these numbers do not include cases of distant metastasis or simultaneous local recurrence/distant metastasis, which account for 65% of recurrences, the overall outcome was not considered to have improved. The development of acute toxicity was also higher in the EBRT group, with a rate of 43% compared to the rate of 27% in the group without radiation therapy.

A meta-analysis[9)] of 2011 cases comprising the PORTEC and GOG99 data was performed in addition to the above ASTEC and EN.5 data. The HR for OS was 1.04 (95% CI, 0.84 to 1.29; P = 0.38), indicating no significant differences depending on whether or not adjuvant EBRT was performed. A sub-analysis divided the patients into what the authors termed intermediate risk and high risk also revealed no significant differences in OS between the ASTEC+EN.5 and the ASTEC+EN.5+PORTEC+GOG99 data.

Because adjuvant EBRT thus failed to improve survival and also resulted in adverse effects in early-stage endometrial cancer patients who had a risk of recurrence, the authors concluded that such treatment could not be recommended for patients with early-stage endometrial cancer.

3. Chemotherapy for advanced or recurrent endometrial cancer

Although adjuvant EBRT can be expected to be effective to a certain extent for advanced or recurrent endometrial cancer, chemotherapy with anti-tumor agents is also being additionally performed in Europe and the US. After many changes in regimens, AP therapy (combining doxorubicin and cisplatin) is currently the standard therapy. The changes in regimens are summarized below.

From the 1970s to the 1980s, doxorubicin monotherapy was reported to result in a response rate of 20% to 42%[10], and a good response rate of 45% to 60% was reported in a subsequent phase II study combining cisplatin with doxorubicin[11]. These two drugs therefore came to be positioned as key drugs in chemotherapy for endometrial cancer. In the 1990s, the Gynecologic Oncology Group (GOG) in the US and the European Organization for Research and Treatment of Cancer (EORTC) conducted phase III randomized comparative studies on "doxorubicin vs. doxorubicin + cisplatin (AP therapy)" in both the GOG107[12] and EORTC55872[13] trials, respectively, and the response rates of 25% vs. 42% in the GOG107 study and 43% vs. 17% in the EORTC55872 study demonstrated the efficacy of AP therapy. Although no significant differences in OS were found in the GOG-107 study, AP therapy was shown to be superior in the EORTC55872 study. On the other hand, CAP (cyclophosphamide + doxorubicin + cisplatin) therapy is also being used for endometrial cancer in Japan, where chemotherapy is more often performed as a postoperative therapy[5]. However, cyclophosphamide was not found to result in significant differences in the response rate in phase II studies of CAP therapy and AP therapy[14], while the GOG48 study on "doxorubicin vs. doxorubicin + cyclophosphamide (AC therapy)" also revealed no significant differences in the response rate, response period, or OS, thus contradicting the usefulness of concomitant cyclophosphamide for endometrial cancer[15];AP therapy has come to be acknowledged as the standard chemotherapy for endometrial cancer in Japan as well.

Radiation therapy and chemotherapy are thus the primary modalities of therapy that should be used after surgery for endometrial cancer. However, the following three questions still need to be answered:

1. Which is more effective for advanced or recurrent cancer: radiation therapy or chemotherapy?
2. Radiation therapy has been shown to be ineffective for early-stage patients classified as being at risk for recurrence, but is chemotherapy effective?
3. Alternatively, is the combination of radiation therapy and chemotherapy effective for early-stage patients classified as being at risk for recurrence?

4. Radiation therapy vs. chemotherapy as adjuvant therapy for endometrial cancer

Three randomized studies have compared radiation therapy and chemotherapy as adjuvant therapies for endometrial cancer (Table 1).

4.1 GOG122

The GOG122[16], reported in the US in 2006, was a randomized study comparing WAI and AP therapy as first-line therapies for stage III and IV cases with residual tumors no greater than 2 cm after surgery. The HR for progression adjusted for stage was 0.71, favoring AP therapy (95% CI, 0.55 to 0.91; $P < 0.01$). At 60 months, 50% of the patients receiving AP were predicted to be alive and disease-free after adjustments for stage, compared with 38% of patients receiving WAI. The stage-adjusted death HR was 0.68 (95% CI, 0.52 to 0.89; $P < 0.01$), favoring AP therapy. Moreover, at 60 months and after adjustments for stage, 55% of the AP patients were predicted to be alive, compared with 42% of the WAI patients. The PFS and OS were both significantly higher in the AP arm, but greater acute toxicity was seen in the

study	phase	year	eligibility	treatment arm	number of cases	compliance rate (%)	percentage of stage I/II/III/IV	percentage of PLN	percentage of PAN	percentage of G3 or serous/clear cell	5-year PFS (%)	5-year OS (%)	hazard ratio (HR) (95%CI)	adverse effects
GOG122 (Randall et al.)	III	2006	stage III and IV cases with residual tumors no greater than 2 cm after surgery	AP(60/50)X7 + P(50)X1, q3w (A: maximum 420 in total)	194	63	0/0/73/27	87	75	52 (serous+clear+ undifferentiated : 26)	42[a]	53[a]	HR of PFS (CT vs. RT): 0.71 (0.55-0.91), HR of OS (CT vs. RT) : 0.68 (0.52-0.89)	hematologic G3/4: 88% (CT) vs. 14% (RT), GI G3/G4: 20% vs. 13%, neurotoxicity 7% vs. <1%, deaths related to Tx: 4% vs. 2%
				WAI + boost EBRT (pelvis +extended field) (45Gy)	202	84					38	42		
Italian study (Maggi et al.)	III	2006	stage IC G3, stage II A to IIB G3 with more than 50% myometrial invasion, stage III disease with no gross residual tumor	CAP(600/45/50) X5, q4w	174	75	26/9/65/0	NA	NA	56 (serous+clear+ undifferentiated : 0)	63	66	HR of PFS (RT vs. CT): 0.92 (0.65-1.30), HR of OS (RT vs. CT): 0.85 (0.72-1.50)	neutropenia G3/4: 35%, radiation proctitis G3: 4%, diarrhea G3: 16%
				EBRT (pelvis ± extended field) 45-50Gy	166	88					63	69		
JGOG2033 (Susumu et al.)	III	2008	stage IC–IIIC with deeper than 50% myometrial invasion, and with no residual tumor.	CAP(333/40/50) X3 or more, q4w	193	97	61/14/25/0	96	29	14 (serous+clear+ undifferentiated : 0)	82	87	HR of PFS (CT vs. RT) : 1.07 (0.65-1.76), HR of OS (CT vs. RT) : 0.72 (0.40-1.29)	G3/4 toxicities: 5% (CT) vs. 2% (RT), treatment-related death: 0%
				EBRT (pelvis ± extended field) 45-50Gy	192	99					84	85		
JGOG2033 (subset analysis: high-intermediate risk)					64						84[a]	90[a]	HR of PFS (CT vs. RT) : 0.44 (0.20-0.97), HR of OS (CT vs. RT) : 0.24 (0.09-0.69)	
					56						66	74		

a: significantly better

Table 1. Randomized trials comparing radiation therapy and chemotherapy as an adjuvant therapy for endometrial cancer.

AP arm. Treatment probably contributed to the deaths of 8 patients (4%) in the AP arm and 5 patients (2%) in the WAI arm, indicating that AP therapy was associated with a somewhat stronger toxicity. However, in view of the survival data, AP chemotherapy appeared to be better than radiation therapy as a first-line postoperative therapy for advanced endometrial cancer. This was the first trial to reveal the positive effects of chemotherapy over radiation therapy. A subgroup analysis revealed that significantly lower HRs regarding OS were recognized in patients younger than 60 years old, cases with microscopic residual tumors, cases with a pathological subtype of endometrioid adenocarcinoma, and stage III cases. After the results of this study were reported, chemotherapy tended to be more often incorporated into adjuvant therapy for endometrial cancer.

4.2 Italian study

Maggi R et al. [17] reported a multicenter randomized trial comparing five courses of adjuvant chemotherapy with CAP (cyclophosphamide, 600 mg/m^2; doxorubicin, 45 mg/m^2; and cisplatin, 50 mg/m^2) and external radiation therapy (45 Gy) for mainly high-risk endometrial cancer patients, including stage IC grade 3, stage IIA to IIB grade 3 with more than 50% myometrial invasion (stage I/II: 36%), and also stage III disease. The pathological subtype was restricted to endometrioid type. Selective pelvic and paraaortic node sampling were performed; however, the percentage of patients undergoing a lymphadenectomy was not stated. More than 60% of the cases were stage III and had a high risk of recurrence. The 3-, 5-, and 7-year OS rates were 78%, 69% and 62% in the RT group and 76%, 66% and 62% in the CT group. The 3-, 5-, and 7-year PFS rates were 69%, 63%, and 56% and 68%, 63%, and 60%, respectively. This study revealed no significant differences in the OS or the PFS. Radiation therapy delayed local relapses, and CT delayed distant metastases.

4.3 JGOG2033

In 2008, the Japanese Gynecologic Oncology Group (JGOG) published a paper[18] about a randomized phase III trial (JGOG2033) comparing adjuvant chemotherapy with cyclophosphamide (333 mg/m^2), doxorubicin (40 mg/m^2), and cisplatin (50 mg/m^2) (CAP) administered every four weeks for three or more cycles with radiotherapy administered using pelvic EBRT (PRT) at 50 Gy in 385 patients with endometrioid adenocarcinoma and myometrial invasion deeper than 50%, myometrial invasion, most of whom had an intermediate -risk but a small proportion of whom had a high -risk of recurrence after the initial operation for endometrial cancer. No statistically significant differences in the PFS or OS were recognized between the patient groups treated with the two modalities. However, in the high intermediate-risk (HIR) group consisting of (1) patients with stage IC disease who were over 70 years of age and/or had G3 endometrioid adenocarcinoma and (2) patients with stage II or IIIA disease (positive cytology), the CAP treatment was associated with a significantly higher PFS rate (83.8% vs. 66.2%) as well as a higher OS rate (89.7% vs. 73.6%). Adjuvant chemotherapy was emphasized as being a useful alternative to radiotherapy for patients with intermediate-risk endometrial cancer.

In this study, a pelvic lymphadenectomy was performed in 96% of the cases and a paraaortic lymphadenectomy was performed in 29% of the cases; furthermore, the ratio of stage I or II cases was higher (75% vs. 35%) and the ratio of grade 3 tumors was lower (14% vs. 56%). Most of the cases in JGOG2033 study had an intermediate risk, while most of the cases in the Italian study[17] had a high risk. Although both of these studies used the CAP regimen, the doses of cyclophosphamide and doxorubicin were lower and the number of chemotherapy cycles was fewer in the JGOG2033 study (Table 2). In fact, the incidence of

study	phase	year	eligibility	treatment arm	number of cases	compliance rate (%)	percentage of stage I/II/III/IV	percentage of PLN	percentage of PAN	percentage of G3 or serous/clear cell	5-year PFS (%)	5-year OS (%)	hazard ratio (HR) (95%CI)		adverse effects
JGOG2041 (Nomura et al.)	II	2011	Patients with measurable disease derived from histologically confirmed stage III/IV or recurrence	DP (70/60), q3w until progression or adverse events	29	72	0/0/31/31/38[a]	NA	NA	NA (serous+clear+undifferentiated : 14)	median PFS: 232 d	median OS: 629 d	response rate: 52%	(95% CI: 33-71)	neutropenia G3/4: 83%, anorexia G3/4: 17%
				DC (70/AUC6), q3w until progression or adverse events	29	69	0/0/21/21/59[a]	NA	NA	NA (serous+clear+undifferentiated : 14)	median PFS: 238 d	median OS: 731 d	response rate: 48%	(95% CI: 30-68)	neutropenia G3/4: 90%, anorexia G3/4: 10%
				TC (180/AUC6), q3w, until progression or adverse events	30	90	0/0/17/43/40[a]	NA	NA	NA (serous+clear+undifferentiated : 23)	median PFS: 289 d	median OS: 854 d	response rate: 60%	(95% CI: 41-77)	neutropenia G3/4: 77%, anorexia G3/4: 10%, motor neuropathy: 7%
JGOG2043	III	accrual finished	stage I/II intermediate risk (G2/3 and myometrial invasion >50%), stage III/IV high risk with residual tumors no greater than 2 cm after surgery	AP(60/50) x 6, q3w	estimated 780										
				DP(70/60) x 6, q3w											
				TC (180/AUC6) x 6, q3w											

a: recurrent tumor

Table 2. Randomized trials comparing chemotherapy regimens as an adjuvant therapy for endometrial cancer.

G3/4 adverse effects was lower in the JGOG2033 study. The CAP regimen in the JGOG2033 study, therefore, represented a more modest therapy than that used in the Italian study. Nevertheless, the 5-year PFS rate and OS rate of the high-intermediate risk (HIR) subgroup of the JGOG2033 study were significantly improved by this modest CAP regimen. This means that the cases in the high-intermediate risk (HIR) subgroup of the JGOG2033 study may be good candidates for answering the question, "Which patients with endometrial cancer may benefit from adjuvant chemotherapy?" To answer this question definitively, further evidence is needed from randomized studies investigating the efficacy of adjuvant chemotherapy designed for patients with intermediate- or high-risk endometrial cancer. The modest adjuvant chemotherapy regimen of CAP was superior to pelvic radiotherapy in HIR patients, as defined above; however, this chemotherapy did not have a sufficient efficacy to improve the prognosis of patients with stage III advanced endometrial cancer.

The Italian study[17)] revealed no significant differences in the PFS or OS rates among high-risk patients even when a higher-dose CAP regimen was used. The dose of doxorubicin was 60 mg/m^2 in the GOG122 study[16)], 45 mg/m^2 in the Italian study, and 40 mg/m^2 in the JGOG2033 study[18)].

4.4 What is the best adjuvant chemotherapy for endometrial cancer?

Then, what is the best adjuvant chemotherapy for endometrial cancer? First, let me look back to some studies for advanced or recurrent endometrial cancer.

The response rates to paclitaxel in phase II studies for advanced or recurrent endometrial cancer were reported to be 37.5%[19)] and 30.4%[20)] in 1996 and 2004, respectively, and the response rates to docetaxel in phase II studies for advanced or recurrent endometrial cancer were reported to be 33%[21)] and 31.3%[22)] in 2002 and 2005, respectively. These numbers are comparable to the response rates obtained with doxorubicin alone.

In the GOG163 phase III randomized study[23)] of AP vs. concomitant doxorubicin + paclitaxel (AT) + G-CSF reported in 2004 on the effects of combining a taxane with doxorubicin or cisplatin, the response rates of 40% vs. 43% revealed no significant differences when compared with the concomitant use of cisplatin, and the median OS was 12.6 months vs.13.6 months, with a HR of 1.00. Furthermore, AT therapy had more disadvantages, such as the need for G-CSF support, compared with AP therapy, and no advantage was found in switching from cisplatin to paclitaxel as the concomitant drug to be used with doxorubicin.

On the other hand, the GOG177 phase III randomized study[24)] of AP vs. concomitant paclitaxel + doxorubicin + cisplatin (TAP) + G-CSF reported in the same year (2004) showed that the results of TAP therapy were superior, based on response rates of 34% vs. 57%. The median PFS (8.3 months vs. 5.3 months) and the median OS (15.3 months vs. 12.3 months) were significantly improved in the TAP group. However, in the TAP arm, the incidence of neurotoxicity was significantly higher, and congestive heart failure or treatment-related deaths occurred. Compliance was therefore considered to be poor in view of the toxicity, and TAP therapy has not widely replaced AP as a standard therapy in clinical practice.

Based on the results of the GOG163 study, it seemed that the next steps should be to study the significance of replacing doxorubicin, which has been considered a key drug for a long time, with a taxane and to study which of the two platinum agents should be used. There was thus a need to first study whether or not a regimen combining two agents (taxane + platinum agent) would be better than AP. As there are two taxanes and two platinum agents, whether these regimens or AP therapy would be more effective was investigated in Japan.

Out of the various combinations of the two taxanes and two platinum agents, i.e., TC (paclitaxel + carboplatin), DP (docetaxel + cisplatin), DC (docetaxel + carboplatin), and TP (paclitaxel + cisplatin), the efficacy and safety of the TC, DP, and DC regimens were first compared in JGOG2041, a phase II randomized study[25)] (Table 2). TP therapy had already been eliminated, as the results of clinical trials for ovarian cancer revealed a strong neurotoxicity, and a shift from TP to TC therapy had occurred[26-28)]. The results revealed the response rates of the three regimens to be in no way inferior to AP therapy, and the toxicity was also within an acceptable range[25)].

Based on the results of the JGOG2041 study, a phase III randomized study (JGOG2043) was conducted to compare AP therapy with chemotherapy combining platinum and taxanes in groups with a high risk for the recurrence of endometrial cancer. The results of the JGOG2041 study revealed the response rate of DC therapy (48%) to be somewhat lower, although not significantly, than that of TC therapy (60%) and DP therapy (52%), and TC and DP therapy were therefore selected for comparison with AP therapy in the JGOG2043 study. The groups with a high risk for the recurrence of endometrial cancer in the JGOG2043 study included advanced cases with residual tumors of no greater than 2 cm, and stage I and II cases with invasion to more than half of the myometrium and histological grade 2 or 3 (including serous or clear cell adenocarcinoma), thus allowing the effects on advanced cases and intermediate risk cases to be analyzed separately using sub-analyses. Enrollment in this study was closed at the end of 2010.

In the phase II study, the TC response rate was 60% and the compliance was high (90%). The response rate of TC is therefore being compared with that of TAP (which had the highest response rate in the GOG177 study but had problems in compliance) in patients with advanced or recurrent cancer. The results of the JGOG2041 study, in conjunction with the results of a comparison of the efficacies of TC, DP, and AP in the JGOG2043 study, should prove to be useful for research on the most effective and appropriate chemotherapy regimens. Randomized studies, such as GOG 209 (TAP vs. TC for advanced or recurrent disease) and JGOG 2043 (AP vs. TC vs. DP for adjuvant therapy) are now underway. The TC regimen is widely used both in practical treatment and in research trials for endometrial cancer, based on the promising efficacies reported by various phase II studies, although no evidence of a phase III trial level that certifies TC as a truly standard regimen for endometrial cancer has been obtained.

Chemotherapy has been the mainstream treatment in Japan, but postoperative therapy in Europe is now shifting from the formerly preferred radiation therapy alone to radiation therapy plus chemotherapy. In the US as well, the GOG194 study (closed) for WAI vs. WAI followed by paclitaxel + doxorubicin + cisplatin (TAP therapy) is being conducted to test the effects of combining chemotherapy with radiation therapy as a postoperative treatment regimen for intermediate-risk or high-risk cases.

5. Comparison of radiation therapy alone and the combination of radiation therapy and chemotherapy

Several randomized studies have compared radiation therapy alone and the combination of radiation therapy and chemotherapy as an adjuvant therapy for endometrial cancer (Table 3).

study	phase	year	eligibility	treatment arm	number of cases	compliance rate (%)	percentage of stage I/II/III/IV	percent age of PLN	percent age of PAN	percentage of G3 or serous/clear cell	5-year PFS (%)	5-year OS (%)	hazard ratio (HR) (95%CI)	adverse effects
GOG34 (Morrow et al.)	III	1990	clinically staged I or II (occult) cases who had greater than 50% myometrial invasion, pelvic or aortic node metastasis, cervical involvement, or adnexal metastases	EBRT (pelvis ± extended field) 50Gy	89	NA	NA (clinically staged)	100	NA	39 (clear cell 2)	NA	not significant (almost 60% in both arms)	NA	small bowel obstruction: 9%, treatment-related death: 2%
				EBRT (pelvis ± extended field) 50Gy followed by A(45-60)x8 , q3w (up to max cumulated dose of 500mg)	92	69% (2 or more cycles)	NA (clinically staged)	100	NA	27 (clear cell 5)	NA			small bowel obstruction: 4%, treatment-related death: 3%
Finnish study (Kuoppala et al.)	III	2008	stage IA-B G3, stage IC-IIIA G1-3	EBRT 28Gy (pelvis) x 2 cycle q3w	72	94	69/13/13/0	78	1	33 (serous+clear+ undifferentiated: 0)	median DFS: 18 months	disease-specific OS: 85	HR of OS (CT+RT vs. RT) : 1.21 (0.56-2.65)	intestinal obstruction: 2% (requiring resection)
				CEP(500/60/50) → EBRT 28Gy (pelvis) → CEP → EBRT28Gy →CEP	84	93	63/25/12/0	82	4	35 (serous+clear+ undifferentiated: 0)	median DFS: 25 months	disease-specific OS: 82		nausea G3/4: <8%, leukopenia G3/4: 17%, intestinal obstruction: 10%(requiring resection)
GOG184 (Homesley et al.)	III	2008	initially stage III or IV with disease limited to the pelvis and abdomen (extrapelvic diseases excluded after 2003, except for paraaortic metastasis)	volume-directed radiation followed by AP(45/50) with optional G-CSF x 6 cycles, q3w	288	83	0/0/88/12	NA[a]	NA[a]	40 (serous+clear+ undifferentiated: 19)	3-y RFS: 62	NA	HR of RFS (RT+TAP vs. RT+AP): 0.90(0.69-1.17) In subgroup analysis of cases with gross residual disease, HR of RFS or death (RT+TAP vs. RT+AP): 0.50 (0.26-0.92).	neutropenia G3/4: 47%, thrombopenia: 10%, febrile neutropenia: 0%, sensory neuropathy: 2%, myalgia G3/4: 0%
				volume-directed radiation followed by TAP(160/45/50) with G-CSF x 6 cycles, q3w	298	78	0/0/88/12	NA[a]	NA[a]	43 (serous+clear+ undifferentiated: 17)	3-y RFS: 64	NA		neutropenia G3/4: 68%, thrombopenia: 25%, febrile neutropenia: 5%, sensory neuropathy: 9%, myalgia G3/4: 3%
(1)+(2) combined NSGO/EORTC and MaNGO/ILAIDE (Hogberg et al.)	III	2010		RT alone	267						69	75 (CSS:78)	HR of PFS (RT+CT vs. RT) :0.63 (0.44-0.89), HR of OS (RT+CT vs. RT) : 0.69 (0.46-1.03), HR of CSS (RT+CT vs. RT): 0.55 (0.35-0.88)	
				RT+CT	267						78[b]	82 (CSS:87[b])		

study	phase	year	eligibility	treatment arm	number of cases	compliance rate (%)	percentage of stage I/II/III/IV	percent age of PLN	percent age of PAN	percentage of G3 or serous/clear cell	5-year PFS (%)	5-year OS (%)	hazard ratio (HR) (95%CI)	adverse effects
(1)NSGO/EORTC55991 (Hogberg et al.)	III	2010	stage I, II, IIIA (positive peritoneal fluid cytology only), or IIIC (positive pelvic lymph nodes only)	EBRT (pelvis 44 Gy) ± vaginal brachytherapy	196	95	90/5/2/0	15	4	48 (serous +clear 40)	72	76 (CSS:79)	HR of PFS (RT+CT vs. RT) :0.64 (0.41-0.99), HR of OS (RT+CT vs. RT) : 0.66 (0.40-1.08), HR of CSS (RT+CT vs. RT): 0.51 (0.28-0.90)	treatment-related death: 0.5%, SAE; intestinal reaction with diarrhea: 0.5%
				CT was given before or after RT;. either CT regimen x4, q3-4w , AP(83%), EP(50 or 75/50) (4%), TEC (175/60/AUC 5) (3%), TC (175/AUC 5-6) (10%).	186	73	91/5/2/0	19	3	58 (serous+clear+anaplastic 35)	79[b]	83 (CSS:88[b])		SAE (4%): diarrhea: 1%, neutropenia: 0.5%, neutropenia:1.5%, allergic reaction to paclitaxel, 0.5%, atrial fibrillation:0.5%, pulmonary emboli:0.5%
(2)MaNGO-ILAIDEIII	III	2010	stage IIB, IIIA–C disease (stage IIIA with positive cytology alone without other risk factors was not included)	EBRT (pelvis 45 Gy) ± vaginal brachytherapy (if cervical stromal involvement) ± EBRT (paraaortic, if paraatotic metastases)	76	88	0/29/67/0	54	9	45 (anaplastic 1)	61	73 (CSS:76)	HR of PFS (RT+CT vs.RT) :0.61(0.33-1.12), HR of OS (RT+CT vs. RT) : 0.74 (0.36-1.52), HR of CSS (RT+CT vs. RT): 0.65 (0.30-1.44)	no
				AP (60/50)x3, q3w, followed by EBRT (pelvis 45 Gy) ± vaginal brachytherapy ± EBRT (paraaortic)	80	88	0/37/63/0	45	9	34 (serous+clear+anaplastic 4)	74	78 (CSS:82)		leukopenia G3/4: 16%, neutropenia G3/4:30%, nausea and vomiting G3/4: 5%
RTOG-GOG9905	III	accrual finished	endometrioid adenocarcinoma, 1) stage IC and IIA, G2-3, with ≥50% myometrial invasion, 2) stage IIB, G2-3, <50% serous or clear cell	EBRT	estimated 436									
				CCRT (P: 2 cycles with pelvic EBRT) followed by TC x 4										
PORTEC III	III	on-going	1) IB G3 with LVSI, IC or IIA G 3, IIB, IIIA or IIIC (IIIA based on cytology alone, only eligible if G3), 2) IB or IC, II or III with serous or clear cell histology	RT arm: EBRT (pelvis 48.6Gy)	estimated 500									
				RT+CT arm: CCRTcisplatin 50mg/m^2, 2 cycles) +TC (175/AUC5) x 4										
GOG249	III	on-going	1) stage I, IIA with high-intermediate risk[c], 2) stage IIB(occult)(any histology) with/without risk factors[c], 3)stage I-IIB(occult) serous or clear cell w/wo other risk features	RT arm: EBRT (pelvis n 45Gy in 25Fr - 50.4Gy i 28Fr) (stageI/II clear/serous:optional vaginal cuff boost)	estimated 562									
				RT+CT arm: brachytherapy followed by TC (175/AUC6) x 3										

a: sampling of PLN or PAN was not required.
b: significantly better
c: 1) G2/3 with LVSI and outer-third myometrial invasion, 2) age of 50 years or greater in addition to any two factors listed above, or 3) age of 70 years or greater with any risk factor listed above.

Table 3. Randomized trials comparing radiation therapy with combination of radiation therapy and chemotherapy as an adjuvant therapy for endometrial cancer.

5.1 GOG34

This study was the first randomized trial to compare radiation alone and radiation followed by chemotherapy[29]. The subjects were comprised of patients with clinical stage I or II (occult) disease in whom surgical-pathologic evaluation had revealed one or more risk factors for recurrence: a greater than 50% myometrial invasion, pelvic or aortic node metastasis, cervical involvement, or adnexal metastases. The patients received 50-Gy EBRT with or without paraaortic radiation and were then randomized into two arms: no further therapy or additional doxorubicin (45 - 60 mg/m^2) every three weeks to a maximum cumulative dose of 500 mg/m^2. No statistically significant difference in the OS or PFS was observed between the two arms. Unfortunately, because of protocol violations, the small sample size, and the number of patients lost to follow-up, this study was unable to determine what effect the use of doxorubicin as an adjuvant therapy had on recurrence, progression, and survival.

5.2 Finnish study

For the Finnish study[30], surgically staged IA-B G3 cases or stage IC-IIIA G1-3 cases were enrolled and randomized to receive pelvic EBRT alone (28 Gy x 2 cycles) or a unique combination of alternating EBRT and chemotherapy, namely, a first cycle of CEP (cyclophosphamide 500 mg/m^2; epirubicin, 60 mg/m^2; and cisplatin, 50 mg/m^2) followed by a first cycle of EBRT (28 Gy), a second cycle of CEP, a second cycle of EBRT (28 Gy), and finally a third cycle of CEP. However, this study failed to reveal an improvement in the OS or PFS by the addition of chemotherapy to radiation therapy. Moreover, adverse events such as severe bowel obstruction requiring surgery tended to occur more frequently in the combined treatment arm.

5.3 GOG 184

For the GOG184 study[31], surgically staged III or IV cases were enrolled and treated with volume-directed irradiation of the pelvic/para-aortic lymph nodes. The patients were subsequently randomized to compare the recurrence-free survival (RFS) and toxicity between two chemotherapy regimens. Treatment was randomized between six cycles of cisplatin (50 mg/m^2) and doxorubicin (45 mg/m^2) with or without paclitaxel (160 mg/m^2). The accrual of stage IV patients was completed in June, 2003. Approximately 80% of the subjects completed six cycles of chemotherapy. Three deaths resulted from bowel complications, and one death was caused by renal failure. Hematologic adverse events, sensory neuropathy, and myalgia, were more frequent and severe in the paclitaxel arm ($P < 0.01$). The percentage of patients alive and recurrence-free at 36 months was 62% for RT + AP vs. 64% for RT + TAP. The hazard of recurrence or death relative to the RT + AP arm and stratified according to stage was 0.90 (95% CI, 0.69 to 1.17; $P = 0.21$). However, in a subgroup analysis, RT + TAP was associated with a 50% reduction in the risk of recurrence or death among patients with gross residual disease (95% CI, 0.26 to 0.92). This study showed that the addition of paclitaxel to cisplatin and doxorubicin following surgery and radiation was not associated with a significant improvement in RFS but was associated with increased toxicity.

5.4 NSGO 9501/ EORTC 55991 study and MaNGO ILIADE III study

Hogberg et al. reported a paper[32], presenting two randomized clinical trials (NSGO EC9501 /EORTC55991 and MaNGO ILIADEIII). The former study was reported at the ASCO 2007 meeting[33]. These two studies were undertaken to clarify whether the sequential combination of chemotherapy and radiotherapy improves the PFS in high-risk subjects with endometrial cancer. These studies had similar designs; however, some differences existed regarding the distribution of stages and the rates of pelvic or paraaortic lymphadenectomy. Most of the enrolled cases were stage I in the former study, while all the cases were stage II or III in the latter study; in addition, the rate of pelvic or paraaortic lymphadenectomy was higher in the ILIADEIII study. In total, patients (n = 540) with surgically resected endometrial cancer stage I - III and with no residual tumor or prognostic factors implying a high -risk were randomly allocated to an adjuvant radiotherapy group with or without sequential chemotherapy.

In the NSGO/EORTC study, patients with stage I, II, IIIA (positive peritoneal fluid cytology only), or IIIC (positive pelvic lymph nodes only) diseases were enrolled. The chemotherapy modalities included AP (doxorubicin, 50 mg/m^2 + cisplatin, 50 mg/m^2; 83%), EP (epirubicin, 75 mg/m^2; 4%), TEC (paclitaxel, 175 mg/m^2 + epirubicin, 60 mg/m^2 + carboplatin, AUC 5; 3%), and TC (paclitaxel, 175 mg/m^2, carboplatin, AUC 5 - 6; 10%). The radiation arm consisted of pelvic EBRT (44 Gy) with or without brachytherapy. The combined modality treatment was associated with a 36% reduction in the risk of relapse or death (HR, 0.64; 95% CI, 0.41 - 0.99; P = 0.04); two-sided tests were used. In the MaNGO ILIADEIII study, only the AP therapy was used as a chemotherapy regimen. The results from the MaNGO ILIADEIII study pointed in the same direction (HR, 0.61) as those of the NSGO/EORTC study, but were not significant. In both studies, adverse effects were more severe in the combined modality group.

In the combined analysis, the estimate of the risk for relapse or death was similar but with narrower confidence limits (HR, 0.63; 95% CI, 0.44 - 0.89; P = 0.009). Neither study showed significant differences in the OS. In the combined analysis, the OS approached statistical significance (HR, 0.69; 95% CI, 0.46 - 1.03; P = 0.07) and cancer-specific survival (CSS) was significant (HR, 0.55; 95% CI, 0.35 - 0.88; P = 0.01). Thus, the addition of adjuvant chemotherapy to radiation improved the PFS and CSS in surgically treated endometrial cancer patients with no residual tumor and a high-risk profile. Regarding the pathological subtypes, combined therapy offered a superior benefit to patients with endometrioid type and grade 1 or 2 diseases, but not to patients with serous or clear cell types and grade 3 diseases. Several remaining questions need to be further investigated in future trials.

6. Ongoing trials comparing radiation therapy alone and radiation therapy plus chemotherapy

At present, there are several ongoing studies comparing radiation therapy alone and radiation plus chemotherapy (Table 3). The RTOG-GOG9905 study finished accrual in 2004; however, its results have not yet been presented. Accrual for the PORTECIII and GOG249 trials is ongoing. These three trials are phase III randomized trials comparing a radiation alone group and a combined radiation and chemotherapy group. Two of them are examining concurrent chemoradiotherapy followed by four cycles of TC, and the third trial is examining brachytherapy followed by three cycles of TC.

7. Conclusions

As described above, many problems regarding adjuvant therapy for endometrial cancer remain. (1) Which patients receive the highest benefit from adjuvant therapy? (2) Is there a definite consensus regarding the criteria for grouping patients according to the risk of recurrence? (3) Which chemotherapy regimen should be certified as the gold standard regimen for adjuvant therapy based on the results of phase III randomized trials? (4) Which combination of radiation therapy and chemotherapy is best? To answer these questions, before designing a trial concept, a worldwide consensus on the criteria for risk groups needs to first be obtained. In addition, to interpret the results of various adjuvant therapy trials, careful attention to the kind of surgery that the patients have received and the percentages of grade 3 endometrioid adenocarcinoma and aggressive pathological subtypes (serous, clear cell, undifferentiated, and so on) is needed. In this review, as shown in Tables 1, 2, and 3, we have collected information regarding the percentages of pelvic lymphadenectomy, paraaortic lymphadenectomy, grade 3 endometrioid adenocarcinoma or aggressive pathological subtypes, and informations about surgical stage distribution, treatment compliance, and adverse effects. Before arguing the results of clinical trials, sufficient information regarding the patient conditions after surgery and just before receiving adjuvant therapy is needed. For example, some trials with low percentages of pelvic or paraaortic lymphadenectomy, trials with high percentages of G3 or aggressive pathological subtypes, and trials with high percentages of advanced stage patients tend to favor chemotherapy, since these patient groups tend to have higher possibilities of micrometastases that cannot be identified using imaging.

The results of ongoing studies, such as GOG0237 (TAP vs. TC, advanced or recurrent disease, phase III) and JGOG2043 (AP vs. DP vs. TC, adjuvant, phase III) may provide important information regarding question (3) above, and the results of the RTOG-GOG9905, PORTECIII, and GOG249 studies may help to answer question (4). Further studies are needed to resolve question (1).

8. References

[1] Creasman WT, Odicino F, Maisonneuve P, Beller U, Benedet JL, Heintz AP, Ngan HY, Sideri M, Pecorelli S. Carcinoma of the corpus uteri. J Epidemiol Biostat. 2001;61:47-86.

[2] Morrow CP, Bundy BN, Kurman RJ, Creasman WT, Heller P, Homesley HD, Graham JE. Relationship between surgical-pathological risk factors and outcome in clinical stage I and II carcinoma of the endometrium: a Gynecologic Oncology Group study. Gynecol Oncol. 1991 ;40:55-65.

[3] Boronow RC, Morrow CP, Creasman WT, Disaia PJ, Silverberg SG, Miller A, Blessing JA. Surgical staging in endometrial cancer: clinical-pathologic findings of a prospective study. Obstet Gynecol. 1984;63:825-32.

[4] Mariani A, Webb MJ, Keeney GL, Aletti G, Podratz KC. Endometrial cancer: predictors of peritoneal failure. Gynecol Oncol. 2003;89:236-42.

[5] National Comprehensive cancer Network: Clinical practice guideline in oncology. Uterine cancers. Version1. 2012; http://www.nccn.org/professionals/physician_gls/pdf/uterine.pdf

[6] Aalders J, Abeler V, Kolstad P, Onsrud M. Postoperative external irradiation and prognostic parameters in stage I endometrial carcinoma: clinical and histopathologic study of 540 patients. Obstet Gynecol. 1980;56:419-27.

[7] Creutzberg CL, van Putten WL, Koper PC, Lybeert ML, Jobsen JJ, Wárlám-Rodenhuis CC, De Winter KA, Lutgens LC, van den Bergh AC, van de Steen-Banasik E,

Beerman H, van Lent M. Surgery and postoperative radiotherapy versus surgery alone for patients with stage-1 endometrial carcinoma: multicentre randomised trial. PORTEC Study Group. Post Operative Radiation Therapy in Endometrial Carcinoma. Lancet. 2000;355:1404-11.

[8] Keys HM, Roberts JA, Brunetto VL, Zaino RJ, Spirtos NM, Bloss JD, Pearlman A, Maiman MA, Bell JG; Gynecologic Oncology Group. A phase III trial of surgery with or without adjunctive external pelvic radiation therapy in intermediate risk endometrial adenocarcinoma: a Gynecologic Oncology Group study. Gynecol Oncol. 2004 ;92:744-51.

[9] ASTEC/EN.5 Study Group, Blake P, Swart AM, Orton J, Kitchener H, Whelan T, Lukka H, Eisenhauer E, Bacon M, Tu D, Parmar MK, Amos C, Murray C, Qian W. Adjuvant external beam radiotherapy in the treatment of endometrial cancer (MRC ASTEC and NCIC CTG EN.5 randomised trials): pooled trial results, systematic review, and meta-analysis. Lancet. 2009;373:137-46.

[10] Thigpen JT, Buchsbaum HJ, Mangan C, Blessing JA. Phase II trial of adriamycin in the treatment of advanced or recurrent endometrial carcinoma: a Gynecologic Oncology Group study. Cancer Treat Rep. 1979 ;63:21-7.

[11] Tropé C, Johnsson JE, Simonsen E, Christiansen H, Cavallin-Ståhl E, Horváth G. Treatment of recurrent endometrial adenocarcinoma with a combination of doxorubicin and cisplatin. Am J Obstet Gynecol. 1984 ;149:379-81.

[12] Thigpen JT, Brady MF, Homesley HD, Malfetano J, DuBeshter B, Burger RA, Liao S. Phase III trial of doxorubicin with or without cisplatin in advanced endometrial carcinoma: a gynecologic oncology group study. J Clin Oncol. 2004 ;22:3902-8.

[13] Aapro MS, van Wijk FH, Bolis G, Chevallier B, van der Burg ME, Poveda A, de Oliveira CF, Tumolo S, Scotto di Palumbo V, Piccart M, Franchi M, Zanaboni F, Lacave AJ, Fontanelli R, Favalli G, Zola P, Guastalla JP, Rosso R, Marth C, Nooij M, Presti M, Scarabelli C, Splinter TA, Ploch E, Beex LV, ten Bokkel Huinink W, Forni M, Melpignano M, Blake P, Kerbrat P, Mendiola C, Cervantes A, Goupil A, Harper PG, Madronal C, Namer M, Scarfone G, Stoot JE, Teodorovic I, Coens C, Vergote I, Vermorken JB; European Organisation for Research and Treatment of Cancer Gynaecological Cancer Group. Doxorubicin versus doxorubicin and cisplatin in endometrial carcinoma: definitive results of a randomised study (55872) by the EORTC Gynaecological Cancer Group. Ann Oncol. 2003;14:441-8.

[14] Dunton CJ, Pfeifer SM, Braitman LE, Morgan MA, Carlson JA, Mikuta JJ. Treatment of advanced and recurrent endometrial cancer with cisplatin, doxorubicin, and cyclophosphamide. Gynecol Oncol. 1991;41:113-6.

[15] Thigpen JT, Blessing JA, DiSaia PJ, Yordan E, Carson LF, Evers C. A randomized comparison of doxorubicin alone versus doxorubicin plus cyclophosphamide in the management of advanced or recurrent endometrial carcinoma: A Gynecologic Oncology Group study. J Clin Oncol. 1994 ;12:1408-14.

[16] Randall ME, Filiaci VL, Muss H, Spirtos NM, Mannel RS, Fowler J, Thigpen JT, Benda JA; Gynecologic Oncology Group Study. Randomized phase III trial of whole-abdominal irradiation versus doxorubicin and cisplatin chemotherapy in advanced endometrial carcinoma: a Gynecologic Oncology Group Study. J Clin Oncol. 2006 ;24:36-44.

[17] Maggi R, Lissoni A, Spina F, Melpignano M, Zola P, Favalli G, Colombo A, Fossati R. Adjuvant chemotherapy vs radiotherapy in high-risk endometrial carcinoma: results of a randomised trial. Br J Cancer. 2006 ;95:266-71.

[18] Susumu N, Sagae S, Udagawa Y, Niwa K, Kuramoto H, Satoh S, Kudo R; Japanese Gynecologic Oncology Group. Randomized phase III trial of pelvic radiotherapy versus cisplatin-based combined chemotherapy in patients with intermediate- and high-risk endometrial cancer: a Japanese Gynecologic Oncology Group study. Gynecol Oncol. 2008;108:226-33.

[19] Ball HG, Blessing JA, Lentz SS, Mutch DG. A phase II trial of paclitaxel in patients with advanced or recurrent adenocarcinoma of the endometrium: a Gynecologic Oncology Group study. Gynecol Oncol. 1996 ;62:278-81.

[20] Hirai Y, Hasumi K, Onose R, Kuramoto H, Kuzuya K, Hatae M, Ochiai K, Nozawa S, Noda K. Phase II trial of 3-h infusion of paclitaxel in patients with adenocarcinoma of endometrium: Japanese Multicenter Study Group. Gynecol Oncol. 2004 ;94:471-6.

[21] Gordon AN, Hart DJ, Bailey C, Anthony S, Surwit EA. Phase II trial of docetaxel in recurrent or advanced endometrial carcinoma. Ann Oncol. 2002 ;13: (suppl 5):109.

[22] Katsumata N, Noda K, Nozawa S, Kitagawa R, Nishimura R, Yamaguchi S, Aoki D, Susumu N, Kuramoto H, Jobo T, Ueki K, Ueki M, Kohno I, Fujiwara K, Sohda Y, Eguchi F. Phase II trial of docetaxel in advanced or metastatic endometrial cancer: a Japanese Cooperative Study. Br J Cancer. 2005 ;93:999-1004.

[23] Fleming GF, Filiaci VL, Bentley RC, Herzog T, Sorosky J, Vaccarello L, Gallion H. Phase III randomized trial of doxorubicin + cisplatin versus doxorubicin + 24-h paclitaxel + filgrastim in endometrial carcinoma: a Gynecologic Oncology Group study. Ann Oncol. 2004;15:1173-8.

[24] Fleming GF, Brunetto VL, Cella D, Look KY, Reid GC, Munkarah AR, Kline R, Burger RA, Goodman A, Burks RT. Phase III trial of doxorubicin plus cisplatin with or without paclitaxel plus filgrastim in advanced endometrial carcinoma: a Gynecologic Oncology Group Study. J Clin Oncol. 2004;22:2159-66.

[25] Ozols RF, Bundy BN, Greer BE, Fowler JM, Clarke-Pearson D, Burger RA, Mannel RS, DeGeest K, Hartenbach EM, Baergen R; Gynecologic Oncology Group. Phase III trial of carboplatin and paclitaxel compared with cisplatin and paclitaxel in patients with optimally resected stage III ovarian cancer: a Gynecologic Oncology Group study. J Clin Oncol. 2003 ;21:3194-200.

[26] du Bois A, Lück HJ, Meier W, Adams HP, Möbus V, Costa S, Bauknecht T, Richter B, Warm M, Schröder W, Olbricht S, Nitz U, Jackisch C, Emons G, Wagner U, Kuhn W, Pfisterer J; Arbeitsgemeinschaft Gynäkologische Onkologie Ovarian Cancer Study Group. A randomized clinical trial of cisplatin/paclitaxel versus carboplatin/paclitaxel as first-line treatment of ovarian cancer. J Natl Cancer Inst. 2003;95:1320-9

[27] Neijt JP, Engelholm SA, Tuxen MK, Sorensen PG, Hansen M, Sessa C, de Swart CA, Hirsch FR, Lund B, van Houwelingen HC. Exploratory phase III study of paclitaxel and cisplatin versus paclitaxel and carboplatin in advanced ovarian cancer. J Clin Oncol. 2000;18:3084-92.

[28] Nomura H, Aoki D, Takahashi F, Katsumata N, Watanabe Y, Konishi I, Jobo T, Hatae M, Hiura M, Yaegashi N. Randomized phase II study comparing docetaxel plus cisplatin, docetaxel plus carboplatin, and paclitaxel plus carboplatin in patients

with advanced or recurrent endometrial carcinoma: a Japanese Gynecologic Oncology Group study (JGOG2041). Ann Oncol. 2011 ;22:636-42.

[29] Morrow CP, Bundy BN, Homesley HD, Creasman WT, Hornback NB, Kurman R, Thigpen JT. Doxorubicin as an adjuvant following surgery and radiation therapy in patients with high-risk endometrial carcinoma, stage I and occult stage II: a Gynecologic Oncology Group Study Gynecol Oncol. 1990;36:166-71.

[30] Kuoppala T, Maenpaa J, Tomas E, Puistola U, Salmi T, Grenman S, Lehtovirta P, Fors M, Luukkaala T, Sipila P. Surgically staged high-risk endometrial cancer: randomized study of adjuvant radiotherapy alone vs. sequential chemo-radiotherapy. Gynecol Oncol. 2008;110:190-5.

[31] Homesley HD, Filiaci V, Gibbons SK, Long HJ, Cella D, Spirtos NM, Morris RT, DeGeest K, Lee R, Montag A. A randomized phase III trial in advanced endometrial carcinoma of surgery and volume directed radiation followed by cisplatin and doxorubicin with or without paclitaxel: A Gynecologic Oncology Group study. Gynecol Oncol. 2009 ;112:543-52.

[32] Hogberg T, Signorelli M, de Oliveira CF, Fossati R, Lissoni AA, Sorbe B, Andersson H, Grenman S, Lundgren C, Rosenberg P, Boman K, Tholander B, Scambia G, Reed N, Cormio G, Tognon G, Clarke J, Sawicki T, Zola P, Kristensen G. Sequential adjuvant chemotherapy and radiotherapy in endometrial cancer--results from two randomised studies. Eur J Cancer. 2010;46:2422-31.

[33] Hogberg T, Rosenberg P, Kristensen G, de Oliveira CF, de Pont Christensen R, Sorbe B, Lundgren C, Salmi T, Andersson H, and Reed NS. A randomized phase-III study on adjuvant treatment with radiation (RT) ± chemotherapy (CT) in early-stage high-risk endometrial cancer (NSGO-EC-9501/EORTC 55991) J Clin Oncol. 2007; 25 (18 suppl): #5003 (ASCO Annual Meeting Proceedings)